At the Heart of Medicine

Essays on the Practice of Surgery and Surgical Education

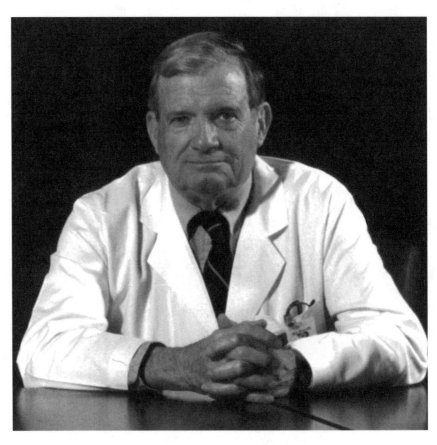

David C. Sabiston, Jr., M.D.

At the Heart of Medicine

Essays on the Practice of Surgery and Surgical Education

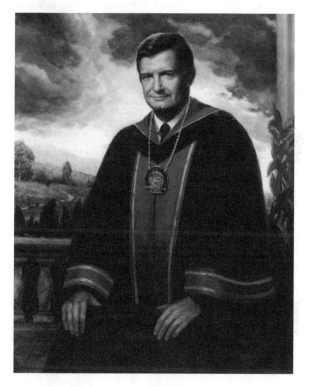

By

David C. Sabiston, Jr., M.D.

Edited and with an Introduction and Epilogue by
Barton F. Haynes, M.D.

CAROLINA ACADEMIC PRESS

Durham, North Carolina

Grateful acknowledgement is made to the following publishers, editors, or authors for permission to reproduce previously published work: Alpha Omega Alpha Honor Medical Society, American Journal of Cardiology, American Surgeon, Association of American Medical Colleges, Journal of Neurosurgery, Annals of Surgery, Annals Thoracic Surgical, Surgery, Bulletin of the American College of Surgeons, Clinical Cardiology, Caduceus, Circulation, American College of Surgeons, Johns Hopkins Medical Journal, Duke University Press, Journal of Thoracic Cardiovascular Surgery, Proceedings of the Rockefeller Archive Center, Radiology, North Carolina Medical Journal, New England Journal of Medicine, Dr. David C. Sabiston, Jr, Lippincott, Williams & Wilkins.

Library of Congress Cataloging-in-Publication Data

Sabiston, David C., 1924–
    At the heart of medicine : essays on the practice of surgery and surgical education / by David C. Sabiston, and edited by Barton F. Haynes.
    p. cm.
    ISBN 1-59460-163-1
    1. Surgery--Philosophy. 2. Surgery--Study and teaching. 3. Duke University. Medical Center. Dept. of Surgery--History. I. Haynes, Barton F. II. Title.
    [DNLM: 1. Duke University. Medical Center. 2. Surgery--Collected Works. 3. Academic Medical Centers--history--Collected Works. 4. Surgery--history--Collected Works. 5. Surgical Procedures, Operative--Collected Works. WO 7 S113a 2005]
    RD31.5.S33 2005
    617'.0071'1756563--dc22

                    2005020786

Carolina Academic Press
700 Kent Street
Durham, North Carolina 27701
Telephone (919) 489-7486
Fax (919) 493-5668
E-mail: cap@cap-press.com
www.cap-press.com

Dedication

To the surgeons of the United States for dedicated patient care, and to Aggie Sabiston, my wife, for dedicated care of our family.

Contents ⌒

Part IV   *Surgical Education*

Part V   *The Heart*

Part VI   *The Lungs*

Part VII   *The Practice of Surgery*

Acknowledgments ⌒

I am grateful to a number of individuals for their assistance with this book. Thanks to Walter Wolfe, Ted Pappas, James Lowe, R. Randal Bollinger, and Robert Jones for comments on the book. Kim McClammy created the electronic version of the manuscript and made countless revisions. Aggie Sabiston oversaw the project and added important facts and perspective. I thank David Sabiston for allowing his words to be edited and compiled in this book, and as well, for his unwavering support of my career at Duke during the past twenty-five years. David C. Sabiston, Jr., is not only a surgeon's surgeon; he is also a supporter and mentor to people throughout the Duke family.

Barton F. Haynes, M.D.
June 2005

Introduction ⌒

This book is a compilation of essays by David C. Sabiston, Jr., one of the great American surgeons of the twentieth century. A protégé of Alfred Blalock at Johns Hopkins Medical School, Sabiston became Chair of Surgery at Duke University School of Medicine in 1964, and for the next thirty years, shaped American Surgery by the force of his intellect, by his teaching, and by his editorships and national leadership. His seminal research accomplishments led in the development of surgical methods to revascularize the heart, and, as well, led to development of radionuclide scanning of the lung for the diagnosis of pulmonary embolus.

He patterned the Duke Department of Surgery training program after Blalock's program at Johns Hopkins. Early in Sabiston's career, Blalock sent Sabiston to work with Donald Gregg at the Army Institute of Research in Washington, D.C. to perform basic research on coronary blood flow, an experience that shaped Sabiston's career. After becoming Chair of Surgery at Duke, Sabiston provided the means for every surgery resident to spend two years in basic research during clinical training. Sabiston's philosophy was that the best surgeons were curious and competent scientists as well as technically proficient surgeons.

David C. Sabiston, Jr. also influenced a generation of surgeons worldwide by his thirty-five years of editorship of *Sabiston's Textbook of Surgery*, numerous other surgical textbooks, and as editor in chief of the *Annals of Surgery* for over thirty years. His leadership in American Surgery was recognized by his peers with his election as President of the American College of Surgeons.

Although traditional in his views on training surgeons, Sabiston was a visionary who could recognize important future opportunities. He was the administrative leader at Duke who recognized the importance of the AIDS epidemic in 1983. David Sabiston invested $5 million dollars and, with a gift from the DuPont company, built the Surgical Oncology Research Facility, a 30,000 square foot Biosafety Level-3 laboratory for AIDS research. From the Department of Surgery program in AIDS, led by Dani Bolognesi, Kent Weinhold, and Thomas Matthews, came two AIDS drugs—AZT and the fusion inhibitor, Fuzeon. David Sabiston never wrote about his contributions to AIDS research, so I have told this story in my epilogue.

His interest in his students and residents earned him every teaching award at Duke, and, as well, earned him the National Teacher of the Year Award from Alpha Omega Alpha. More than one former student has told me long after graduating from Duke that "the greatest thrill of my medical school time was being personally taught surgery in the laboratory by Dr. Sabiston." Thus, the Sabiston work ethic and his professional values will live on in every Sabiston trainee.

One of the most decorated and honored surgeons of our time, Sabiston has received numerous awards and honorary degrees. However, a major lasting legacy is the legion of surgeons trained from 1964–1994, many of whom have gone on to become division chiefs and departmental chairs around the United States.

Finally, David Sabiston established a tradition of excellence at Duke University that permeated every department in the medical center for thirty years, and this tradition continues even after his retirement.

The purpose of this book is to create a volume that presents representative samples of David Sabiston's major scientific works, and, as well, presents a series of essays on topics that are important to various aspects of surgical medicine. I have edited David Sabiston's scientific papers by not including the methods sections and many of the scientific graphs and charts. This was done to preserve the content of the classic message of the text, while making the chapter more readable to the non-researcher. I hope these essays remind current and future generations of doctors of the levels of excellence and commitment he expected in good physicians.

The book starts with chapters on his background and early development in Sabiston's own words, "David Sabiston on David Sabiston."

Next, we hear of his views on the development of surgery at Duke University School of Medicine and how the Hopkins traditions were transplanted to Duke. Seven chapters in the book are Sabiston's treatises on the history of surgery and reveal that Sabiston was an avid historian.

An additional seven chapters teach us his philosophy for training students and residents in surgical medicine and should be required reading for surgical educators today. One of the most striking lessons in these seven chapters is the clear message of how much time and teaching it takes to make a good surgeon.

Next come reprints of portions of Sabiston's classic papers on revascularization of the heart and diagnosis of pulmonary embolism, followed by three chapters on Sabiston's views on important professional issues such as professional liability, animal rights activism, and national health insurance. Finally, the epilogue tells the story of the Surgery Department and early AIDS research at Duke.

Taken together, Sabiston's essays on surgical practice and life in medicine reflect a long and richly productive body of work that has touched the lives of physicians and patients worldwide for nearly half a century. They are timely and are written in a style that reflects the man himself—insightful, thoughtful, straight-forward, and gracious.

Barton F. Haynes, M.D.
June 2005

At the Heart of Medicine

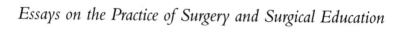

Essays on the Practice of Surgery and Surgical Education

I

Background and Early Days

I think everyone would agree that the step between being a fourth-year senior medical student and a first-year intern is the biggest single step one takes in one's career.

Chapter 1 ☞

David Sabiston on David Sabiston[1]

I was born in eastern North Carolina on my grandfather's farm in Onslow County in 1924, and later lived in Jacksonville, North Carolina, and went to school in the public schools. Quite early, I became interested in science and history because my mother, Marie Jackson, was a teacher and a great mentor to me to become an academic. So rather early on I developed an interest in medicine, and that was furthered by my association with my father's brother, who was an otolaryngologist. I used the summers in high school to spend a good bit of time with my uncle, so by the time I went to college at the University of North Carolina-Chapel Hill, I had made up my mind that I was going into medicine.

I look back on my days in Chapel Hill and recognize that it was very fortunate for me to have selected the University of North Carolina. My otolaryngologist uncle had been there, as had several members of my family. It was recognized at that time as not only the first state university in the nation, having been founded in 1793, but also as having very good faculty and a very good reputation for research and teaching. My time there was extremely pleasant, both socially and educationally, and I look back upon that as a very fine initial part of

---

1. Edited composite of two interviews with David Sabiston. One interview was conducted by Dr. Paul A. Ebert, formerly a member of the faculty in the Department of Surgery at Duke, Professor and Chairman of the Department of Surgery at the University of California in San Francisco. Dr. Sabiston spoke with Dr. Ebert on November 30, 1994, at Duke University Medical Center. This interview is one of a series entitled, "Leaders in American Medicine," by Alpha Omega Alpha, Honor Medical Society. The other interview was conducted by William C. Roberts, the editor of the *American Journal of Cardiology* and was published in the *Journal* in 1998.

educational life. Dr. Edwin Calyle Markham was an important and influential teacher at Chapel Hill, as were Dr. James Talmage Dobbins, Professor of Chemistry, and Dr. John N. Couch, a well-known botanist. While I was at UNC-Chapel Hill, I applied to medical school at Chapel Hill, because it had a two-year school at that time. Many of us were interested in starting medical school at UNC-Chapel Hill, and after two years going on to take the final two years in another school. Later, in 1952, the University of North Carolina developed its own four-year school. But at the time I was applying in 1942, it had only a two-year school, and I applied there. My roommate, Dotson Palmer, suggested to me to also apply to Johns Hopkins School of Medicine. At that time it was considered the paramount place. I applied, and I was never more surprised in going to the mailbox one day at Old East Hall and finding a letter from Johns Hopkins that I had been accepted. I had not expected it, but I wrote to my parents immediately and told them how pleased I was. I entered Johns Hopkins School of Medicine in the fall of 1943.

The highlights of my medical school education were being introduced to the great Johns Hopkins Hospital and to all of the eminent individuals who were our teachers, and then, of course, the emergence of Dr. Alfred Blalock was all very exciting for me. He had recently come there two years before, as the new Professor and Chairman of the Department of Surgery, and was very interested in research as well as in clinical surgery. I was just entering my sophomore year in November 1944 when he did the first Blalock operation for tetralogy of Fallott. And, of course, we saw large numbers of very cyanotic children come into the hospital at that time, with very cyanotic purple lips and purple nailbeds. They were transported in wheelchairs because they didn't have enough energy to walk. They were desperately ill, and he took these children to the operating room and gave them the Blalock operation, and they awakened pink and had great exercise ability. It was a very special time. It was then that my interest focused upon surgery. I had known it was medicine that I wanted to go into, but the exact field was uncertain until my sophomore year in 1944, when surgery became my definite choice. It was interesting because we recognized that Dr. Blalock had worked six years before that, beginning with the experimental operation of anastomosing the subclavian artery with the pulmonary artery in the experimental laboratory, and it was now successful clinically. Dr. Blalock's success made a big impression on me.

Actually, as a medical student I got to know Dr. Blalock pretty well. He had just performed the first blue baby operation, and he had filmed his very early operations on them. He needed to show these films to foreign visitors, and he did not have anyone on the house staff at that time who knew how to operate a motion picture machine. He found out that I knew how to use one. He would call me when visitors were there from England or France and ask if I would mind showing the film for them that afternoon. He would always ask what time would be convenient for me. Actually, I wanted it to be convenient for him. He got accustomed to me because previously he had had several of his films chewed up in the machine when it was run by people who did not know how to use it. That was very annoying to him. Every time I ran a film for him I would put it back just like it came. He got to know me by my first name when I was a third-year medical student. That is how we got close. I have often thought how smart it was that I knew how to run a motion picture machine, because otherwise I probably would not have had that relationship with him.

Another influential teacher who caught my imagination and desire to be like him was Dr. Arnold Rich, an accomplished scholar and professor of pathology at Hopkins. He knew each name of every medical student in my class, and at a medical student weekly conference, he would go around the class and ask each one of us, by our names, what the answer was to this or that question.[2]

My residency time was exciting during that period in the development of cardiac surgery at Hopkins, and I reflect back on those years as being extremely significant for my own development. Of course, the step between being a fourth-year senior medical student and a first-year intern was tremendous. I think everyone would agree that's the biggest step one takes in one's career. It certainly was that way at Hopkins, because we were working day and night. We were on call

2. The practice of learning each student's name is a method of teaching that David Sabiston used for thirty years at Duke.

seven days a week, much the same as when we were residents, some years later, and if we got off at night, we had to sign out to someone else, never more than once a week for an evening. We lived in the hospital day and night. It was a very demanding experience, but we thought nothing of it really, because everybody else was doing it. We learned a great deal and were obviously very grateful for having been appointed at Hopkins, because it was a highly competitive appointment and also quite a pyramidal system. We knew we would be cut down. Dr. Blalock took in our class twelve interns, and ten of them left at the end of the first year, and only two stayed on. So it was a very competitive time.

When I was a third-year medical student, I went to Dr. Blalock and told him that I would like to do research, and we tied it into his background. I had remembered, of course, that he had done the original work in shock and had been the individual who showed that in trauma there was loss of fluid in the local tissues at the site of trauma that was the pathogenesis of shock. And then the blue-baby operation came along, and he had done all that in the laboratory, too. So he encouraged me to start working. My first experience was with Dr. Willian Longmire, who was then the surgery chief resident. At that time, there was only one chief resident, and he did all of the major operations, and the only time he had to operate in the laboratory was on Saturday afternoon. That was when the Hunterian laboratory at Hopkins was cold. There was no heat in the Hunterian laboratory on weekends, but we went over there, even in the winter, and did the work. I prepared the animals, and he was very interested at that time in producing experimental lymphedema of the limb; we worked on that, and I enjoyed it. He was an excellent operator, a very skillful clinical surgeon, and I learned a tremendous amount from him in that experimental study. Longmire soon went on to join the faculty and became busy with other things, and Dr. Mark Ravitch[3] next took me on. I worked in the laboratory with him, and it was there that the first ileoanal anastomoses were done. The two of us worked together on that procedure, perfecting it, and by the time we had finished the laboratory work, it had also been done on a human at Hopkins. And so I

---

3. Chief Resident of Surgery at Johns Hopkins School of Medicine.

saw the fruition of the lab work go right into the clinical setting. The first paper that I ever published was on that work; it appeared in June of the year that I graduated from medical school. I can remember taking my parents to the Welch Library and showing them that issue of *Surgery Gynecology and Obstetrics,* and they saw that I had done that, and it was very nice. Later on in the residency, Dr. Blalock appointed me to the Cushing Fellowship, and I continued research by working with Dr. Hanlon and Dr. H. William Scott. I finished the residency and went on to further work at Walter Reed Graduate School with Donald Gregg in coronary physiology, and later on with Sir Howard Florey, who was Professor of Pathology at Sir William Dunn School of Pathology in Oxford, where we studied experimental atherosclerosis. I also had the privilege of working with Philip Allison,[4] who was Professor of Surgery at Oxford, on experimental pulmonary embolus. And that led to work that we later did in the laboratory in developing radionuclide diagnosis of pulmonary embolus and radionuclide scans of the lung.

In 1952, while I was a resident, Dr. Blalock took me on a tour of England and France for one month and I thoroughly enjoyed that.[5] What I did then was carry his slides and projector. I was his handyman, but he introduced me to everybody and he knew them all. It was amazing. It was an honor for me for him to introduce me to those people. To be introduced by him might mean they would remember me. Dr. Blalock always gave everyone else more attention than he gave to himself, and we all respected him for that. He knew it was so important to us, and he was so genuine about it. He also would say, "This work was Dave's idea or Hank's idea." It made an impression on everyone. There were very few professors in those days who would say that such and such work was not all theirs. Dr. Blalock was very modest. He always gave his colleagues credit.

The development of coronary bypass surgery is an interesting story, and it is based upon several events. When I finished the residency training program at Hopkins, Dr. Blalock called me to the office

---

4. Sabiston was sent by Blalock to Oxford University in England to study for a year with Allison and Florey to broaden his research experience.

5. See photograph on page 128.

one day. It was May of the year that I was to finish on the first of July, and he said, "You know you are going to stay on the faculty," and I didn't know anything about it until that time. I and my fellow residents had been very apprehensive, but we just waited to see if we might stay on, and we didn't ever ask him beforehand, and so I was very relieved and very happy. He could see that I was overjoyed by this, and then he said, "I have a specific plan for you; I want you to develop coronary artery surgery at Hopkins," and with that I am sure my jaw fell, and he saw a different expression on my face, and I paused, and he said, "I know what you're thinking." He said, "There's not much you can do, is there, in the field, because there is really nothing objective you can do that we know about that has been proven to increase myocardial blood flow". So he said, "Well, what do you do when you're faced with a problem for which there is no immediate answer?" And, of course, knowing his background, I said, "Well, I know what you mean; I should do more research in that field and get to know more about it." Then he arranged that I would spend the time with Dr. Donald Gregg, who was the Chief of Cardiorespiratory Physiology at the Army Institute of Research in Washington. So it was through Dr. Blalock that I got the appointment and spent two full-time years working with Dr. Gregg on the physiology and metabolism of the coronary circulation. Gregg was a meticulous scientist, and he taught me a tremendous amount about the myocardium. Working with him was a real experience. One of the first things he set me to doing was to show that during systolic contraction of the heart, coronary blood flow comes nearly to zero. We were able to identify that as one of the cardinal features that was quite different from that of any other organ in the body. Of course, when peak systole comes, that indicates the highest blood flow for most organs, except for the head. So that was the beginning. From that work, I recognized that at the end of those two years I knew much about the basic problem of coronary atherosclerosis.

In 1958 Dr. Blalock told me, "You know a lot about the physiology of the coronary circulation, but you have not had any real research experience in coronory artherosclerosis. I want you to work with a person who has had a great deal of experience in experimental atherosclerosis." He sent me to Oxford to work with Howard W. Florey.

Howard Florey will be remembered, of course, as the man who won the Nobel Prize for penicillin back in 1945. But in 1960 he was interested in atherosclerosis, having said that he had done about all he could do in antibiotics, and he wanted to do something else that he thought was more important.

We worked on coronary atherosclerosis with Sir William Dunn in the Dunn School of Pathology at Oxford. I signed on to work with him and with Dr. Phillip Allison, the Professor of Surgery there. Those two were my chief mentors while I was at Oxford. Dr. Blalock had said, "You need some support while you are over there. I recommend that you apply for a Fulbright Fellowship." I was fortunate to receive one because research money was hard to come by in those days, particularly if you trained abroad. One might get an NIH scholarship in the United States, but it was not honored if one went abroad. The Fulbright scholarship, of course, allowed me to go to Oxford for a year.

There we worked on the development of experimental atherosclerosis in animals, both in primate and canine preparations, with experimental hypercholesterolemia, and watched the development of atherosclerosis. It was possible to operate on some of these animals and to do endarterectomies and see that they would not only survive but the suture lines and the lumen would be patent.

Florey said, "We must put our attention on the endothelium. I think it is more than just a plastic lining. A man cannot know too much about the endothelium and how many enzymes it makes." I think how wise he was. Florey told me that the endothelium did a lot more than just line the vascular system. He did not know any facts but he knew how to get them. He was a brilliant man.

I knew why Florey was so interested in angina. He had it himself, but he had kept it a secret from almost everyone. People would not often let it be known that they had angina in those days because it had such a bad prognosis. He did not want that condition to be associated with him. When I got back to Baltimore, he called me and said, "If I come over, will you do a vascular operation on my heart? I have severe angina and I don't think I will live very long." Because the outcome of a vascular operation was not certain in those days, I said, "Let me do a little more on this, and I will call you." Unfortunately, he had a heart attack before I got back to him. I don't know how long he had had angina, but it could not have been any worse.

Given that research, I came back from Oxford and first did some coronary thromboendarterectomies. They were successful for about a year. We did about forty-four of those operations. But a year's success was not sufficient, because at the end of the year about half of those patients had rethrombosis and reappearance of their angina. But then, having seen that, we tried some experimental aorta-to-coronary grafts in a dog, and they stayed patent. It was on about the fifth of April, 1962, that we did the first coronary artery bypass operation; we bypassed the obstruction of the right coronary with a graft from the aorta to the distal right coronary. That patient did very well, and we had an artist, Mr. Slossberg, who was always in the hospital, come to the operating room, and he did a nice drawing. That patient developed a stroke, and I thought it was probably due to thrombosis at the site of the aortic anastomosis, part of which might have slipped up into the carotid circulation. Unfortunately, I did not do another such operation until after Favaloro and Johnson had done them about six years later. But that operation was an initial procedure that I think did circulate around the country; the cardiologists spoke well of it, and certainly it set me and others to thinking about how to use surgery to bypass obstructed coronery arteries.

My work on pulmonary embolus originated with our work at Oxford in creating experimental pulmonary emboli in Philip Allison's laboratory. We developed large experimental emboli in the vena cava, got them up into the lungs, set the physiology, but we found very soon that it was very difficult to be certain objectively about the embolization unless we did a pulmonary arteriogram. Pulmonary arteriography, of course, in those days was risky, particularly in patients that had hypotension, low blood pressure from the pulmonary embolus, and so I was fortunate in linking up with Henry Wagner at Hopkins who was a very well-known radionuclide physiologist. We decided that we could get pulmonary scans by heating human serum albumin to a certain degree for a period of time so that the protein molecules would aggregate physically and we would then have something to inject into the circulation and thus map the lungs.

When I was in Dr. Gregg's laboratory, I first started dating Aggie, the wonderful woman who became my wife. Often I would have planned a date and Dr. Gregg would be working late in the lab. It would come time for me to go on my date, and I would have to call her and tell her I was sorry but I had to work. I could not see leaving him in the laboratory by himself. He was so grateful about my dedication to the work. He always believed one should finish everything in one day and not put it off until the next. He worked many nights until midnight. He taught me the discipline of investigation. In spite of the fact that I broke many dates, I must give Aggie credit. She was very understanding. That was not easy because she was still in college. She would make plans to be off on a particular night, and I would have to call her and tell her I could not come over that night. I was in Washington, D.C., and she was in Baltimore. She had a good introduction to medicine.

I met Aggie when I was in Washington. Her father was a United States congressman who had represented the Tidewater section of North Carolina for twenty-six years in the House of Representatives. She lived on campus while she was at Goucher College in Baltimore, but during the summer she would stay at her parents' Washington home. The circumstances of how we first met are funny. I had an aunt who lived next door to me when I was growing up, and she met Aggie at some function her father had taken her to. My aunt wrote me and said, "I met this very attractive lady who is in Baltimore right now. She is the daughter of Congressman Barden and I recommend her to you." I called Aggie for a blind date. First she was busy. She was dating a midshipman from Annapolis and she said, "No, I am sorry, I am tied up." I said, "Well, may I call you some other time?" She said, "Yes, call me again." The next time we had a date. We got married in 1955, when I was thirty-one and Aggie was twenty-two.

I was very pleased to have been selected as Chairman of Surgery at Duke University in 1964. I was coming home back to North Carolina. My wife, Aggie, appreciated that fact so much because she had always wanted to come back to the state. She liked Baltimore, since she had been there as a student at Goucher College, but when she finished college she was ready to come home. We had stayed in Baltimore for about nine years.

Dr. Blalock had carcinoma and died in 1964 at the age of sixty-five. I was already in Durham. I used to go back on weekends to see him in Baltimore when he was in the hospital. He diagnosed his cancer himself; his physician believed that he had hepatitis, but Blalock felt his liver getting bigger and said he had cancer. I saw him on a Saturday before he died the following Tuesday. He told me he thought he had cancer. He had had an operation about six months earlier for a slipped disc, but, in retrospect, the slipped disc was due to a metastasis.

The early chairmen of the various departments at Duke had mainly come from Hopkins. Dr. William Welch was the one that dedicated the medical school and made the initial address here. He was very well liked at Duke. Welch was asked who should be appointed as Chairman of Pathology, and he picked one of his own former residents, Wiley Forbus, who had trained at Hopkins under Welch. Forbus was a Hopkins graduate and Chief Resident under Welch. Then there were other physicians who came to Duke from Hopkins. They all had respect for Hopkins. I always thought my tenure at Hopkins was the reason I got my position at Duke.

Duke had strong chairs and had a system of turning things over to them. Instead of letting the Dean make the decisions, the chairman made the decisions. Welch himself was the first Dean at Hopkins Medical School. He already knew how to pick good people and let them develop. Duke had a great history of that and that is how Davison chose his first chairs; it was an environment where one was allowed to grow, and that environment allowed me to grow, too. I have always been very grateful that I could go to a medical school that had been influenced as much by Hopkins as Duke had.

I enjoyed my work at Duke and worked long hours operating, teaching, administering the Private Diagnostic Clinic, and writing. Aggie gets a lot of credit because she graciously never complained when I spent so much time working at home at night and on weekends. I had to do the work that way, but she always provided a happy expression on her face, and she was always good to me. Also I had good people to work with on the faculty, both at Hopkins and then at Duke. I shared a lot of things with them. I was always happiest when I was working. I did not like to waste time or do things that did not seem productive.

As a faculty member, I became very interested in residency training. It takes a number of attributes to train a good resident. In the first place, one must have a deep interest in residency training and a commitment to it, because it is a full-time process and one must give a great deal of time to it. One needs to think about it continuously and change the training plan as time progresses, and to be certain that all the residents have a large clinical experience. That has to be the first order, I think, in a training program. Putting it another way, a timid surgeon is usually timid because they haven't had much clinical experience. Surgeons with a lot of experience can understand and can take over any complex situation.

The second thing, in my own instance, and I am sure that we are all creatures of our past, I followed Dr. Blalock's example in insisting that they all do research. In my program at Duke through the years, residents took at least two years of basic research, not just going to their laboratory and doing experimental operations but doing basic research and recording their data. Nowadays, the process has gone a step further; they are not only physiologists, biochemists, and bacteriologists, but they have to be molecular biologists. They have to know medical genetics. Molecular oncology today is dependent largely on that field. The developments in cardiology are genetically related; transplantation surgery is the same way. So I think today we must have in our laboratories sophisticated scientists who train our residents in their research fellowships for a period of two or more years.

Regarding changes in residency training in the coming years, I think as it is said, "The more things seem to change, the more they stay the same." I think there will be a great deal of similarity. There will be certain changes; I think the economics are going to force us to reduce the length of the program. That's not going to be easy, but it probably can be done without too much difficulty. I think that we must be certain at all times to give the residents in surgery adequate training, and much of it may come at their own expense. I hope not, but whatever it takes, they should be fully trained before they are doing major work on patients. I also hope very much, as long as we have our wits, for them to do research, because otherwise we will not have advances.

Regarding my honors and awards, I can remember being elected to the various offices in the American College of Surgeons, beginning

with a member of the Board of Governors, later the Chairman of the
Board, and then later a Regent, and then Chairman of the Board of
Regents, and then President of the College. I think the Presidency of
the College has to be the highest post that a surgeon can aspire to in
this country, because the College represents essentially all the major
surgeons in the United States, over 50,000. The opportunities, the
challenges, as well as the honors which that post and those leading to
it, offer to one, would have to be very high. In the same vein, the
members of the foreign surgical organizations in other countries have
been very kind to me, and I would have to acknowledge my appreciation for my election to the Royal Colleges of Surgeons in England,
Ireland, Scotland, and the major organizations in France, Germany,
Spain, Australia, Canada, Brazil, Argentina, and Equador. They have
been exceedingly kind to me. And there have been other honors, for
example, in the field of education. Ranking very high in my own
mind are the honors that I received from the AOA and the American
Association of Medical Colleges. Being the 1992 Distinguished Clinical Teacher in the country was one honor that I greatly appreciated.

My view of the future is bright for surgical medicine. One has
only to look at the past and see that each generation has seemed to
outdo the other, which is certainly the direction that science, medicine, and research should take; I can see this moving ahead at a rapid
pace. We are getting better. The human mind is getting more percep-
tive. We are enlarging fields rapidly, with more depth of understanding
about them, and the technical aspects have increased so vastly in terms
of achieving objective ways to register this understanding. Yes, these
are going to be the reasons why the major remaining problems in
medicine that cause illness and death are apt to be solved in the future.

For the young surgeons of the future, I first encourage them to
emphasize excitement and enthusiasm, because I know they are there.
I think one rarely finds a surgeon who isn't totally, or almost totally,
happy, with his or her own life and what he or she has been able to
do, because every day is different, and one can see a very ill patient
come in and be operated on and then go out essentially well. Second,
I encourage them to be told some of the historical accounts of what
surgery has done in the past and be told how that has resulted in the
the remarkable progress in treating disease today. Third, I encourage

them to commit themselves to a very extensive clinical program and understand the reason for that commitment; they must settle for nothing less than excellence, because it is so important. A certain group of surgeons trained in the university medical centers should be imbued with the necessity of doing research, because they have the responsibility of pushing the frontiers of surgical science back further each year, and that is the only way that progress can be achieved. Then come the teaching opportunities, of course, and armed with that type of background and experience, surgeons are in a position to not only teach in the classroom but to supervise original research in their younger trainees.

These are very turbulent times in medicine today. Each time we pass through one of these phases, it looms very large in our daily experience, because it seems to make one believe things are going to change rapidly. On the other hand, if one looks back in history, such difficulties usually can be conquered and straightened out and medicine returns to an even keel. For example, just shortly after I accepted the appointment here at Duke in 1964–1965, Medicare came along. Many national organizations in medicine decried this, said that it marked the beginning of the end, that with Medicare the government was getting into medicine, that the government would run medicine, that Medicare would mean that 30 percent of all of our patients would be under the thumb of the government, and that both physicians and patients would no longer have any freedom. There were a great number of people who felt very strongly about Medicare. Yet now, thirty years later, if we look at the current situation, we have never had in the history of the world thirty years of greater discovery, better medical care, better patient care, better doctor satisfaction.

So, I think we need to remember these things, and to put them in proper perspective. We should say that we are going to look at the situation and whatever comes, we are going to make the best of it. Intelligent physicians can do this successfully. So I have a positive attitude about the future. I do not see gloom out there; I see that the next thirty years stand very much the same chance of being as successful and productive as the last thirty have been.

Chapter 2 ⌒

Taking Care of Business[1]

*W*hen I went to Duke, I set my sail as near to that as Dr. Blalock had done in trying to make Duke a place for young people to thrive, to give them opportunities, to make sure that they got credit for their accomplishments and rewards, such as being elected to a society. They then got their own appointments elsewhere very soon. They learned that they would be happier in academic work than in private practice. I did try to choose academic-type surgeons from the beginning. It was all a tremendously pleasant experience.

When I first came to Duke, Dr. Deryl Hart, my predecessor and the first Chairman of Surgery at Duke, had for good reason adopted the Hopkins system, starting off with twelve or fifteen interns and then ending up with two chief residents. I soon figured out that that was very hard and, in a way, it made the program too competitive, and negatively so, because the house staff fought against each other to rise to the top. I reduced the entering number down to the same number we finished with to cut out the competition. I had to do that by degrees. I could not do it overnight. My goal was if they were picked for an internship they would probably finish as Chief Resident. When I went to Duke, I always paid particular attention to what the intern applicants said they wanted to do with their futures. I wanted it be crystal clear and unmistakably objective as possible. I listened to what they said, and if they had the right message, that would be the person I appointed.

Without a doubt the single thing I enjoyed most was being a teacher. There is nothing like looking in a student's face and seeing it

---

1. Edited from the two interviews with David Sabiston as in Chapter 1.

light up or observing a student's intense concentration while teaching and have them tell you later something to that effect. It is a tremendous boost. It makes life worth living.

Another activity that gave me pleasure was writing and editing textbooks. The Saunders Company came to me in the late 1950s and said they had been publishing for many years the most popular textbook of surgery by Christopher, who was then Professor of Surgery at Northwestern. They wanted me to edit the next edition. That was a real bonanza. I took it on and was very fortunate to carry it through a number of editions. It was translated into five foreign languages. Just the other day I got a notice from Russia that they wanted to translate some of our texts. I had a good publisher and a good book to start with and tried to build on that. *Surgery of the Chest* was first written by Jack Gibbon, who developed the heart-lung machine. He edited the first three editions. He turned it over to Frank Spencer and me. I was fortunate to be with it for a long time.

For my writing, I wish I did use pencil and paper because I think some of the most productive authors are individuals who write it down. Instead, I dictated. My mind does not keep up with my handwriting. I get way behind when writing. I can talk much better. I have always dictated and had a secretary take it down. I went over it quite intensely afterwards and corrected the dictation.

For my daily activities, I have always gotten up early, had an early breakfast, and arrived at the hospital around 7:30 A.M. Usually, I would have a morning report with the Chief Residents, then make rounds, and then go to the operating room. That was my usual schedule for many years. When I got to be senior, I cut my own operating down to a more reasonable schedule.

I would usually he home by 8:00 P.M. with the family. I did not always make it in time for dinner, but I tried. After dinner, I would go back to my study. Aggie planned our house, and when she did, she planned it so that I would have my study in the corner of the house in the quietest area. I have three doors between my study and the children. They spent a lot of time in the family room, but there was a good distance between my study and the family room. Aggie took care of the children most of the time. That was the way it worked.

I thought it was very important for the Chief of Surgery to operate, so I always started off the day with at least an operation in the morning and sometimes two. I would finish by noon. I would try to leave the afternoons open for appointments (faculty, residents, students, and visitors) and my university and departmental responsibilities. I knew I could not be in the operating room in the afternoons when I should be attending committees, because my people would not get treated right if I were not sitting at the table. I soon learned that there was nothing to be gained by being in the operating room in the afternoon.

I have to spend a lot of time on being editor in chief of the *Annals of Surgery* (over thirty-one years). For a journal to be good, respected, and widely read, it has to merit it. A journal cannot live on reputation for long. You have to have something there going for it. I always have given the journal prime time, each issue my best effort. It has been very valuable for me as a learning experience, and also hopefully for what I have been able to do for the authors. Again, it is just like so many things; it does not run by itself. It just takes hard work.

I have always thought surgeons ought not wear gowns outside the operating room because of the unsterile environment. You should not be walking around in "pajamas" because that is just not the image I think we should be showing. You can carry that too far, of course, by making a scene out of every issue, but I think in the end it is the proper thing to do and my house staff, I believe, usually kept the habit.

In summary, the major things in surgery that have caught my attention and that I have enjoyed the most have been training the residents to become surgeons, to see them progress in their contributions both clinically and in experimental research, and to see them get into outstanding positions in this country, both in academia and in the practice of surgery in communities. Those that have taken on major teaching responsibilities, of which there a very large number, perhaps three-quarters of the residents for the past thirty years here at Duke, are now in teaching positions and academic positions. These accomplishments of my faculty, residents, and students have brought me the greatest satisfaction.

II

The Duke Department of Surgery

D uke had a system of having strong chairs and turning things over to them, instead of letting the Dean make the decisions.

Chapter 3

The Duke University Medical Center[1]

*I*n December 1924, less than a year before he died, James B. Duke established Duke University with an endowment that was the culmination of many philanthropic contributions by the Duke family. By this action, Mr. Duke converted Trinity College into Duke University in honor of his father, Washington Duke, "whose gifts had made possible the building of Trinity College in Durham, North Carolina, in 1892 (3, 7).

Trinity College and the Duke Family

Trinity College had begun as a rural subscription school, Brown's Schoolhouse, in the village of Trinity, North Carolina. In 1839, as the result of the union of purpose of Quaker and Methodist groups, this neighborhood school became Union Institute. The Institute was incorporated by the state as Normal College in 1849; ten years later the name was changed to Trinity College. The total enrollment reached a high of 238 students before the Civil War, but hard times followed and only 107 students were enrolled in 1875 (7).

Trinity College attracted a new president. John Franklin Crowell, in 1887, and there was renewed interest in the school by the Methodist Church. Changes occurred at the instigation of President Crowell that invigorated the faculty and students. For example, the curriculum was revised and expanded, and a campaign was launched to acquire books for the library and equipment for the laboratories (7). However, the college continued to experience a shortage of funds that

---

1. Coauthored by R. H. Williams of the Duke Divison of Neurosurgery.

impeded its development. President Crowell persuaded the Board of Trustees to investigate the possibility of moving Trinity College to an urban location. Although several cities expressed interest, a group from Durham made the best offer. This group included Washington Duke, who became the main benefactor of the struggling college (3, 7). Mr. Duke and his sons were Methodists and had previously contributed to Trinity College. Furthermore, one of the sons, Benjamin, had been elected to the Board of Trustees in 1889. The offer made by the Durham group included land donated by Julian S. Carr, but the key to the relocation of Trinity College to Durham in 1892 was the provision of sufficient funds by Washington Duke (3, 7).

Washington Duke had been a farmer near Hillsborough, North Carolina, when at forty-three years of age he was drafted into the Confederate Navy during the Civil War. He had been married twice and had been a widower twice. At the time when he was drafted in 1864, he was responsible not only for managing his 300-acre farm but also for rearing a teenage son, Brodie Leonidas Duke, and three small children, Mary Elizabeth Duke, Benjamin Newton Duke, and James Buchanan Duke. Washington Duke arranged for the care of his children and reported for duty in Charleston, South Carolina. A year later he was captured by Union troops in Richmond, Virginia. After the war, Washington Duke was released in New Bern, North Carolina, and walked some 130 miles home to his children and what was left of his farm (3).

"Possessing in ready cash only a fifty-cent coin... Washington Duke found his farm stripped and bare — save for a quantity of dried leaf tobacco.... Washington Duke, aided by ten-year-old Ben and nine-year-old 'Buck,' proceeded to launch his manufacturing career. In a crude log shed which stood close by the dwelling, they beat the tobacco with wooden flails, sifted it by hand, and packed it in cloth bags labelled 'Pro Bono Publico.'"

"Although every member of the family worked hard, the children received some schooling too. Ben and Buck Duke attended sessions at the academy in nearby Durham.... And in 1871 Washington Duke enrolled Mary and Ben Duke in the New Garden School (later Guilford College).... Buck Duke,... who was sent to New Garden in 1872, missed the farm and factory.... Coming home from New Garden before the term was half completed, Buck Duke later attended the Eastman Business College in Poughkeepsie, New York...." (3).

"The first member of the family to move into Durham...was Brodie Duke. In 1869, at twenty-three years of age, he purchased a small frame building on Durham's Main Street, and while living in the upstairs room began to manufacture in the ground-floor room his own brands of smoking tobacco.... Inspired by Brodie Duke's move and lured by the larger business opportunities offered by bustling little Durham, Washington Duke sold his farm and moved his family into town in 1874.... Washington Duke and his sons built their frame factory on the south side of Main Street...but the business from the first was a family affair, with Washington Duke selling goods for his son Brodie and *vice versa*.... Through the labors and skill of Washington Duke and his three sons..., they built a modestly successful business in the 1870's.... But they were only one of about a dozen tobacco manufacturers in Durham—and the firm that stood far ahead of all others ...was W. T. Blackwell and Company, with its globally-famed 'Bull Durham' smoking tobacco" (3).

As a way of beating the competition, W. Duke, Sons, and Company entered the cigarette-manufacturing business in 1881 and introduced the newly invented Bon-sack cigarette-making machine to their enterprise in 1885. W. Duke, Sons, and Company was reorganized in 1885 as a joint-stock company and, led by its young president, James B. Duke, forged to the top of the cigarette industry by 1890. At that point, James H. Duke engineered the affiliation of his company with the nation's four other major cigarette manufacturers as a new entity, the American Tobacco Company, and became its first president (3).

Although the initial Duke fortune came from the tobacco industry, the family later diversified its interests. Led by Benjamin Duke, the family became involved in textile production starting in 1892. The Dukes then became interested in the potential of hydroelectric energy in the Carolinas as an economical source of power for their factories. After several years of preliminary experience, James and Benjamin Duke formed the Southern Power Company (later the Duke Power Company) in 1905 and subsequently were key figures in the creation of an electric railroad, the Piedmont and Northern Railway. Other business ventures involved hydroelectric power plants in other locations, including Canada, and factories to produce various chemicals (3).

After Trinity College moved to Durham in 1892 and while James and Benjamin Duke were developing the family's businesses, the little college passed through a series of turbulent events. As it matured, Trinity College continued to receive periodic financial support from the Duke family. But it took the perseverance of a far-sighted Trinity College president, William Preston Few, to take full advantage of the Duke philanthropy and transform the college into a university. It was President Few who gradually convinced James B. Duke to make a sufficient endowment in 1924 to permit the major institutional changes that followed, including the establishment of a medical school and hospital (3, 4, 7).

The hope for a medical school in Durham had surfaced five times between 1889 and 1923, but each time a plan had been put forward, it had failed because of political or economic factors (4). Success was finally achieved as the result of the 1924 and 1925 gifts from James B. Duke. The Duke Endowment of December 1924 provided benefit to many institutions, especially educational institutions, hospitals, and the Methodist Church. The newly established Duke University received 32 percent of the initial gift of $32 million. Then, at the time of his death in October, 1925, Mr. Duke bequeathed an additional $10 million for Duke University, of which $4 million was to be expended for a medical school, hospital, and nurses' home (2).

As the endowment was being planned and put into effect, more than 5,000 acres of woodland near the site of Trinity College were quietly obtained for expansion of the new Duke University (3, 7). The Tudor Gothic buildings that were to be built on this West Campus included a medical school facing the main quadrangle and an attached 400-bed hospital (2,4). Trial walls of stone from various quarries in the United States were erected to permit James B. Duke and the trustees of the endowment in March 1925 to select the stone from which the new Duke University buildings would he constructed (2, 3). Interestingly, they selected stone from a location in Hillsborough, near the original Duke farm. The university purchased the quarry and constructed railroad tracks so that the stone could be brought to the building site.

The initial Duke medical faculty was recruited primarily from the Johns Hopkins University School of Medicine, beginning with the appointment in 1927 of the Dean, Wilburt C. Davison, who had been a pediatrician and assistant dean at Johns Hopkins (2, 4, 6). Dr. Davison also took on the chairmanship of the Duke University Department of Pediatrics. As an interesting footnote, Wilburt Davison had become friends with Wilder Penfield[2] during their student days (1, 5). Both were Rhodes scholars who had studied physiology at Oxford with Charles Sherrington. Both were admitted in the fall of 1916 as transfer students to the Johns Hopkins University School of Medicine, and they roomed together that year.

After the selection of the Chairman of the Department of Medicine, the third individual appointed to the Duke medical faculty was Deryl Hart, a Johns Hopkins-trained surgeon, who accepted the appointment as Professor and Chairman of the Department of Surgery in 1929 (6). After Duke Hospital opened on Monday, July 21, 1930, Dr. Hart and his associate, Dr. Clarence F. Gardner, Jr. (who came to Duke from Johns Hopkins in 1932), included neurosurgery in their daily practice. The seventy-third patient to register at the new facility presented with headaches and papilledema. On July 24 a ventriculogram was performed through bilateral occipital trephine openings, and a right frontal cyst was aspirated by Dr. Hart. This cystic glioma was then successfully resected two days later by Dr. Hart.

In September 1937, Barnes Woodhall came to Durham after completing his surgical training at the Johns Hopkins Hospital where he had been a favorite resident of Walter Dandy (8, 10). Dr. Woodhall was given the charge of forming a Division of Neurosurgery, but his work was interrupted when he volunteered for military service in 1943 (6). Later in 1943, Guy L. Odom, who had received his training in neurosurgery under Wilder Penfield and William Cone at the Montreal Neurological Institute, was recruited to the Duke faculty by Dr. Hart.

---

2. Wilder Penfield (1891–1976) was one of the great neurosurgeons of the twentieth century at the Montreal Neurological Institute. He is credited with the discovery of the functions of the temporal lobes of the brain and for the development of the motor homunculus, a portrayal of the motor function of the brain.

Dr. Woodhall returned to Duke University after his discharge from the Army in 1946, and he and Dr. Odom founded the Duke University Division of Neurosurgery, including the establishment of a residency program. In 1960, Dr. Woodhall resigned his position as Chief of the Division to start a second career in medical and university administration that culminated in a term as Chancellor pro tem of Duke University in 1969 and 1970. Dr. Odom succeeded Dr. Woodhall as Chief of the Duke University Division of Neurosurgery, serving from 1960 to 1976 and establishing many of the patterns of practice and instruction used today by those who have followed in his path.

Many individuals and many events led to the formation and development of the Duke University Medical Center, but a few stand out because of their primary importance. Washington Duke overcame recurrent personal adversity to establish finally a successful family business by 1880. Trinity College demonstrated the same tenacity in surviving decades of financial drought before it began to receive major support from Washington Duke and his sons in 1892. In 1924, toward the end of his life, James B. Duke felt the need to leave a worthwhile legacy that would benefit others in perpetuity. Finally, William Preston Few had the foresight and patience to bring substance to Mr. Duke's dream.

The seed that was planted by James B. Duke in 1924 has grown into an outstanding medical center. In many ways it has eclipsed the various other significant achievements that he realized during his lifetime.

References

1. Brown, I. W., Jr. A classmate's tribute to Dean Wilburt C. Davison. A recently discovered and previously unpublished memorial note by Wilder G. Penfield, M.D. *NC Med. J.* 1:164–166. 1990.
2. Davison, W. C. *The Duke University Medical Center (1892–1960).* Durham: Duke Endowment, 1966.
3. Durden, R. F. *The Dukes of Durham, 1892–1929.* Durham: Duke University Press. 1987.

4. Gifford, J. F,. Jr. *The Evolution of a Medical Center: A History of Medicine at Duke University to 1941.* Durham: Duke University Press, 1972.

5. Grant, R. *Charles Scott Sherrington: An Appraisal.* London: Thomas Nelson & Sons, 1966.

6. Hart, D. *The First Forty Years at Duke in Surgery and the P. D. C.* Durham: Duke University Press, 1971.

7. Porter, E. W. *Trinity and Duke, 1892–1924: Foundation of Duke University.* Durham: Duke University Press.

8. Wilkins, R. H. Barnes Woodhall, M.D.: A biographical sketch. *Clin. Neurosurg.* 18: xvii–xx. 1971.

9. Wilkins, R. H. Guy L. Odom, M.D.: A biographical sketch. *Clin. Neurosurg.* 22: 16–21. 1975.

10. Woodhall, B. Neurosurgery in the past—The Dandy era. *Clin. Neurosurg.* 18: 1–15. 1971.

Chapter 4 ⌒

Deryl Hart: Leader in the Development of the Duke University Medical Center

*W*ith the passage of time and reflection upon the origin of the Duke University Medical Center, it has become increasingly apparent that of its founders none deserves more recognition than Deryl Hart. He served for more than thirty years as Professor of Surgery and Chairman of the Department, and was then appointed President of the University by the Board of Trustees. In addition to creating a strong department with primary emphasis upon excellence in clinical surgery, Dr. Hart turned his innovative mind to the structuring of the Private Diagnostic Clinic, a concept that has since become the foundation upon which the Duke University Medical Center is based and one that has also served as a model for many similar institutions throughout the nation. Together with Wilburt C. Davison[1] and Frederic M. Hanes,[2] Deryl Hart was a key figure in this triumvirate that within a very short time placed Duke among the foremost medical centers in the nation.

Several years before his death, in response to a reporter's question concerning his philosophy of life, Deryl Hart replied, "Set your goal high, if you think you can do it, and finish what you start." In this succinct statement, he embraced a life-long emphasis upon hard work, and in a unique way, related the pleasures and rewards that it brought. It was obvious from the beginning that he had set high standards for

---

1. Wilbert C. Davison was the first Dean of Duke University School of Medicine.

2. Frederic M. Hanes was the first full-time Chair of Medicine at Duke University School of Medicine.

himself, and his entire life was an example of the admirable completion of each goal he set. Born of industrious parents in Buena Vista, a
cotton-growing region in Georgia, he went to Emory University and
graduated cum laude with election into Phi Beta Kappa. After receiving a master's degree in mathematics, he entered the Johns Hopkins
Medical School and achieved an outstanding record, graduating in the
class of 1921. His dedication, hard work and achievement was rewarded by being selected for one of the highly coveted internships in
surgery under William Stewart Halsted at Johns Hopkins Medical
School, generally recognized as America's greatest surgeon of this century. He progressed upward through the program, ultimately becoming Chief Resident.

It is interesting to reflect upon the method by which Deryl Hart
was chosen to be the first Professor and Chairman of the Department
of Surgery at Duke. By his own account, while in his second year of
Chief Residency at Johns Hopkins, he was approached in the hospital
corridor by the Chief of Otolaryngology, Dr. Samuel J. Crowe, who
invited him to his home for dinner. During the evening Dr. Crowe
casually mentioned the new medical school being built in North Carolina as a result of a generous gift from the famed industrialist, James
Buchanan Duke. He asked whether or not Dr. Hart might have an
interest in being Chief of Surgery. Sometime earlier, Dr. Hart had
agreed to remain on the faculty at Johns Hopkins and therefore wished
to give the matter additional thought before responding. A week later,
another invitation came from Dr. Crowe to come for dinner, and that
evening Dr. Hart expressed a definite interest in the position. Shortly
thereafter, Dean Wilburt C. Davison offered him the position of Professor and Chairman of the Department of Surgery, an offer he accepted on March 9, 1929, at the age of only thirty-five. In this decision he
had the strong support of Dean Lewis, the Surgeon in Chief at Johns
Hopkins, as well as that of the noted John M. T. Finney. It is interesting, however, that the Director of the hospital, Winford M, Smith,
strongly advised him to remain at Hopkins, saying that the many hospitals being developed in the Carolinas through the Duke Endowment
would prevent sufficient clinical material being referred to Durham,
and further commented that it would be "easier for you to obtain private patients from North Carolina at Hopkins than at Duke."

The Duke Hospital was opened on July 21, 1930, and the following day Dr. Hart did the first operation, performing bilateral repair of inguinal hernias on a seventy-two-year-old patient. He later emphasized the low cost of hospitalization in the early days, with the average daily cost per bed at Duke Hospital in 1936 being $4.57, and somewhat apologetically added there was a "subsequent gradual rise to $5.73 per day by 1942."

Shortly after his arrival at Duke, in the midst of the Great Depression, Dr. Hart, together with Dean Davison and Frederic Hanes, Professor and Chairman of the Department of Medicine, laid the foundations for the development of the Private Diagnostic Clinic. The basic principles upon which the Clinic was established were that all clinical appointments in the University would he on a part-time basis and that each department would develop its own geographic full-time clinical faculty. Moreover, each department would have maximal independence as long as cooperation for the general development for Duke Medical Center was maintained. As a result of that careful and thoughtful plan, these principles remain in effect to this day, and the contributions to the University Medical Center from the private practice of its faculty have been vital in the development of Duke Hospital and Medical School. As one example, through the Duke Medical Center building fund and departmental contributions, the clinical faculty at Duke provided $10 million toward the construction of the new Duke University Hospital. In addition, some $2 million is currently contributed annually toward the Medical Center Building Fund by the clinical faculty.

Dr. Hart was respected not only in the Department of Surgery but throughout the entire Medical Center and indeed the country. Shortly after his arrival, one of the new members of the faculty in the Department of Medicine, who had been recruited from Harvard, said, "I know of nobody in Boston within ten years of his age whose opinion I would rather have on any surgical condition." Of that early era, one of his Chief Residents was later to write "I wish to acknowledge on behalf of our group the fine example of craftsmanship and sound surgical judgment and knowledge personified by Dr. Hart. During his active teaching days, which corresponded to my period of training, he was the one surgeon that the staff looked to as the example of how a surgical procedure should be properly carried out. In endeavoring to emulate his technique, I am sure we all became much better surgeons. His vast fund of knowledge of surgery and recall was a source of awe, as well as an inspiration." The faculty were also aware of his immense contributions and one summarized by saying, "Dr. Hart literally devoted his life to the development of this school and his department, combining qualities of leadership, surgical skill, business acumen, personal integrity, and judgment, and an ability to pick an able staff to build one of the leading departments of surgery in this country."

In 1960, Duke University found itself in a difficult administrative controversy, and Dr. Hart responded to the Trustees' call that he lead the institution as President through that turbulent era. As a result of his determination, his sound judgment, and hard work, he rapidly reversed the divided campus and firmly united it. With a series of bold strokes, he greatly enhanced the character and image of Duke throughout the nation. Under his leadership, faculty salaries quickly rose to rank among the top few universities in the nation, and the number of distinguished professorships was doubled. Fortunately, his masterful achievements were recognized at the time, and one of the senior Duke Board of Trustees confidently commented, "I believe there is no one who, during the particular time Dr. Hart served as President, could have accomplished so much for the advancement of Duke University."

At the time of his appointment as President of Duke University, The *Raleigh News and Observer* interviewed Dr. Hart and quoted him in its "Profile of a Tarheel" as saying that he originally came to Duke because "...I wanted to help build the medical school—its future looked bright, and so I decided to make my future with the school. After coming here, I found that my confidence was justified. After I once started here, I knew that I would rather stay here than go anywhere....Everyone has been cooperative and is pulling together. They help me to meet the problems as they arise and get me through, somehow." It was in this milieu that Deryl Hart built a strong clinical surgical service, developed in an extraordinary way the specialties of surgery at Duke, organized an outstanding residency program, and trained a number of leading practitioners of surgery as well as a distinctive group in academic surgery.

Later in his life, Dr. Hart said, "In retrospect, it is my opinion that if I have made any contribution to the development of this Medical Center and to the Department of Surgery, it is based upon my complete freedom and encouragement to think, to plan, and to propose and then to receive the support of the Dean in decisions to act."

All who know the full story of Deryl Hart's success recognize the very supportive and highly important role played by Mary Johnson Hart, his wife for half a century. Dr. Hart himself acknowledged this fact in the introduction to his book *The First Forty Years at Duke in Surgery and the PDC* when he said, "This book is dedicated to my wife, Mary Johnson Hart, whose encouragement, suggestions, and help account for many of the accomplishments for which credit has been given to me" (1).

As Daryl Hart's close colleague and friend of many years, Clarence E. Gardner, said of him posthumously, "It is impossible to know the extent of Dr. Hart's influence on the thousands who knew him, his patients, his students, the residents whom he trained, his staff, and the University community. His life will surely carry on in the lives of many of them. Certainly his life leaves a permanent imprint on his Department and on Duke University."

Finally, as was said of him at the memorial service held in the Duke University Chapel shortly after his death in June 1980, "As we reflect upon this man, and this hour, we recognize and cherish all that he leaves us. These combine to assure his continuing presence as his shadow lengthens into the future, as surely it will."

Reference

1. Hart, D. *The First Forty Years at Duke in Surgery and the PDC.* Duke University Press, 1971.

Chapter 5 ☞

The Department of Surgery of
Duke University Medical Center[1]

T he Duke Hospital is the clinical teaching unit for the Duke University School of Medicine. This complex, together with the School of Nursing and the School of Hospital Administration, comprises the Duke University Medical Center. It contains 802 beds of which 128 ward and 170 private beds are devoted to general surgery and the surgical specialties. The Hospital admits approximately 22,000 patients each year, of whom about half are surgical admissions. The Hospital has an operating suite consisting of eighteen rooms and three hyperbaric oxygen operating rooms and treatment chambers in the Clinical Research Building.

The Veterans Administration Hospital with 489 beds is located immediately adjacent to the Duke University Medical Center, and is supervised by a Dean's Committee of the School of Medicine. The Chiefs of Clinical Departments at Duke are responsible for the respective services at the Veterans Hospital. Its residency program is completely integrated with the Duke program both in General and Cardiothoracic Surgery as well as those of the surgical specialties, with some 200 beds devoted to Surgery and its Divisions. Residents rotate through the various surgical services of the Veterans Hospital, and a portion of the chief residency is taken at the Veterans Hospital. This service is an important supplement to surgical services at Duke Hospital. The residency programs of each of the surgical specialties also include rotations through the services of the Veterans Hospital.

---

1. This article was written in 1970.

The Department of Surgery owes much to its founder, Dr. Deryl Hart, the first Professor and Chairman of the Department, who laid a firm foundation in the selection of an outstanding faculty and resident staff over a twenty-year period. He was largely responsible for the formation of the Private Diagnostic Clinics at Duke, and the impact of this contribution has been of much benefit to the Medical Center and to the entire University. Moreover, the concept of providing excellence in medical care for private patients while simultaneously yielding support for an academic Department has spread to other institutions. In 1966 the Deryl Hart Pavilion, in which are located the surgical clinics, general operating rooms, and surgical wards, was dedicated in his honor.

The second Professor and Chairman of the Department of Surgery, Dr. Clarence F. Gardner, considerably furthered the original aims and accomplishments. Dr. Gardner was the first Chief Resident in Surgery at Duke and throughout his teaching career here was regarded as an exceptionally able teacher of students and residents. In his teaching rounds he often placed considerable emphasis on the importance of the historical aspects of surgery, and he is annually honored jointly by the Department of Surgery and the Medical Center Library in the "Clarence L. Gardner Lecture in the History of Surgery." In 1968 the new Surgical Out-Patient Clinic was dedicated in his honor.

Several of the previous Chiefs of Divisions, each of whom was originally appointed at an early age and is now a Professor Emeritus, have contributed heavily to the image of the Medical Center. Dr. Edwin P. Alyea, the first Professor of Urology, built an impressive clinical service and residency program, as did Dr. W. Banks Anderson in Ophthalmology and Dr. Watt W. Eagle in Otolaryngology. Dr. Lenox Baker, the leader of an outstanding Division of Orthopaedics, has recently been succeeded as Chairman of the Division, but remains quite active in teaching and clinical orthopaedics. Dr. Barnes Woodhall was the first head of the Division of Neurosurgery and remained in the post until his appointment as Dean of the School of Medicine in 1960. He later became Associate Provost and is currently Chancellor pro tem of the University. Dr. Woodhall's impact on clinical and investigative neurosurgery as well as in the training of young leaders in the field is well known.

The Department of Surgery sponsors a surgical internship and a first-year assistant residency of one year each. Eighteen interns are appointed each July 1 through the National Intern Matching Plan and are promoted later to first year residents. Eight of the appointees are selected as potential candidates for the Residency Program in General and Cardiothoracic Surgery and in this group are also included any appointees who are undecided about the specific residency to be pursued in the future. Ten of the internships are available for candidates who have already decided upon a career in one of the surgical specialties (Neurosurgery, Orthopaedics, Otolaryngology, Plastic Surgery, or Urology). These appointments are made in conjunction with and upon approval of the chief of the respective division with the tentative understanding that the applicant will continue training in that specialty.

The Department of Surgery has two principal aims in its graduate program of training in General and Cardiothoracic Surgery. First, all residents are provided a thorough experience in the diagnosis and operative management of an adequate number of patients with disorders which comprise the entire field of general surgery. Second, each resident is provided an opportunity to obtain depth in a specific area of general surgery such that upon completion of the program he not only is a qualified general surgeon but has obtained particular skills and recognition in an area which he selects. Moreover, each resident is expected to spend a year in experimental or clinical investigation. The program is directed by the Chairman of the Department together with Dr. William W. Shingleton, Chief of the Division of General Surgery, and Dr. Will C. Sealy, Chief of the Division of Thoracic Surgery.

The clinical facilities and large number of patients at the Duke Hospital and the Veterans Hospital provide a broad basis for residency training. In order to accomplish depth in a selected part of general surgery, the resident is encouraged to choose the field of his interest such that quite early in his training it can be arranged for him to observe, assist at operations, and actually perform the procedures in this field. For example, special interests might include one or more of the following: abdominal surgery, peripheral vascular surgery, thoracic surgery, children's surgery, homotransplantation, surgery of endocrine disorders, cardiac surgery, and similar fields as chosen by the resident. Thus, with the primary emphasis being on training in general surgery, each resident has the opportunity to select a special field of interest. The time devoted to original investigation is expected to be closely related to the clinical field previously selected.

The Department of Surgery has a number of established laboratories in which investigative interests are being pursued. For example, specific laboratories are available for a) homotransplantation, b) hyperbaric medicine and surgery, c) studies on the pulmonary circulation, d) shock and homeostasis, e) cancer research, f) thrombosis and blood coagulation, g) wound infections and healing, h) gastrointestinal research, and i) cardiovascular research. Following the internship, the Residency Program in General and Cardiothoracic Surgery is designed as a five year program. Three additional years of senior assistant residency (including one year in the laboratory) are then devoted to gradually increasing responsibilities in preparation for the final year as Chief Resident. Positions are available for several Chief Residents in the final year by rotations as Chief on the Duke General Surgical Service, on the Duke Cardiothoracic Service, and on the corresponding Services at the Veterans Administration Hospital. The Department of Surgery has an affiliation with the Oteen Veterans Hospital in Oteen, N.C., that is also a cardiothoracic center and provides unusual opportunities for those interested in obtaining qualifications for cardiothoracic surgery. In addition, a senior resident is assigned to the Watts Hospital in Durham, N.C., and to the North Carolina Tuberculosis Hospital. At the completion of the five-year program, all candidates are eligible for the American Board of Surgery. For those candidates who are interested in simultaneously qualifying for the Board of Thoracic Surgery, special rotations may be selected in advance to provide ample clinical experience for application to this board.

At the completion of the Chief Residency, one or two of those finishing the program may be appointed for an additional year as Teaching Scholar in Surgery. Such appointees should have an interest in remaining in academic surgery. The responsibilities of this position consist mainly of additional and selected experience in the field of choice both in the operating room and in a teaching and consultant capacity to the resident staff. Moreover, considerable administrative responsibility is delegated to these appointees who hold the rank of an Instructor in the School of Medicine. In this year opportunity is available for extended operative experiences in special fields such as cardiac surgery and advanced general surgery. These teaching scholars act as consultants to Chief Residents, are independent investigators, and also perform selected operations of their choice.

During the past decade the impact of the basic sciences on the surgical disciplines has become quite forceful. With specific goals in mind, the Department of Surgery has mounted sizable investigative programs in cardiovascular disease, homotransplantation, biology, neoplastic disease, hyperbaric oxygenation, and gastrointestinal research. The Scholar in Academic Surgery Program is supported by a grant from the National Institutes of Health. Currently nine senior residents are in this program and each is committed to a minimum of two years' study in experimental and clinical investigation. In addition, a fundamental feature of this program is that each Scholar will be thoroughly trained in clinical surgery and is a part of the regular Surgical Residency Program. It is for these young investigators, who will ultimately be appointed to faculty posts to further their careers, that numerous opportunities are available.

The Department is fortunate in having strong divisions in the specialties of surgery, each of which has a separate Residency Training Program directed by the division. These programs are as follows.

The Residency Program in Neurosurgery is under the direction of Dr. Guy L. Odom, Professor and Chairman of the Division, and is a five-year program following surgical internship qualifying the resident for certification by the American Board of Neurosurgery. Two candidates each year are appointed to the program. The first year is spent in the Neuropathologic Laboratory and includes participation in the research program of the division. The second year includes a primary study program in Neurology with a secondary interest in Neuroanatony and Electroencephalography. The last three years include clinical training in Neurosurgery at both the Veterans Hospital and

Duke Hospital. Throughout the training period, individuals are encouraged to pursue research projects of clinical and basic science interests.

The Residency Program in Orthopaedics is under the direction of Dr. J. Leonard Goldner, Professor and Chairman of the division. The senior staff includes six full-time orthopaedic surgeons who actively participate in all phases of residency training. Rotations occur through clinical and basic science services at Duke Hospital, the adjacent Veterans Hospital, and Watts and Lincoln Hospitals, which are county-supported institutions. Additional rotations for training in children's orthopaedics are offered at the North Carolina Orthopaedic Hospital in Gastonia, the Shriners Hospital for Crippled Children in Greenville, South Carolina, and the North Carolina Cerebral Palsy Hospital in Durham. Basic science and research rotations are planned in keeping with the trainee's particular interests.

The Residency Program in Otolaryngology is a fully approved program under the direction of Dr. William R. Hudson, Professor and Chairman of the Division. Two residents are appointed yearly upon completion of an approved internship. The program is four years in length and includes a year of General Surgery. Responsibility is graduated during the program, and the senior resident has the ultimate responsibility of all public cases under the direct supervision of the senior staff. A comprehensive teaching program is provided by means of frequent teaching rounds, conferences, and journal clubs, with time alloted for research. Basic science instruction is provided with the assistance of other departments.

The Residency Program in Plastic and Maxillofacial Surgery is under the direction of Dr. Kenneth L. Pickrell, Professor and Chairman of the division, and is designed for board certification in Plastic Surgery. Candidates are accepted after completing at least three years of certified training in General Surgery beyond the internship. Two trainees are accepted each year and the period of training is three years in length, encompassing graded responsibility and independent experience in excisional and reparative surgery of the scalp, face, orbit, nose, oral cavity, neck, trunk, and extremities; the surgical treatment of neoplastic lesions of the head, oral cavity, and neck; congenital abnormalities; reconstructive and esthetic surgery; facial trauma; surgery of the hand and extremities; the treatment of burns, etc. Research and investigation are encouraged, and each resident must work on one or more problems simultaneously. The residents in training spend approximately one-half time on the Plastic Surgery Service at the Veterans Hospital. The division is closely associated with Orthodontics, Dr. Galen Quinn, Chief, and with Medical Speech Pathology under the direction of Dr. Raymond Massengill. The Residency Program in Urology is under the direction of Dr. James F. Glenn, Professor and Chairman of the division.

An internship and one year of assistant residency in General Surgery are minimum prerequisites to the appointment of two residents each year. In addition, applicants may be appointed to a one-year Fellowship in Investigative Urology. Research activities include extensive programs of investigation of urinary physiology, urologic rehabilitation, and urologic malignancies and are coordinated in the facilities of Duke University Medical Center and the adjacent Veterans Hospital. Residents are encouraged to participate in research and teaching activities as well as to acquire progressive proficiency in patient care and surgery. Rotation between Duke Hospital with active private and ward services, the Veterans Hospital, and the Watts-Lincoln community Hospitals insures a broad spectrum of training advantages.

In summary, since its founding in 1930, the Department of Surgery has grown from an original faculty of five members and a resident staff also numbering five to its present roster of 110 members of the senior faculty and 122 interns, fellows, and residents. Despite the progressive increase in the size of the staff and of the supporting research facilities, the primary aim of all members of the Department continues as it was originally: the best possible care of the surgical patient.

III

History of Surgical Medicine

C learly, high standards and understanding the past represent our best hope for the future.

Chapter 6

Major Contributions to Surgery from the South

*I*n presenting a review of outstanding contributions to surgery from the South, I intend to emphasize the importance of the past in the development of achievements of the future. In other words, it is not my intent to present a solely historical account, but rather emphasis is placed upon the relationship of these major contributions to the present and future. My personal experiences in the teaching and practice of surgery have led to the firm belief that Santayana captured an enduring truth when he said, "Those who cannot remember the past are condemned to repeat it." It is from our appreciation of earlier contributions that incentive springs for new discoveries, and in turn, provides a continuing stimulus for each new generation of physicans.

It is of considerable significance that, upon the organization of the Southern Surgical in 1887, Ephraim McDowell was chosen as its exemplary patron and his likeness appears in gold on the first issue of the *Transactions* of this association. It becomes clear in pursuing the life and work of this surgical pioneer that he was descended from a courageous and public-spirited family. His father represented Augusta County in Virginia at the Convention of 1775 in Williamsburg. Ephraim was born in 1771 and later moved with his parents to Kentucky and entered the Transylvania Seminary at the age of fifteen. He studied medicine in Edinburgh where he fell under the strong influence of John Bell, the famed surgical teacher of the day. Returning from Edinburgh in 1795, he entered practice in his hometown of Danville, Kentucky, which at the time was described as "containing upwards of 150 homes and some tolerable good buildings."

The records indicate that McDowell's practice extended over a radius of fifty miles from the town of Danville, and most of his calls were made on horseback and on many occasions through trackless regions. He was not only a medical practitioner but also a surgeon, being noted in the region for having performed thirty-two operations for removal of bladder stones (lithotomy) without the loss of a single life. One of his most celebrated lithotomy patients was James Knox Polk, the eleventh president of the United States, upon whom McDowell operated in 1812 and who remained a friend for life.

On December 13, 1809, some fourteen years after he had entered practice, Dr. McDowell was called to the home of Mrs. Jane Todd Crawford, who lived about sixty miles from Danville. Mrs. Crawford had suffered for some time with massive enlargement of the abdomen, first thought to be a pregnancy. But when the mass persisted and the diagnosis could not be confirmed, McDowell stated:

> Having never seen so large a substance extracted, nor heard of an attempt, or success attending any operation, such as this required, I gave to the unhappy woman information of her dangerous situation. She appeared willing to undergo an experiment, which I promised to perform if she would come to Danville. (20)

It is interesting to note the choice of word "experiment," for indeed this was clearly the situation. Until that time there had not been a successful opening of the peritoneal cavity for removal of an intraabdominal tumor, and this was well known to the thoughtful practitioner in the backwoods of Kentucky.

McDowell's first report of this historic case is to be found in the *Eclectic Repertory and Analytical Review* in 1817. It can be seen that he waited until he had managed three such cases before reporting the first. In this paper, he states that Mrs. Crawford undertook the journey from her home in Danville on horseback, which required several days. On Christmas Day 1809, McDowell performed the now famous operation in his home. The following is McDowell's description of the procedure on Mrs. Crawford:

> With the assistance of my nephew and colleague, James McDowell, M.D., I commenced the operation, which was concluded as follows: Having placed her on a table of the ordinary height, on her back, and removed all her dressing which might in any way impede the operation, I made an incision about three inches from the musculus rectus abdominis, on the left side, continuing the same nine inches in length, parallel with the fibres of the above named muscle, extending into the cavity of the abdomen, the parts of

which were a good deal contused, which we ascribed to the resting of the tumor on the horn of the saddle during her journey. The tumor then appeared full in view, but was so large that we could not take it away entire. We put a strong ligature around the Fallopian tube near to the uterus, we then cut open the tumor, which was the ovarium and fimbrious part of the Fallopian tube very much enlarged. We took out fifteen pounds of a dirty, gelatinous looking substance. After which we cut through the Fallopian tube, and extracted the sac, which weighed seven pounds and one half. As soon as the external opening was made, the intestines rushed out upon the table; and so completely was the abdomen filled by the tumor, that they could not be replaced during the operation, which was terminated in about twenty-five minutes. We then turned her upon her left side, so as to permit the blood to escape: after which, we closed the external opening with the interrupted suture, leaving out, at the lower end of the incision, the ligature which surrounded the Fallopian tube. Between every two stitches we put a strip of adhesive plaster, which, by keeping the parts in contact, hastened the healing of the incision. We then applied the usual dressings, put her to bed, and prescribed a strict observance of the antiphlogistic regimen. In five days I visited her, and much to my astonishment found her engaged in making up her bed. I gave her particular caution for the future; and in twenty-five days, she returned home as she came, in good health, which she continues to enjoy. (20)

For this operation there was, of course, no anesthetic, and Mrs. Crawford's grandson later reported that she read the Psalms throughout the procedure. It is remarkable that this historic achievement, the first successful of its kind in the history of medicine, was ever performed in the first place, was successful, was performed without anesthesia, and was completed in twenty-five minutes. Mrs. Crawford lived in excellent health with no evidence of return of her disease until her seventy-ninth year. Her son, Thomas H. Crawford, became a successful businessman and ultimately was elected Mayor of Louisville.

In 1829, the year before his death, McDowell wrote a letter to a medical student, Robert Thompson, describing a total of eleven patients upon whom he had operated for ovarian tumors, with ten survivors (24). Fortunately, McDowell received considerable praise for these achievements during his life, and in 1825 he was awarded an Honorary Degree from the University of Maryland. In dedicating the McDowell monument some years later, the noted Samuel D. Gross of Philadelphia stated:

He achieved that renown which so justly entitles him to be ranked among the benefactors of his race...an operation which, in its aggregate results in the hands of different surgeons, has already added upwards of forty thousand years to woman's life, and which is destined, as time rolls on, to rescue thousands upon thousands of human beings from premature destruction. (7)

Of all the contributions to surgery, none ranks higher than the introduction of anesthesia, representing a landmark achievement in the progress of medicine. Throughout the history of man, attempts have been made to find appropriate means for alleviation of pain, and while a number of drugs had been successful in part, the challenge remained to find a safe method of producing a state of unconsciousness.

On November 1, 1815, a son was born to the James Long family in Danielsville, Georgia. Young Crawford, as he was named, was a quiet, studious boy who was fond of horses, swimming, and fishing. He entered the University of Georgia at the age of fourteen and was graduated in 1835. His roommate in college was Alexander H. Stephens, who was to become governor of Georgia and later vice president of the Confederacy. Following graduation, Long remained for a year in Danielsville, since his father thought he was too young at nineteen to enter medical school. He first matriculated at Transylvania University of Lexington, Kentucky, in 1836, but then transferred to the University of Pennsylvania, where he graduated in 1839.

In 1799, Sir Humphry Davy had written, "As nitrous oxide in its extensive operation appears capable of destroying physical pain, it may he used with advantage during surgical operations." However, this gas was used primarily by those who wished to demonstrate its more humorous and comical effects and was employed by traveling showmen, one of whom appeared in Jefferson, Georgia, during the winter of 1841. It was in that village that Dr. Crawford W. Long had settled, having only two years previously been graduated from the University of Pennsylvania. Also in this town was a private academy, and a number of the students there attended the session given by the visiting showman. The students were impressed that when under the influence of nitrous oxide they did peculiar things, including the most ridiculous of antics. Since they knew and related well to Dr. Long, a young man of only twenty-six, they approached him to obtain some laughing gas.

He told them that he had none but mentioned the similar effects of ether. He recalled to them a lecture he attended in Philadelphia, where a showman induced inebriation, not with laughing gas but with ether. The students returned to school with the news, and this marked the beginning of the now famous ether parties, which were held two or three evenings each week in Crawford Long's office. As a matter of fact, the young ladies of the community soon heard of these sessions and finally were successful in persuading Dr. Long to allow them to attend. As might be expected, he was reluctant to let them inhale ether, saying one could not predict what might happen while they were under the influence and he would not want them to do anything which they might later regret. Instead of diminishing their interest, this apparently increased it, and they jointly replied that they didn't care what happened and wouldn't notice it. Moreover, they assured him that it would not be his fault but the fault of the ether should anything untoward occur. One writer said of this event, "Never had such a course of promises been heard under one roof in Georgia and with the utmost of solemnity."

The actual story of the first patient to whom ether was given as a planned anesthetic for a surgical procedure is carefully and authentically described (2). One of the students in the local academy in Jefferson, James Venable, consulted Crawford Long about a tumor on the back of his neck, which was causing considerable discomfort. He had attended some of the ether parties, and after a long discussion they agreed that it should be removed, using ether as an anesthetic. For historical purposes, it is interesting that the student permitted several of his classmates to see the procedure. Moreover, in order to lend proper respectability to the occasion, the principal of the academy was invited as well. On March 30, 1842, James Venable appeared in the office of Dr. Long together with three of his student friends and the principal of the academy. Venable was described as being rather nervous as he lay down on the sofa while Long reached for the ether bottle which had been their companion in so many earlier sprees. He poured ether on a towel as he had done many times before, but on this occasion, it was under different circumstances, for he realized he was making an important experiment. The spectators gathered in a group at the back of the room and watched as the patient inhaled both ether and air intermittently. Long pricked his friend with a pin, and when Venable no longer felt it, he reached for the scalpel and removed the tumor. The entire operation took approximately five minutes, and when the towel was removed from his face, Venable awakened in good condition. In fact, he had to be shown the specimen to be convinced that it had been removed.

In Crawford Long's account book for the year 1842, one finds a fascinating entry which was later published in the *Boston Medical and Surgical Journal*. It is interesting to note that the fee of this pioneering country doctor for the anesthetic was $25 and for the surgical procedure was $2.

Further search into these interesting original reports reveals that appropriate skepticism of anything new was just as true in 1842 as it is today, for there were many who said that the ether anesthetic was not directly responsible for the absence of pain in this historic case. It is clear that Long was an objective observer, since after this criticism he had a patient in whom it was necessary to amputate two fingers. One amputation was performed under anesthesia during which there was no pain. The other amputation was done in the usual manner of the day, that is, without anesthesia and the young boy cried loudly. To confirm this further, Long removed three tumors from the same patient in one day, the second with ether and the first and third without. Again, the procedure performed with ether was painless as opposed to the excruciating discomfort associated with the removal of the other two lesions.

When the state of Georgia was asked to select its two most distinguished citizens to be placed in Statuary Hall of the United States Capitol in Washington, Crawford W. Long and another famed historical figure, Alexander H. Stephens, the vice president of the Confederacy, were chosen.

In addition to relief of pain, another major impact of this contribution can best be appreciated by citing the fears that surgeons had of the inadvertent movement of the patient during a critical part of an operation prior to the advent of anesthesia. For example, one of America's greatest surgeons, Valentine Mott, said:

When operating in some deep, dark wound, along the course of some great vein, with thin walls, alternately distended and flaccid with the vital current—how often I have dreaded that some unfortunate struggle of the patient would deviate the knife a little from its normal course and that I, who fain would be the deliverer, should involuntarily become the executioner, seeing my patient perish in my hands by one of the most appalling forms of death.

In 1912, Long received a medallion from his alma mater, the University of Pennsylvania, with the inscription:

To Crawford W. Long. First to use ether as an anesthetic in surgery, March 30th, 1842, from his Alma Mater.

The proper credit due William T. G. Morton and his associates in Boston is a matter of record, and it is unnecessary to emphasize the importance of their role in broadly disseminating the use of anesthesia throughout the practice of medicine. Nevertheless, the point seems historically clear that the first anesthetic ever to he intentionally administered to man for painless surgery occurred in Jefferson, Georgia, on March 30, 1842. In 1902, when King Edward VII of England awoke from the anesthetic which had been administered during an operation for appendicitis, he asked the surgeon, Sir Frederick Treves, "Who discovered anesthesia?" Sir Frederick answered immediately. "It was an American, your Majesty, Crawford W. Long" (2).

One of the greatest of the Southern surgeons, J. Marion Sims, has been celebrated worldwide for more than a century. Born in 1813 in Lancaster County, South Carolina, he received early education in Charleston and later was graduated from the Jefferson Medical College in Philadelphia. Sims originally began medical practice in his native town of Lancasterville but soon left to settle in Alabama. For a short period he practiced in Mount Meigs and later moved to Montgomery. In the summer of 1845 some rather unique experiences occurring in swift succession were to greatly influence his professional career. In his autobiography, *The Story of My Life*, Sims said:

Early in the month of June (1845) Dr. Henry asked me to go out to Mr. Wescott's, only a mile from the town, to see a case of labor which had lasted three days and the child not yet born. He said, "I am thinking that you had better take your instruments along with you, for you may want to use them. (26)

Sims found a young woman about seventeen years of age who had been in labor for seventy-two hours with impaction of the head in the pelvis such that labor pains had almost entirely ceased. It was evident that matters could not remain in this condition without the pressure producing a sloughing of the soft parts of the mother, and so forceps were chosen for delivery. She recovered from the immediate effects of the delivery, but because of the prolonged engagement of the head, pressure necrosis and a fistula between the bladder and vagina developed. As Sims said:

> Of course, aside from death, this was about the worst accident that could have happened to the poor young girl. I went to see her, and found an enormous slough, spreading from the posterior wall of the vagina, and another thrown off from the anterior wall. The case was hopelessly incurable. (26)

Sims made a thorough investigation of the literature concerning vesicovaginal fistulas and continued in his autobiography:

> Then, seeing the master of the servant the next day, I said: Mr. Wescott, Anarcha has an affection that unfits her for the duties required of a servant. She will not die, but she will never get well, and all you have to do is to take good care of her so long as she lives....Mr. Wescott was a kind-hearted man, a good master, and accepting the situation, made up his mind that Anarcha should have an easy time in this world as long as she lived. (26)

Sims considered the condition a medical curiosity since he had been in practice for ten years and had not seen a single patient with a vesico-vaginal fistula. Strange to say, within a month Dr. Harris from Lowndes County referred Sims another seventeen-year-old girl, Betsy, who according to Sims, "had a baby about a month ago. Since then she had not been able to hold a single drop of water." As fate would have it, the following month he was referred still a third similar patient, an eighteen-year-old girl, Lucy, who since childbirth two months previously had been unable to retain urine. Thus, Sims was faced with three young girls who were destined to be social outcasts because of the constant leakage of infected and malodorous urine. He became intrigued with the challenge to help these pitiful young victims and spent the next three years working diligently on each of them, collectively performing more than forty operations, all of which failed.

Gradually, however, Sims learned from each successive procedure some additional points. He obviously maintained an excellent rapport with his patients, since he states that "one of them alone submitted to more than twenty operations, not only cheerfully but with thanks." Rather poignantly, he summarized these experiences saying "The history of these three cases is truly interesting in many points, and particularly, as exhibiting the slow degrees by which my originally clumsy mechanical apparatus was gradually improved and brought to its present state of simplicity." He finally recognized the significance of several general features of the operation, including adequate exposure. In the first procedure he used a silver spoon as a retractor, but to improve this situation he later developed the Sims retractor, now a classic instrument in surgical practice.

The two surgical principles which Sims ultimately found to be essential for success were as follows: first, after the fistula had been established, epithelium grew from the bladder into the rectum across the granulation site, and he finally seized upon the concept that this tissue must be removed in a circumferential manner such that when approximated there would not be bladder epithelium within the rectal suture line.

The second basic surgical principle was the use of special sutures, since he had tried all known forms of suture material, but in each instance erosion and infection of the sutures were serious problems. Finally, he seized upon the idea of using a metallic suture and obtained the aid of a jeweler to make a wire of silver drawn as thin as a horsehair. Then arose the problem of tying such a suture in the limited space and awkward exposure available in the closure of a vesicovaginal fistula. During the course of a sleepless night, when he was pursuing in his mind for the thousandth time the problem of tying such sutures he suddenly conceived the idea of placing the sutures through a perforated bird shot pellet, pulling the threads tightly and then compressing the malleable shot to stabilize the suture.

Sims' dedication, both to his patients and to his dream, is illustrated by the fact that all of these developmental operations were performed in his own small hospital and at his own expense. Thus, in May 1849 he prepared Anarcha for her thirtieth operation. On this occasion the circumference of the fistula was excised and the edges

were approximated with four of his fine, flexible new silver wires passing through small strips of lead to prevent cutting into the tissue. The
wires were tightly fixed by securing each with a perforated lead shot.
A catheter was placed in the bladder, and Sims spent a tedious week
awaiting the outcome. On many earlier occasions he had been certain
that when the week came to a close he would witness a successful
cure, and he was filled with anxiety and dread. This time, however,
the operation was successful. He had shown clearly that the final
answer had been achieved by the combination of excision of the circumference of the fistula and the use of silver wires. In rapid succession similar cures were achieved in Lucy and Betsy. Soon the success
of his procedure on Anarcha and the others became known throughout Montgomery and surrounding areas.

Despite the medical aid he provided others, Sims himself fell victim to chronic diarrhea and became quite ill. His son contracted the
same problem and succumbed from the condition. Sims naturally
became alarmed and, thinking a change in climate might be beneficial, spent three months in New York. Upon return to Montgomery,
however, he fell ill again. He then sought the curing waters at Cooper's Well in Mississippi, which had gained a reputation for being quite
helpful for victims of chronic diarrhea. After trying several other
places, he returned north and spent part of the summer in New York
and part in Connecticut. Some of his Southern patients followed him
to New York for treatment. Dr. Valentine Mott, the noted Professor
of Surgery at Columbia, invited him to operate on a patient with a
vesicovaginal fistula, and within a short time Sims' fame had justly
spread throughout the North as well as abroad.

Indeed, Sims received a call to attend the most prestigious royal
family in Europe. Napoleon III urgently summoned him to his wife
Eugenie, the beautiful and sensitive empress, who had fallen ill. The
imperial family was in residence at St. Cloud, and Sims was provided a
suite there for his entire stay. He restored the empress to health, for
which she was deeply grateful. Napoleon III was also extremely kind
to Sims and made him a member of the Legion of Honor, a rare
honor for a foreigner. Following this royal achievement, Sims experienced a quantum leap. The Emperor Napoleon invited him to serve as
Surgeon in Chief of the Ambulance Corps in the Franco-Prussian

War, and from these experiences he learned much about perforated wounds of the abdomen. His paper, "The Careful Aseptic Invasion of the Peritoneal Cavity Not Only for the Arrest of Hemorrhage, the Suture of Intestinal Wound, and the Cleansing of Peritoneal Cavity But for All Intraperitoneal Conditions," signaled a new era in the field of abdominal surgery. For this reason, when President Garfield became the victim of a gunshot wound in 1881, a cable was sent to Sims in Paris for advice. He replied as follows:

> If the President has recovered from the shock, and if there is undoubted evidence that the ball has traversed the peritoneal cavity, his only safety is in opening the abdomen, cleaning out the peritoneal cavity, tying bleeding vessels, suturing wounded intestine, and treating the case as we would after ovariotomy, using drainage or not as circumstances require. (14)

Although his advice was not followed and the president succumbed, his reply was obviously eloquent as well as succinct. Moreover, these comments are as contemporary today as a century ago.

Fortunately, Sims was honored not only in Europe but in his native country. A statue of Sims stands in New York in Central Park at Fifth Avenue opposite the New York Academy of Medicine, and another stands on the capitol grounds in Columbia, South Carolina. In February 1855, Sims began his drive to found the Woman's Hospital of New York, which became a reality, much to his delight. As Wyeth concluded in his Southern Surgical Address in 1895:

> It is safe to say that Marion Sims attained the highest position ever achieved in the history of our profession. He stands alone in this; his reputation as a surgeon was so world-wide that in any capital, in any country within the domain of civilization, he could command at any time a lucrative practice. In New York, London, Paris, Brussels, Berlin, Vienna, Rome, Madrid, Lisbon, St, Petersburg, he found himself everywhere sought after, not only by the patients he could benefit, but by the leading members of his own profession, who were anxious to pay tribute to his wonderful genius. (28)

Many interesting contributions in the development of vascular surgery originated in the South. In the early experiences, both in this country and abroad, ligation of arteries both for hemorrhage and in the management of aneurysms was fraught with much danger. Ligation of the innominate artery was first attempted by Valentine Mott in New York in 1818, but subsequent infection and ultimate hemorrhage resulted in the death of the patient. The operation was repeated by

Hall in Baltimore in 1830 and again by Cooper of San Francisco in 1859, but both attempts ended fatally.

The first successful ligation of the innominate artery was performed in New Orleans in 1864. In the first issue of the *New Orleans Medical Record*, Dr. Andrew W. Smyth of the Charity Hospital of Louisiana reported a thirty-two-year-old male with an aneurysm of the right subclavian artery (27). The tumor was the size of an orange, pulsated vigorously, and produced considerable pain as well as numbness in the forearm and hand. For two months the patient had been unable to lie down or to stand erect but was compelled to lean forward continuously for relief of the severe pain and to sleep sitting in a chair with his head resting on the side of the bed. Smyth placed a ligature on the innominate artery a quarter of an inch below its bifurcation and another on the carotid an inch above its origin. On tying the former, the pulsations in the aneurysm ceased. In the postoperative period, a severe hemorrhage from the wound occurred on the fourteenth day, producing syncope. With continuing hemorrhage, Smyth elected to place lead shot in the wound in hope that compression produced by the weight of the shot would stop the bleeding. Despite this, the bleeding persisted and on exploration was found to originate from the right vertebral artery, which was ligated. The wound healed with subsequent recovery of the patient, and thus another milestone in the history of surgery was achieved. The significance of this contribution is perhaps best described in Samuel Gross's own words when, in a superb monograph entitled "A Century of American Medicine," he said of this feat:

> The case of Dr. Smyth is replete in interest, not only as illustrative of extraordinary ability of the operator, but as showing how recovery may occasionally occur under, apparently, the most desperate circumstances. It is proper to add, that, in all the other cases amounting to upwards of a dozen, in which the innominate artery was tied, the result was unfavorable, the immediate cause of death being secondary hemorrhage. (6)

In 1852 a leader was born who was to greatly alter the course of surgery, in the United States and the world. William S. Halsted entered Yale where he was not only a scholar but captain of the varsity football team. He attended the College of Physicians and Surgeons at Columbia and chose Bellevue for house training in surgery. Quite early he was struck by the important contributions being made in Europe where he spent the years of 1878, 1879, and 1880, attending the clinics of Billroth, Mikulicz, Von Bergniann, Volkmann, Schede, Esmarch, and others. On return to New York he began the practice of surgery and in 1889, at the age of thirty-seven, was invited to become Surgeon in Chief at the newly opened Johns Hopkins Hospital. There his attention was immediately drawn to the close relationship of laboratory investigation and clinical surgery, and many of his brilliant operations were performed in the amphitheater before students and surgeons from all parts of the world.

Shortly after his arrival at Hopkins, Dr. Halsted met Miss Caroline Hampton, who soon became his nurse assistant in the operating room. She was descended from the famous Hampton family of South Carolina and was born in the ancestral home of Millwood near Columbia, where she spent her early life. Her father, Frank Hampton, was a Confederate officer who was killed at the Battle of Brandy Station in 1863. Caroline was left in the care of her aunts and uncles, including her father's brother, General Wade Hampton, who was on General Lee's staff and who later became governor and United States senator from South Carolina. Dr. Halsted became an adopted Southerner both by his move to Baltimore and through his marriage to Caroline Hampton. Moreover, he and Mrs. Halsted spent from May until October each year in Cashiers, in the mountains of western North Carolina, at the original summer estate of the Hampton family. Halsted often commented that the time he spent at their mountain home was the most productive part of his career, since it was there that he wrote and generated new ideas.

Mrs. Halsted, who had earlier been the professor's scrub nurse, was quite prominent in the development of rubber gloves. According to Halsted's own account:

> In the winter of 1889 and 1890—I cannot recall the month—the nurse in charge of my operating room complained that the solution of mercuric chloride produced a dermatitis of her arms and hands. As she was an unusually efficient woman, I gave the matter my consideration and one day in New York requested the Goodyear Rubber Company to make as an experiment two pairs of thin, rubber gloves with gauntlets. On trial these proved to he so satisfactory that additional gloves were ordered. In the autumn, on my return

to town, the assistant who passed the instruments and threaded the needles was also provided with rubber gloves to wear at the operations. At first, the operator wore them only when exploratory incisions into joints were made. After a time, the assistants became so accustomed to working in gloves that they also wore them as operators and would remark that they seemed to be less expert with the bare hand than with the gloved hands. (10)

It is an interesting fact that Halsted not only introduced the meticulous surgical approach as a fundamental principle of surgery but also used his practical mind to attack the greatest clinical challenges facing surgery in his day. For example, the simple inguinal hernia had resisted a successful operative approach for many years, and in the first report of his unique operation for its correction, he quoted Shuh, who had said, "If no other field were offered to the surgeon for his activity than herniotomy, it would be worth while to become a surgeon and devote an entire life to this service." In the current edition of *Keen's Textbook of Surgery* of that day, it was recommended that operation *not* be performed for hernia if it could be reduced, since the recurrence rate was 27 to 42 percent within the first year following operation. In his report to the Medical and Chirurgical Faculty of Maryland in 1892, without knowledge of the report by Bassini, Halsted described fifty-eight cases without a single recurrence in those cases which healed per primum in a study covering a three-year period beginning in 1889.

Halsted also directed his attention to the management of carcinoma of the breast, which at the time had an amazingly high local recurrence rate. For example, Billroth reported a local recurrence of 82 percent in the first year following operation, whereas with the Halsted procedure, it was reduced to 6 percent. When Halsted reported his series of 210 patients in 1907, there was a 1.7 percent mortality and a 75 percent survival when the axillary nodes were negative, and a 25 percent survival rate when they were positive. These were remarkable achievements, especially in a day when the vast majority of patients had advanced lesions at the time of first examination.

In writing about carcinoma of the breast in 1890, Halsted stated that he began eight years earlier "not only to clean out the axilla in all cases of cancer of the breast but also to excise in almost every case the pectoralis major muscle or at least a generous portion of it to give the tumor all sides an exceedingly wide berth" (9).

Halsted also was quite interested in the healing of intestinal anastomoses, since in that day breakdown of such anastomoses was common. In early animal experiments, he demonstrated that in small intestinal anastomoses in which the sutures were taken only through the muscularis but did not penetrate into the submucosa, frequent dehiscence occurred producing suppurative peritonitis and death (12). However, when sutures included the submucosa, the anastomoses healed perfectly. Dr. Halsted summarized these studies as follows:

> It is impossible to suture the serosa alone, as advised by authors. It is impossible to suture unfailingly the serosa and muscularis alone unless one is familiar with the resistance offered to the point of the needle by the coats of the intestine. Furthermore, stitches which include nothing but these two coats tear out easily and are, therefore, not to he trusted. Each stitch should include a bit of the submucosa. A thread of this coat is much stronger than a shred of the entire thickness of the serosa and muscularis. It is not difficult to familiarize oneself with the resistance furnished by the submucosa, and it is quite as easy to include a bit of this coat in each stitch as to suture the serosa and the muscularis alone. (9)

Halsted was a master of all forms of surgery and in 1899 was the first to successfully remove a carcinoma of the ampulla of Vater.[1] He resected a part of the duodenum, pancreas, and a portion of the common bile duct with successful reanastomosis (13). The patient survived but ultimately succumbed to metastases. In 1884, he had shown that nerve trunks could be blocked with cocaine (11), the first clear demonstration of the use of local infiltration anesthesia, and for this the American Dental Association gave him its Medal of Acknowledgment.

Of all his contributions, many consider the training of surgeons the most significant achievement. Although he was Professor and Head of the Department for thirty-three years, only seventeen Chief Residents completed his program during the entire period. This was due to the long tenure upon which he insisted, particularly in the early days. One is reminded of Mont Reid who, having been in the residency for eleven years, asked Dr. Halsted if he did not think it was time for him to finish the program. Dr. Halsted replied, "Reid, what's

---

1. The ampulla of Vater is a duct that enters the duodenum, and is made up of ducts from the liver and pancreas.

the rush?" If one considers the second generation of Halsted residents, one finds an equally impressive number with 37 professors, 14 clinical professors, 18 associate professors, and 80 others in academic appointments, with 99 in the practice of surgery. In his text on the history of surgery, Meade summarizes Halsted's career with this statement: "His teachings have had a greater effect on operating techniques in this country than those of any other person" (21).

Few surgeons have achieved the worldwide acclaim accorded Rudolph Matas. He was born in Bonne-Carre near New Orleans in 1860. At the age of four he was taken to Paris, where his father pursued postgraduate work at the Sorbonne. Thus, early in life he was exposed to a scholarly and academic environment and became a man of letters as well as science. Extremely well educated, he spoke English, Spanish, and French fluently and could also read several other languages. He entered Tulane in 1877 and graduated in 1880. In 1882 he became editor of the *New Orleans Medical and Surgical Journal*, a rare achievement for one of his age, and in 1886 was elected President of the New Orleans Medical and Surgical Society.

The year 1888 was to become a very important one for Matas, for in that year Manuel Harris, a plantation worker, was admitted to Charity Hospital with a pulsating mass in his left arm, which had steadily increased in size following a hunting accident two months previously. At that time, the standard procedure for the treatment of such an aneurysm was proximal and distal ligation of the main arteries supplying the lesion. This was the procedure chosen, but Matas was quite disappointed some ten days later to note that the aneurysm continued to pulsate as vigorously as before operation. Therefore, at the end of the second week he reoperated and, upon opening the aneurysm, noted three large openings at its base, each bleeding retrograde into the sac. These were then separately closed with sutures, with cessation of the bleeding. The procedure was successful, and Matas carefully stored this observation in his mind for future use (18).

More than a decade passed, and as the year 1899 drew to a close, Matas was busily engaged in the preparation of a paper for the Southern Surgical Society on the use of positive pressure apparatus for pulmonary insufflation during surgery. At this time he was asked to see a patient who had suffered a gunshot wound in the thigh while deer hunting. A large femoral aneurysm had resulted, which was quite painful and was enlarging rapidly. Following standard practice, Dr. Matas ligated the femoral artery both above and below, with immediate cessation of the pulsation in the aneurysm. However, the note states that "gangrene occurred immediately after the ligature," and a hasty amputation was required as a lifesaving measure (3). It is of interest that within a month an identical situation developed in another patient and Dr. Matas noted again, "Gangrene of the toes occurred as a sequel to the ligation" (30). These events led him to consider again the possibilities of the procedure he had performed in 1888. The impact of this procedure was emphasized by a third patient, who sustained a gunshot wound to the brachial artery followed by an aneurysm which steadily increased in size and discomfort. Following ligation of the proximal brachial artery in the patient's home, all pulsations immediately arrested and the wound healed per primum. However, within two months the aneurysm returned and was as large as ever. He was fearful of ligating the vessel distally and stated, "I decided to incise the sac and suture the orifices as I had done in the previous case" (of Manuel Harris twelve years before) (3). Since the patient would not be operated upon in a hospital, the procedure was done in his home. Two sawhorses were placed with two ironing boards atop them and the patient was strapped securely. The house did not have electricity, so it was done by daylight with chloroform anesthesia. An Esmarch tourniquet was placed just below the shoulder to occlude the proximal brachial artery, and an incision was then made over the aneurysm and the upper pole exposed. The sac was incised longitudinally and a large mass of mixed clot was evacuated. Two large orifices, one the inlet and the other the outlet of the artery, were now seen in the interior of the sac-orifices large enough to admit the tip of the little finger. These were quickly sealed with a fine continuous silk suture which penetrated the entire thickness of the sac wall, and these sutures held perfectly. After this, the tourniquet was removed and he was pleased to see that not a drop of blood escaped. In the same year, another patient, a married saloon keeper, aged twenty-seven, had a similar procedure on a popliteal aneurysm, with cure by the newly described Matas endoaneurysmorrhaphy (19). With these contributions, the modern era of the direct approach to the management of vascular problems was initiated, and Matas formally presented this feat to the American Surgical Association in 1902.

One of the finest and best known surgeons of this century, the late John M. T. Finney, was born on a plantation near Natchez, Mississippi, in 1863, just three weeks before the Battle of Gettysburg. His father, the Reverend Ebenezer Dickey Finney, was a Presbyterian minister who also served as principal of a school for boys. Dr. Finney was fortunate in being reared in an exemplary environment with a sound religious background which was obviously to influence him and his notable family for many years. He entered Princeton at the age of seventeen and upon graduation went to Harvard Medical School, where he achieved an outstanding record and remained for surgical training at the Massachusetts General Hospital.

Shortly after his arrival in Boston, a close associate told him that he was very fortunate in securing a surgical residency there and confided: "From Dr. Porter you will learn how to operate, from Dr. Cabot you will learn how to take care of your patients after operation, and from Dr. Homans you will learn *what not to do,* and I fancy you will probably learn more from him than from either of the others." Later, when his Chief asked him about his career preference in terms of immediate position, he immediately replied that his first choice would be an appointment with Dr. Halsted at the newly opened Johns Hopkins Hospital.

J. M. T. Finney is particularly well known for his innovative concept of pyloroplasty. In 1902, he performed a gastroduodenostomy without a gastric resection, making a long horeseshoe incision from the lower stomach across the pylorus to the duodenum (5). The two structures were then sutured together so that a large opening resulted between the stomach and duodenum, which he called a pyloroplasty. He emphasized that the advantage of the procedure over gastroenterostomy was the absence of regurgitation of bile and an unaccelerated evacuation of the stomach. It is interesting to reflect upon his own assessment of the procedure at the time he wrote his autobiography in 1940. He said:

> But the contribution which I have made to surgical technique which strikes
> me as the most outstanding is the plastic operation on the pylorus suggested

by me a number of years ago, and known as 'pyloroplasty'.... Certain it is that in selected cases, it is very useful in obviating a much more serious and mutilating operation. (4)

Dr. Finney was chosen as the president of the Southern Surgical Association in 1912 and a year later as the first president of the American College of Surgeons. He also received numerous other honors, including an offer of the presidency of Princeton and one from Hopkins to be Dr. Halsted's successor as Professor of Surgery. Both were declined, the latter primarily because he did not believe in the principle of the full-time system with a fixed, and often inadequate, income. He regarded this of particular significance for those with extensive family commitments.

Clearly, Dr. Finney was one of the most highly respected of all American surgeons, and of his contribution of pyloroplasty, Dr. William J. Mayo was to state before the American Surgical Association that "it constituted the introduction of a new principle in surgery." In retrospect, it is unlikely that either Dr. Finney or Dr. Mayo could have realized at the time the subsequent impact and wide usage that this procedure was to enjoy in the future.

Many contributions to cardiac surgery have their origin in this country, and the first major achievement in this field was made in 1902 by Luther Leonidas Hill, Jr., of Alabama. The son of a Methodist minister who had moved from Warrenton, North Carolina, some years previously, Luther Hill was born in 1862 and was reared on a farm near Montgomery. He became a distinguished student, receiving certificates of distinction in Latin and Greek, and later chose to study medicine and was graduated from New York University. Upon deciding to become a surgeon, he sought further courses at Jefferson Medical College, where he studied under Dr. Samuel D. Gross and was awarded a second M.D. in 1882. He then went to King's College in London where he worked under Lister, a teacher who made a very deep impression upon him.

In the 1896 edition of Stephen Paget's *Surgery of the Chest*, one finds the following statement:

Surgery of the heart has probably reached the limits set by Nature to all surgery: no new method, and no new discovery, can overcome the natural difficulties that attend a wound of the heart. It is true that heart suture has been vaguely proposed as a possible procedure, and has been done on animals: but I cannot find that it has ever been attempted in practice.

In that same year Ludwig Rehn performed the first successful cardiac suture in Germany. As Pasteur noted many years before, "Chance favors the prepared mind," and so it was that about 1900 Luther Hill began an interest in heart wounds and investigated the subject thoroughly. On September 14, 1902, he was called to the home of Henry Myrick, a thirteen-year-old boy who had been stabbed five times in the chest. In his report, printed in the *Medical Record* in 1902, Hill wrote that he was called to see the patient about six hours after a knife blade had been driven into the left fifth intercostal space, about a quarter of an inch to the right of the nipple (15). The radial pulse was almost imperceptible and the heart sounds were heard with difficulty. The young boy was dyspneic, restless, with cold extremities and had to he aroused to answer questions.

Dr. Hill then proceeded to perform an operation which was the first successful closure of a heart wound in this country. Dr. Hill's account is as follows:

"The wound was about three-eighths of an inch in length, and from it came a stream of blood at every systole.... Securing two lamps, I removed the boy from his bed to a table, at one o'clock at night, eight hours after the stabbing, and proceeded to cleanse the field of the operation, and placed the patient in as favorable a condition as my surroundings in the negro cabin would allow. Commencing an incision about five-eighths of an inch from the left border of the sternum, I carried it along the third rib for four inches. A second incision was started at the same distance from the sternum and carried along the sixth rib for four inches. A vertical incision along the anterior axillary line was made, connecting them. The third, fourth, and fifth ribs were cut through with the pleura. The musculo-osseous flap was raised, with the cartilages of the ribs acting as the hinges. There was no blood in the pleural cavity, but the pericardium was enormously distended. I enlarged the opening in the pericardium to a distance of two and one-half inches, and evacuated about ten ounces of blood, the pulse immediately improved and was commented upon by Dr. L. D. Robinson, who so successfully and skillfully administered chloroform. I had my brother Dr. R. S. Hill, to pass his hand into the pericardial sac and bring the heart upward, and, at the same time, steady it sufficiently for me to pass a catgut suture through the center of the wound in the heart and control the hemorrhage. I cleansed the pericardial sac with a saline solution, and closed the opening in it with seven interrupted catgut sutures. The pleural cavity was also cleansed with a saline solution, and drained with iodoform gauze. In September 17 he commenced to improve, and his recovery has been uninterrupted. (15)

Shortly after this remarkable feat, Professor Sherman wrote, "The road to the heart is only 2 or 3 centimeters in a direct line, but it has taken surgery nearly 2,400 years to travel it."

One cannot mention he name of Hill in the United States without recognizing its more recent pertinence in the field of medicine. Dr. Luther L. Hill's son, Lister, named for Joseph Lister, was first sent to the United States Congress from Alabama at the young age of twenty-eight and was later elected to the United States Senate in 1938. He was the original author of the Hill-Burton Act for the building of hospitals, which, together with his strong support of medical research through the National Institutes of Health, has brought the United States to first place among the nations of the world in medicine. Lister Hill served in Congress for forty-five years and was consistently a champion of medical education, research, and patient care. Helen Keller said to him, "My heart grows warm every time I think of you, and that is ever so often."

James A. Shannon, the noted director of the NIH for many years said, "I know that I can express the admiration, respect, and gratitude of the research community for what he has done for medical research in our time" (25). In March of 1968, an appreciation dinner was held for him in Washington, D.C., and it was my privilege to have been in attendance. At the dinner, Russell A. Nelson said of him, "Let no one doubt for even a moment that this great man has done more for the building of hospitals in this country than any other person in his generation" (22). At that time the president wrote, "If any one man could be called the father of our nation's health, it would be Lister Hill."

The final contributor to be discussed had strong affection, respect, and loyalty for this organization and its members. His original contributions to surgery have been recognized throughout the world, and he did much to advance the total image of the surgeon in this country and abroad. Alfred Blalock was educated at the University of Georgia and at Hopkins and later completed a surgical residency under Dr. Barney Brooks at Vanderbilt. Remaining on the faculty in Nashville, he was able to devote large segments of his time to basic investigation and quite early began his fundamental work on the pathogenesis of shock. At that time, the status of this important subject was in a total state of disarray, with many conflicting views concerning its genesis.

The basic experiment which Dr. Blalock designed was performed on the hind limb of an anesthetized animal. The thigh was injured by blunt trauma and eight hours later its weight was compared with that of the control limb after separate dissection. The increased weight of the traumatized limb was shown to account for 66 percent of the circulating blood volume and thus fully explained the state of shock. In this simple, yet clearly brilliant, experimental study, Dr. Blalock showed that shock is due chiefly to the loss of circulating blood and plasma from the vascular compartment, either externally or into the tissues.

From his monograph "Principles of Surgical Care, Shock and Other Problems," Dr. Blalock summarized his work, saying, "Shock was once a surgical complication to be dreaded, but now in the light of recent intensive investigations of its causes it would seem to be largely preventable" (1). For these unique contributions, no less an authority and able critic than Sir James Pickering, the Regius Professor of Medicine at Oxford, said, "The conclusion that emerged from World War I was that shock was a traumatic toxemia produced by the effects of vasoactive substances like histamine released from injured muscles. It needed the genius of your Alfred Blalock and the experience of the Second World War to show that this was not so."

Few investigators make more than one major contribution, but Dr. Blalock continued his research and proceeded to become a prime leader in the development of cardiac surgery with his brilliant operation for tetralogy of Fallot. It is important to emphasize that this major achievement came directly from his basic observations in the experimental laboratory and, in fact, as a result of experiments on an unrelated subject. In the late 1930s he became quite interested in pulmonary hypertension and attempted to produce this condition in an experimental model by creating a subclavian artery to pulmonary artery anastomosis. This was published in 1939 and with some disappointment, since it was not possible to produce an elevated pulmonary arterial pressure by such an anastomosis (16). However, some seven years later, when Helen Taussig approached him about the need to augment blood flow to the lungs in children incapacitated with dyspnea and cyanosis as a result of pulmonary stenosis, he recalled these experimental observations and undertook the identical procedure in a severely ill fifteen-month-old patient on November 30, 1944. The result was superb and from that time forward, cardiac surgery began a period of remarkable progress.

In 1947, Dr. Blalock was invited to Guy's Hospital for a month's visit to introduce cardiac surgery in the British Isles. Concerning his impression of that visit, Evarts Graham was to say of him in a letter to President Isaiah Bowman of the Johns Hopkins University:

> I wish you could have been with me in London last month to have seen the acclaims which Alfred Blalock received. It did my heart good to see it. I could not help recalling some of the correspondence and conversations which you and I had about him a few years ago when he was being considered for his present post. I have always been sure of his ability and I have always been confident that he would go far in surgery if he had a good opportunity. I was tremendously proud of him in Europe, and I could not help getting a great deal of satisfaction out of the thought that my confidence had not been misplaced. There has never been anything quite like Al Blalock's triumphal tour of Europe. The only thing that I can think of that remotely resembles it was a tour made by Marion Sims in the seventies or eighties of the last century. He had devised an operation and was received with great acclaim in the European capitals because of the success of his demonstrations. He came back loaded with honors from the various crowned heads. Al Blalock's tour has been no less dramatic and successful despite the fact that Europe is now down at the heel and there are few crowned heads left. The prestige of Johns Hopkins was enormously increased by Al's visit. All of us Americans were proud to claim him as a fellow American. His unassuming personality captivated everyone as much as his epoch-making surgical accomplishment.

Russell Brock, the noted British cardiac surgeon, wrote of Dr. Blalock's visit to England in 1947:

> Dr. Blalock who presented his surgical contribution with his characteristic, apparently casual, drawl but really a forceful and incisive presentation of his brilliant and impressive results. The silence of the audience betokened their rapt attention and appreciation. The hall was quite dark for projection of his slides which had been illustrating patients before and after operation, when suddenly a long searchlight beam traversed the whole length of the hail and unerringly picked out on the platform a Guy's nursing sister, dressed in her attractive blue uniform, sitting on a chair and holding a small cherub-like

girl of 2 and 1/2 years with a halo of blonde curly hair and looking pink and quite well; she had been operated on at Guy's by Blalock a week earlier. The effect was dramatic and theatrical and the applause from the audience was tumultuous. No audience could fail to have been convinced or satisfied by this summation and no one there could possibly forget it....the outstanding and important result of his visit was the firm introduction and launching of his operation in Great Britain and the Continent, acceptance of the immense possibilities of surgery in the alleviation of congenital heart disease in centres previously unconvinced and reluctant. The large numbers of visitors from the continent and London for the international meeting meant that they were also able to benefit and so the gospel was spread even more widely. (23)

With all of his achievements and international acclaim, those who worked with him closely knew Alfred Blalock's first love. On the occasion of his sixtieth birthday, when a large throng from this country and abroad gathered to honor him, in his closing remarks he expressed his feeling and with unconcealed emotion, saying, "With the exception of my family and close friends of my own vintage, my greatest pleasure in life has come from the resident staff. Most of them are here tonight, much to my delight, and all are fine gentlemen and superb friends." There can be no doubt that this feeling was thoroughly reciprocated on the part of his residents who knew him as exemplary teacher, investigator, clinical surgeon, and loyal friend.

In bringing these remarks to a close, let me emphasize the great surgical heritage which has been ours. Quite clearly, there is much reason to take pride in these accomplishments of our forebears, provided we accept them as challenges for future achievements. While it is a part of our nature to cherish tradition, we must recognize that its most poignant meaning is the standard which it establishes. Clearly, high standards represent our best hope for the future. This concept and its potential relationship to surgery is beautifully expressed in a statement made by the London Times in its edition announcing the successful expedition of Sir Edmund Hillary in the conquest of Mount Everest:

In an age whose heart is dulled by the leveling of standards to the mediocre measure of the masses, here is an aristocracy that all can admire without envy.

References

1. Blalock, A. *Principles of Surgical Care. Shock and Other Problems*. St. Louis: The C.V. Mosby Co., 1940.
2. Boland, F. K. *The First Anesthetic. The Story of Crawford Long*. Athens: University of Georgia Press, 1950.
3. Cohn, I. and Deutsch, H. B. *Rudolph Matas. A Biography of One of the Great Pioneers in Surgery*. Garden City New York: Doubleday & Co., Inc., 1960.
4. Finney, J. M. T. *A Surgeon's Life. The Autobiography of J. M. T. Finney*. New York: G.P. Putnam's Sons, 1940.
5. Finney, J. M. T. A new method of pyloroplasty. *Trans. Amer. Surg. Assoc.*, 20: 165, 1902.
6. Gross, S. D. *A Century of American Medicine. 1776–1876*. Philadelphia: Lea, 1876.
7. Gross, S. D. *Memorial Oration in Honor of Ephraim McDowell, "The Father of Ovariotomy."* Louisville: John P. Morton & Co., 1879.
8. Halsted, W. S. The radical cure of inguinal hernia in the male. *Johns Hopkins Hosp. Bull.*, 4: 17, 1893.
9. Halsted, W. S. The results of operations for the cure of cancer of the breast performed at Johns Hopkins Hospital from June 1889 to January 1894. *Ann. Surg.*, 20: 497, 1894.
10. Halsted, W. S. Ligature and suture material. The employment of fine silk in preference to catgut and the advantages of transfixion of tissues and vessels in control of hemorrhage. Also an account of the introduction of gloves, gutta-percha tissue and silver foil. *JAMA* 60: 1119, 1913.
11. Halsted, W. S. Practical comments on the use and abuse of cocaine; Suggested by its invariably successful employment in more than a thousand minor surgical operations, *Surgical Papers by William Stewart Halsted*, Vol. 1. Baltimore: The Johns Hopkins Press, 1924.
12. Halsted, W. S. Circular suture of the intestine. An experimental study. *Surgical Papers by William Stewart Halsted*, Vol. 1. Baltimore: The Johns Hopkins Press, 1924.

13. Halsted, W. S. Contributions to the surgery of the bile passages, especially of the common bile-duct. *Surgical Papers by William Stewart Halsted*, Vol. II. Baltimore: The Johns Hopkins Press, 1924.

14. Harris, S. *Woman's Surgeon. The Life Story of J. Marion Sims.* New York: Macmillan Co., 1950.

15. Hill, L. L. A report of a case of successful suturing of the heart, and table of thirty-seven other cases of suturing by different operators with various terminations, and the conclusions drawn. *Medical Record*, Nov. 29, 1902, pp. 846–848.

16. Levy, S. E. and Blalock, A. Experimental observations on the effects of connecting by suture the left main pulmonary artery of the systemic circulation. *J. Thoracic Surg.*, 8: 525. 1939.

17. Mahorner, H. Rudolph Matas (1860–1957). *Bull. Amer. Coll. Surg.*, June 1973, pp. 23–26.

18. Matas, R.: Traumatic Aneurism of the Left Brachial Artery. Med. News, 52 and 53:462, 1889.

19. Matas, R. An operation for the radical cure of aneurism based upon arteriorrhaphy: With the report of four cases successfully operated upon by the author. *Trans. Surg. Assoc.*, 30: 396, 1902.

20. McDowell, E. Three cases of extirpation of diseased ovaria. *Eclectic Repertory and Analytical Review*, 7: 242, 1817.

21. Meade, R. H. *An Introduction to the History of General Surgery.* Philadelphia: W.B. Saunders Co., 1968.

22. Nelson, R. A. A tribute to Senator Lister Hill. *Clin. Res.*, 14:483, 1968.

23. Ravitch, M., ed. *The Papers of Alfred Blalock*, Vol. I. Baltimore: The Johns Hopkins Press. 1966.

24. Schachner, A. *Ephraim McDowell. "Father of Ovariotomy" and Founder of Abdominal Surgery.* Philadelphia: J.B. Lippincott Co., 1921.

25. Shannon, J. A. A tribute to Senator Lister Hill. *Clin. Res.*, 14: 483, 1968.

26. Sims, J. M. *The Story of My Life.* (Edited by his son, H. Marion-Sims) New York: D. Appleton and Co., 1886.

27. Smyth, A. W. Successful operation in a case of subclavain aneurism. *New Orleans Med. Record*, 1: 4, 1866.

28. Wyeth, J. A. Dr. J. Marion Sims and his work. *Trans. South. Surg. Assoc.*, 8: 9, 1895.

Chapter 7

The First Hundred Years: The Annals of Surgery and a Century of Progress

T he first issue of *Annals of Surgery* appeared in January 1885, and today it is widely recognized as the oldest journal published in English devoted exclusively to surgery. The Editorial Board has made special plans for the issues during this Centennial Year of 1985 to recognize the accomplishments achieved during the first hundred years. This Centennial is a landmark in the history of surgical literature, and much appreciation is extended to the authors who have submitted their work for publication and to the members of the Editorial Board for maintaining the highest standards together with a complete devotion to multiple responsibilities.

Early in 1885 the *Canada Medical and Surgical Journal* stated editorially: "We have received the prospectus of a new medical monthly called the *Annals of Surgery.* It is to be devoted entirely to surgery and is intended to be representative of the surgical thought and work of the present day. The journal will appear on the first day of each month, simultaneously in the United States and Great Britain. It is in a way a successor of that admirable periodical which appeared for several years, the *Annals of Anatomy and Surgery.* It is to be edited by L.S. Pilcher, M.D., of Brooklyn, N.Y., and C.B. Keetley, F.R.C.S., of London, Eng., assisted by a large staff of collaborators. Among these latter are many well-known British and American surgeons. This is the first attempt, as far as we know, to publish in the English language a periodical exclusively devoted to surgery. We wish the enterprise every success and feel sure that it will be supported by both British and American surgeons" (1).

This issue represents the flagship of a series that will follow during the remainder of 1985. The article, "Lewis Stephen Pilcher, Founding Editor of the *Annals of Surgery:* Editor for 50 Consecutive Years," is of considerable historic significance and is authored by two direct descendants of the first editor. *A* grandson, Dr. Lewis Stephen Pilcher II, is a retired general surgeon in West Newton, Massachusetts, and the co-author, Dr. David Bogart Pilcher, is a great grandson and currently Professor of Surgery at the University of Vermont College of Medicine. This timely biographic presentation reveals the carefully planned foundations of the journal, together with the strong leadership that Lewis S. Pilcher provided as editor until his death at the age of ninety. Much of the information provided is hitherto unpublished and probably will become a classic reference for the future.

It is very fortunate that since 1897 the sole publisher of *Annals of Surgery* has been J. B. Lippincott Company, a firm totally committed to the highest standards of publication together with an established policy of excellence in every aspect of the field. Complete responsibility for the decision-making process has been entrusted to the Editorial Board, and the publisher has been repeatedly supportive of the Board in every way. For these reasons, the Board is particularly pleased to have the publisher's comments in this issue. During 1985, the issues will contain special articles including feature presentations by the members of the Editorial Board. These special contributions can be predicted to become frequently cited references in future literature.

It is fascinating to review the first volume of *Annals of Surgery,* which contains the January-through-June issues for 1885. Lewis S. Pilcher had selected the well-known British surgeon, Charles B. Keetley of London, to serve as coeditor. Keetley provided a paper on the dangers of operative measures for correction of inguinal hernia (2), as well as another presentation on curettement of bone marrow in the management of osteomyelitis (3). Keetley expressed the view held by surgeons at that time concerning surgical correction of hernias, admonishing: "Besides the dangers of a general surgical kind, such as that of a vitally important ligature giving way, or of septic infection, there are certain particular troubles and dangers of which the most constant and serious depend on the relations of the cord to the sac when the hernia is inguinal...the remaining constituents of the cord are, upon the whole, more likely to go with the sac than with the vas deferens to which they more correctly belong. The natural consequence is trouble with the testicle, perhaps orchitis, perhaps suppuration, or even gangrene. And every proceeding which sometimes leads to these will sometimes lead a little further, that is to say, to a fatal result" (2). Also in this volume the importance of surgical contributions from Europe was emphasized by summaries from selected meetings in Germany, the British Isles, and France, each of which provides much insight into the stepwise evolution and progress of surgery in that day.

Pilcher himself was involved in two contributions in this volume: one describing a patient he had presented to the New York Surgical Society who had successful simultaneous management of wounds of the femoral artery and vein (4); the other was a description of two patients with malignant lymphoma (5). Concerning the patient with the vascular injury, Pilcher described an accidental self-inflicted wound in the groin that involved the femoral artery and vein and nearly caused exsanguination. He ligated and divided both vessels above and below the wounds and considered this approach to be the preferred method of management, as it was standard for that day. Problems of infection are emphasized by his comment that the wound was irrigated in order to prevent infection, but then he added: "Suppuration, however, took place, and on the third day the wound was re-opened at its most dependent point, and drainage tubes inserted, and irrigation resorted to. A sharp attack of cellulitis following the line of the sartorius muscle followed, necessitating several counter-openings for drainage for its control."

Another problem of the day was the inability to prevent adequately or treat hemorrhagic shock, as evidenced by a well-illustrated paper describing excision of a large sacrococcygeal cyst in a two-month infant, ending with the comment, "The child survived the operation but a few hours, dying from shock" (6).

In the first six issues of *Annals,* there were a total of fifty-one authors; twenty-two were from the British Isles and Canada. Lewis Atterbury Stimson, the noted Professor of Surgery at Columbia University and Presbyterian Hospital in New York, reviewed the use of the ligature in the treatment of aneurysms (7). He emphasized that

Anel was the first to employ this technique in the management of a brachial arterial aneurysm in a priest with "a very large aneurism of the brachial artery at the bend of the elbow, caused by an unskillful venesection; he exposed the artery above the tumor, and tied it as close to the latter as was possible; the patient made a good recovery."

On the twentieth anniversary *of Annals,* the *Montreal Medical Journal* noted: "The December issue of the *Annals of Surgery* sustains the verdict that it has achieved an undisputed place as the leading exponent of surgery in the English language. This issue signalizes the close of the first twenty years of the publication of this journal, and the publishers have properly marked the event by issuing a festschrift number, which is more than double the usual size, and is remarkable for the value of its contents, the number and authority of its contributors, and the abundance and quality of its illustrations" (8).

In commemorating the fiftieth anniversary, an editorial in *Annals* commented that when the journal first was established, the centers of surgical thought were concentrated largely along the Atlantic coast. It was for this reason that an "entente cordiale" was arranged with the New York Surgical Society and the Philadelphia Academy of Surgery for publication of the papers presented at their meetings. With the passage of time it was recognized that the journal had surpassed its original local influence and that it affected surgical thought not only in this country but around the world. One of the strongest current features of *Annals* is that it is the journal of the American Surgical Association. It is interesting that the affiliation initially began in the year the journal was founded with a publication by Nicholas Senn of Milwaukee of a paper presented at the American Surgical Association meeting in Washington in April 1885. The title of the paper was "An Experimental and Clinical Study of Air-Embolism" (9). In 1931, the relationship was made official and first appeared on the masthead *of Annals.* It is also very fortunate that since January 1936 *Annals* has been the official journal of the Southern Surgical Association. The discussions of these two important annual meetings add much to the significance and scope of the papers presented, especially since the comments of the discussants provide excellent critiques and additional viewpoints for our readers.

As *Annals* enters its second century, it can be said with confidence that the journal has continued a course of steady upward progress. Last year more manuscripts were submitted for publication than ever before, and papers were published from thirty-three foreign countries. The demands upon members of the Editorial Board continue to increase, and thirty-four guest reviewers provided expert advice for highly specialized manuscripts. The total circulation continues to increase, and the international image of *Annals* is emphasized by the fact that it is currently being sent to subscribers in 117 countries. Finally, during the next century the primary goal will continue to be the publication of a journal of the highest quality and one worthy of the respect and support of the entire international surgical community.

References

1. *Can. Med. Surg. J.* 1885; 13: 376.
2. Keetley, C. B. On the dangers of modern operative proceedings for the radical cure of hernia [Editorial]. *Ann. Surg.* 1885; 1: 129.
3. Keetley, C. B. On removal (by scraping out) of the marrow of long bones, and especially on this proceeding as a treatment of osteo-myelitis. Also on the same followed by the local application of corrosive sublimate solution and of iodoform. *Ann. Surg.* 1885; 1: 1.
4. Presentation of patient of Dr. L. S. Pilcher at the New York Surgical Society, November 11, 1884. Simultaneous incomplete wound of femoral artery and vein—ligation of the wound—recovery. *Ann. Surg.* 1885: 1: 167.
5. Pilcher, L.S., Two cases of malignant lymphoma, with remarks. *Ann. Surg.* 1885; 1: 123.
6. Fowler, G. R. Congenital sacral cysts—description of a recent case, with remarks. *Ann. Surg* 1885; 1: 115.
7. Stimson, L. A. An inquiry into the origin of the use of the ligature in the treatment of aneurysm. *Ann. Surg.* 1885; 1: 13.
8. Editorial. *Montreal Med. J.* 1905; 34: 124.
9. Senn, N. An experimental and clinical study of air-embolism. *Ann. Surg.* 1885; 1: 517.

Chapter 8 ☞

Surgeons and the Nobel Prize

A lfred Nobel, the noted Swedish chemist and engineer, created the Nobel Foundation in a will signed in 1895. He provided generously for the annual awarding of prizes to be made "to those who, during the preceding year, shall have conferred the greatest benefit on mankind" in the fields of physics, chemistry, physiology or medicine, literature, and peace. Nobel selected the Royal Swedish Academy of Science to designate the awardees in physics and chemistry, the Karolinska Institute for the awards in physiology or medicine, the Swedish Academy for literature, and the Norwegian Nobel Committee, which is appointed by the Norwegian Parliament, for the peace prize. In 1968 an additional prize in economics was established, and the recipients of this prize are elected by the Swedish Academy of Science.

Alfred Nobel was born in Sweden in 1833. Brilliant and hardworking, he trained in chemistry and engineering and was to spend his life in many countries, including Sweden, Russia, France, Italy, and the United States. Making pioneering discoveries using nitroglycerin as an explosive, he developed dynamite. Because this was such an important part of the expansion of industry in the United States in the construction of many new projects and the building of roads and railroads in the latter half of the nineteenth century, Nobel established the Atlantic Giant Powder Company in New York, which later became a member of the DuPont Corporation.

The royal announcement for the Nobel Prize is made by the statement, "I wish to convey to you our warmest congratulations and now ask you to receive the Prize from the hands of his Majesty the King" (1), at which point the Nobel prize winners stand, go forward to the

King of Sweden, and receive a solid gold medal as well as a diploma. In addition they receive a generous monetary award.

The first Nobel prizes were awarded in 1901, at which time Wilhelm Conrad Róentgen received the first prize in physics "in recognition of the extraordinary services he has rendered by the discovery of the remarkable rays subsequently named after him" (1). In 1990 Joseph E. Murray, the noted Professor of Surgery at Harvard and the Brigham and Women's Hospital, received the Nobel Prize in Medicine for his pioneering work in renal transplantation. The event reawakened the interest of surgeons in this award, which is widely recognized to be the most respected scientific honor worldwide.

In 1909 the Director of the Royal Caroline Institute (Karolinska) rose to say, "Your Majesty, your Royal Highnesses, Ladies and Gentlemen. The Nobel Medical Prize has been awarded this year to the famous surgeon Professor Theodore Kocher of Bern in recognition of his work concerning the physiology, pathology, and surgery of the thyroid gland" (2). He proceeded to review the disorders of the thyroid gland, which occurred with pathologic enlargement, and indicated that for many years the gland had been extirpated to relieve the symptoms of pressure on vital structures such as the trachea. It was recognized that once the gland was removed, the patient's symptoms dramatically improved; however, with the passage of time, additional problems appeared. These included muscular weakness, swelling of the extremities and face, anemia, dementia, and finally death from exhaustion. It was then recognized that thyroid function was essential for life and that severe degenerative processes occurred in its absence.

The Nobel award was given to Kocher because of his excellence in surgical extirpation of the thyroid with very low morbidity and mortality rates and also because "he has also carried out extensive investigations into the causes of the endemic occurrence of goitre in certain regions and into the cretinism connected with disturbances in thyroid function. In the thyroid...other diseases can occur in addition to those which arise with the ordinary goitre. To these as well, Kocher has devoted successful work, as a result of which it has been possible to define with more and more certainty the method of treatment best suited to each case; in addition, on the basis of Kocher's work a broader, deeper knowledge of the pathology of the thyroid has been achieved" (2).

In his lecture that followed, Kocher stated, "Murray and Howitz's finding, which seemed simple and yet is so exceedingly important, that the administration of thyroid juice was quite sufficient to compensate for the deficiency of thyroid function, was of great significance for the theory of thyroid function." He went on to state, "We are indebted to Baumann's brilliant discovery of the thyroid's iodine content for providing a more precise justification of this interpretation" (2). In a masterful essay on the various manifestations of hypothyroidism, Kocher then described the characteristic features of myxedema as it progressed from the mildest form to total disability and death. He noted cessation of growth in young individuals and emphasized the skeletal changes that occurred. He stressed the bloated condition of these patients as well as the increased corpulence of the body and declining mental status. Paresthesias were common, as were areas of pigmentation and dryness of the skin as well as flakiness and coldness of the hands as an expression of defective circulation. He also recognized the hormonal changes, with periods of dysmenorrhea and menorrhogia in women. He published beautiful illustrations of patients receiving thyroid extract with resolution of the physical changes and their return in several months after cessation of therapy, followed by improvement again after resumption of therapy.

It is obvious that Kocher was not only a master surgeon but also a physiologist who understood the combined role of basic science and clinical surgery. He was honored widely throughout Europe and in the United States was elected an honorary member of the New York Academy of Medicine, the College of Physicians of Philadelphia, and the American Surgical Association.

In 1912 Alexis Carrel of the Rockefeller Institute of New York was awarded the Nobel Prize "for his work on suturing of vessels and transplantation of organs" (2). Of Carrel it was said,

> You have achieved great things! You have invented a new method of suturing lesions in blood-vessels. By virtue of this method, you ensure a free flow at the site of the suture, and at the same time, you prevent post-operative haemorrhage, thrombosis and secondary stricture. Thanks to the same

method, you are able to reconstruct the vascular pathway, to replace a segment removed from the patient with another segment taken from another part or from another person. You have examined what useful ways and means there are of preserving the sections of blood vessel in a condition such that they may be used later. Thanks to your method, you transplanted whole organs— a lobe of thyroid, the ovaries, the spleen, a kidney, both kidneys indeed, and you have proved that these transplanted organs can survive and carry out their special functions. In addition, you have transplanted whole limbs.... You are successful with the boldest and most difficult operations. You have increased the scope for surgical intervention in humans, and proved once more that the development of the applied science of operative surgery depends on the lessons it learns from animal experiments. What then are the causes of your success? First, you have set yourself a definite target, and have pursued it without respite and by all means. Then your steady, sensitive fingers have acted as very sure, obedient instruments for your intellect, and all the procedures you have used for these complex operations are distinguished by their astonishing appropriateness and simplicity. Finally, the clear, bright intelligence which was the patrimony you received from your country, from France, and in whose debt humanity stands for so much that is valuable, was allied to the bold, resolute energy of your adopted country, and these marvelous operations, of which I have just spoken, are the manifest result of this happy collaboration. Sir, The Caroline Institute, and, I dare say, the whole medical world, offers you today, through the medium of my voice, its congratulations and compliments." (2)

In a very carefully and thoughtfully prepared address, the new Nobel Laureate then reviewed the steps that led to his monumental contributions, feats that were to change the entire field of surgery. Quite understandably Carrel was honored throughout the world for his masterful and innovative contributions. In the United States he received honorary degrees from Princeton, the University of California, New York University, Brown University, and Columbia University.

In 1923 Dr. Frederick C. Banting of Toronto shared the Nobel Prize with Professor John J. R. Macleod for the discovery of insulin. In announcing the award in Stockholm, it was said, "Although the disease which has received the name of diabetes mellitus has evidently been known from immemorial time—Celsus and Araeteus in their writings in the first century described an illness which was characterized by an enormous secretion of urine, an unquenchable thirst and a considerable loss of flesh" (3). In 1889 Mering and Minkowski succeeded in performing a total pancreatectomy and noted that these animals secreted large amounts of sugar in the urine and became the victims of a wasting disease that appeared to have all the characteristics of diabetes, including hyperglycemia. Furthermore, if a part of the gland was left behind, or even "if a bit of it was sewn under the skin, diabetes failed to develop" (3).

The problem was in this state when a young orthopedic surgeon, Dr. Frederick C. Banting, thought the ability to find an effective pancreatic extract should be successful in correcting the hyperglycemia. Therefore he thought ligation of the pancreatic duct would result in atrophy of the exocrine function of the pancreas and thereby eliminate the production of trypsin. He proceeded to perform this procedure in the laboratory and the experiments were successful. After the exocrine cells became atrophied and died, he made an extract if the remaining islet cells. This extract lowered the blood glucose in animals made diabetic and reduced the amount of sugar excreted in the urine. The first injection of insulin was given in 1922 to a fourteen-year-old youth suffering from severe diabetes. The patient's blood sugar decreased to a normal level and the sugar in the urine was reduced to a minimum. Furthermore the state of acidosis that had been previously present was reversed. It was said of this discovery that "there would seem to be cause to remember Pasteur's words: 'Chance favors the prepared mind'" (3). In his Nobel address, Banting stated,

On April 14, 1921, I began working on this idea in the Physiological Laboratory of the University of Toronto. Professor Macleod allotted me Dr. Charles Best as an associate. Our first step was to tie the pancreatic ducts in a number of dogs. At the end of seven weeks these dogs were chloroformed, The pancreas of each dog was removed and all were found to be shriveled, fibrotic, and about one-third the original size. Histological examination showed that there were no healthy acinus cells. This material was cut into small pieces, ground with sand, and extracted with normal saline. This extract was tested on a dog rendered diabetic by the removal of the pancreas. Following the intravenous injection, the blood sugar of the depancreatized dogs was reduced to a normal or subnormal level, and the urine became sugar-free. There was a marked improvement in the general clinical condition as evidenced by the fact that the animals became stronger and more lively, the broken-down wounds healed more quickly, and the life of the animal was undoubtedly prolonged. (3)

Banting closed his address stating,

> Insulin enables the severe diabetic to burn carbohydrate, as shown by the rise
> in the respiratory quotient following the administration of glucose and insulin.
> It permits glucose to be stored as glycogen in the liver for future use. The
> burning of carbohydrate enables the complete oxidation of fats, and acidosis
> disappears. The normality of blood sugar relieves the depressing thirst, and
> consequently there is a diminished intake and output of fluid. Since the tis-
> sue cells are properly nourished by the increased diet, there is no longer the
> constant calling for food, hence hunger pain of the severe diabetic is replaced
> by normal appetite. On this increased caloric intake, the patients gain rapidly
> in strength and weight. With the relief of the symptoms of disease, and with
> the increased strength and vigor resulting from the increased diet, the pes-
> simistic, melancholy diabetic becomes optimistic and cheerful. (3)

In 1956, Werner T. O. Forssmann received the Nobel Prize in
Physiology or Medicine with Andre F. Cournand and Dickinson W.
Richards, Jr., "for their discoveries concerning heart catheterization
and pathological changes in the circulatory system" (4). The Nobel
citation called attention to the fact that as late as 1928 there were good
reasons for a statement in a textbook indicating that humans were naturally confined to use indirect methods in examining the heart.
Therefore it was highly surprising that in the following year a young
intern in surgery who was later to become a urologist, Werner Forssmann, fired with a brilliant concept and with the determination to
pursue it thoroughly, performed a by no means harmless experiment
on himself by introducing a catheter in his own anticubital vein and
passing it into the right atrium. Of these experiments by Forssmann
on himself the citation read,

> It must have required firm conviction of the value of the method to induce
> self-experimentation of the kind carried out by Forssmann. His later disap-
> pointment must have been all the more bitter. It is true that the method was
> adopted in a few places—in Prague and in Lisbon—but on the whole Forss-
> mann was not given the necessary support; he was, on the contrary, subjected
> to criticism of such exaggerated severity that it robbed him of any inclination
> to continue. This criticism was based on an unsubstantiated belief in the dan-
> ger of the intervention, thus affording proof that—even in our enlightened
> times—a valuable suggestion may remain unexploited on the grounds of a
> preconceived opinion. A contributory cause in this substance was presumably

that Forssmann was working in a milieu that did not clearly grasp the great value of his idea. (4)

In 1941, working at New York University, Cournand and Richards, making detailed studies of circulation, decided to reperform Forssmann's daring achievement on a patient after much deliberation and planning. At the ceremony in 1956 in Stockholm, Forssmann heard the citation,

> As a young doctor you have had the courage to submit yourself to heart catheterization. As a result of this, a new method was born which since that time has proved to be of very great value. It has rot only opened up new roads for the study of physiology and the pathology of the heart and the lungs, it has also given the impetus for important researches on other organs. We are glad to be able to welcome you in this country where once your ancestors worked. (4)

After receiving the Nobel Prize, Forssmann's fame increased rapidly and stimulated much interest in his original description of the daring experiment he performed on himself. As published in *Klinische Wochrenschrift* in 1929 (translated from German), Forssmann said,

> After the first trials had been successful on cadavers, I tried the first experiments in living man on myself. In a pre-experiment I had a colleague of mine puncture my right elbow vein with a thick needle, then introduced as in the experiments on the cadavers a very well lubricated ureteral catheter having the diameter of '4 Charriers'. This catheter could be inserted easily and advanced up to 35 cm. Because my colleague thought that a continuation of this experiment was too dangerous, we discontinued this trial. Nevertheless, I felt completely well all of the time. After one week I undertook another experiment. Under local anesthesia, I performed on myself a venous section in my left elbow because it is very difficult to puncture yourself with a thick needle. It was then very easy to put the catheter into the vein in its whole length which was 65 cm. This length seemed adequate to me after having measured on the body surface the approximate distance from the left elbow to the heart. After having introduced the catheter I had only very slight sensations mostly that of warmth similar to what you feel after intravenous injections of calcium chloride. Using pushing movements the catheter buckled on the upper and dorsal wall of the subclavian vein and I felt an especially intense warmth behind the clavicle behind the insertion of the sternocleidomastoid, At the same time I felt a stimulus to cough, possibly by stimulation of vagal branches. The

position of the catheter could be checked on the fluoroscreen....I watched the advancement of the catheter myself in the mirror which was held by the nurse who handled the fluoroscopic screen....There were no other than the above mentioned sensations, and even though I paid close attention to possible cardiac irregularities, I could not find any. Even the quite distant walk from the Operating Room to the X-ray Department, where I had to climb the stairs did not lead to any kind of bad sensations. Even later I could not find any disadvantages besides a slight infection, where I made the venous section. Apparently, this resulted because of lacking asepsis during this kind of self-operation. My method seems to have some advantages as to the possibilities to infuse drugs in a central part of the circulation and very rapidly. It is not necessary, therefore, to use the dangerous path through the thoracic wall and the cardiac muscle. Concluding then I want to point to the possibility that this method opens up several possibilities for studying metabolism and the activity of the heart. (5)

In 1966 Peyton Rous, the first to show that a virus could be the etiologic agent of cancer, and Charles Huggins a urologist, shared the Nobel Prize in Physiology or Medicine. Of Huggins it was said,

It took almost half a century for Rous's discovery to advance to its dominant place in modern experimental cancer research. In contrast, the discovery of Charles Huggins was of immediate practical applicability and has already given many valuable and relatively symptom free years to gravely ill cancer patients throughout the civilized world. At first glance, the contributions of Rous and Huggins may appear as of entirely different nature. They have, however, a common denominator. Both were concerned with the question, is the cancer cell completely self-sufficient and independent of all normal regulating mechanisms of the organism, or does it still maintain some of the responsiveness of the normal cell? Rous showed that there are some tumour cells that do not grow by their inner tendencies but rather due to the outside influence of virus or chemical agents. Huggins found that other tumour cells could show a similar dependence towards certain natural hormones of the body. He started to study the normal prostatic gland in dogs and found that its function and growth were stimulated by male sex hormones and inhibited by female sex hormones. This was the starting point for the hormone therapy of human prostatic cancer, based on the assumption that the human prostate may react to hormones essentially in the same way as the dog prostate, and that cancer cells of the prostate may retain part of the hormonal responsiveness of the normal cell. This reasoning suggested treatment by eliminating the male sex hormones through castration, and/or antagonizing them by introducing female sex hormones. (6)

Remarkably good therapeutic results were obtained, showing that the basic assumptions were correct. More than one-half of patients with advanced prostatic cancer, already beyond a stage accessible to surgical therapy, due to cancerous invasion of neighboring normal tissues, or even metastases to distant organs, showed an objective reduction in size, or disappearance of the tumours, including those which had spread to other organs. These patients who would not have had more than a short time to live without this treatment, became frequently free of symptoms for many years. This was a completely new type of cancer therapy, capable of helping a previously unaccessible category of patients, by the administration of non-toxic, naturally occurring hormones rather than by toxic or radioactive agents, and with few side effects. In addition to the therapy for prostatic cancer Huggins has also introduced the hormonal treatment of human breast cancer. The clinical value of this treatment is more limited, due to the fact that breast cancer cells have often lost the hormone responsiveness of their normal ancestor cell. Even this treatment has given symptomatic relief and long tolerable periods to otherwise incurable patients. (6)

Surprisingly enough, Peyton Rous was among the first to recognize the importance of Huggins' discovery. He wrote that the importance of this discovery far transcends its practical implications; for it means that thought and endeavor in cancer research have been misdirected in consequence of the belief that tumor cells are anarchic. "No one else has clarified the causes and limitations of this anarchy better than Rous and Huggins" (6).

In his opening remarks in Stockholm, Huggins stated,

The natural course can be utterly different in various sorts of malignant disease. Some tumors grow without any apparent restraint whatever. When man harbors a neoplasm of this kind, an increase in the size of the cancer is readily evident from today and death ensues in, say, six weeks. Conversely some malignant growths disappear spontaneously. Both of these antipodal effects are rare. Mostly, man with cancer lives one year or a little longer after the neoplasm becomes manifest, and it would appear that some inhibition of growth of the tumor takes place to produce this protracted course. (6)

Huggins emphasized that following orchiectomy, the prostate gland shrinks and the oxidative phase of carbohydrate metabolism diminishes and prostatic secretion ceases. These effects are corrected by administration of testosterone. He noted that the cells in the prostate do not actually die in the absence of testosterone but rather become shrunken. However, a prostatic cancer cell, which is hormone dependent, is entirely different because it grows in the presence of supporting hormones but dies in their absence and for this reason cannot participate in growth cycles. In addition Huggins found that administration of estrogen caused a rapid shrinking of experimental prostatic tumors. Quite significantly he showed that the activities of acid and alkaline phosphatases in the blood were reliable indicators of prostatic metastases. The level of acid phosphatase indicates activity of the disseminated cancer cells that had metastasized, while the level of alkaline phosphatase corresponded with function of the osteoblast as influenced by prostatic cancer. In accepting the Nobel prize, Huggins concluded, "Cancer is not necessarily autonomous and intrinsically self-perpetuating. Its growth can be sustained and propagated by hormonal function in the host which is not unusual in kind or exaggerated in rate but which is operating at normal or even subnormal levels." He added,

> Hormones, or synthetic substances inducing physiologic effects similar thereto, are of crucial significance for survival of several kinds of hormone-responsive cancers of man and animals. Opposite sorts of change of the hormonal status can induce regression and, in some instances, cure of such cancers. These modifications are deprivation of essential hormones, and hormone interference by giving large amounts of critical compounds. The control of cancer by endocrine methods can be described in three propositions. Some types of cancer cells differ in a cardinal way from the cells from which they arose in their response to change in their hormonal environment (2). Certain cancers are hormone-dependent and these cells die when supporting hormones are eliminated (3). Certain cancers succumb when large amounts of hormones are administered. (6)

These pioneering achievements by Huggins opened an entirely new vista for the treatment of cancer. Today these principles are responsible for achieving significant palliation in many patients with malignant disease and actual cure in others.

In 1990, Dr. Joseph E. Murray and Dr. E. Donnall Thomas were chosen for the Nobel Prize in Physiology or Medicine for their contributions in renal transplantation and transplantation of bone marrow, respectively. On this occasion it was stated, "During the 19th century, the association between disease symptoms and organ damage was well understood. Trouble with the urine could be caused by damage of the kidney, and if the skin was yellow the cause could be in the liver. Damage to the kidney was most often incurable." Therefore, it was thought very early that perhaps a new undamaged organ from somebody else could cure the disease. Thus, at the turn of the century many heroic attempts were made to transplant kidneys from swine, sheep, and goats, however without success. In 1902 attempts were made to transplant a kidney from one human being to another, again with no success. Very soon it was learned that it was possible to transplant an organ or tissue within an individual without harm, but not between individuals. In 1912, Alexis Carrel received the Nobel Prize among other things for his discoveries concerning transplants of blood vessels and organs. However, this success was limited to transplants within an individual. Carrel concluded that there was a biological force that prevented transplantation between individuals, and he believed that it would never be possible to succeed in having an organ from one individual function in another. He received support for his belief, among others, from the 1960 Nobel Prize winner, Peter Medawar, who discovered the role of the immune defense system in rejection of a graft and also showed that the biological force defined by Carrel was of an immunological nature (7).

Joseph Murray was not discouraged by this knowledge. There were reasons to believe that the immunological barrier was lacking between identical twins. Joseph Murray developed a surgical technique for kidney transplantation in dogs and showed that a kidney that was transplanted from one dog to the other could be induced to function. He used the technique in the first successful kidney transplant between identical twins in December 1954. Richard Herrick, who had incurable kidney damage was the first candidate. In order to make sure that he and his brother Ronald were identical twins, Joseph Murray asked the police in Boston to document their fingerprint patterns. During a routine review of police records, journalists found out about the investigation and its confidentiality was breached. However, Richard Herrick appeared to take this leakage to the press calmly. He became the darling of the media. The operation worked out perfectly and the kidney functioned well. Richard Herrick married his recovery room nurse and became the father of two children. He lived happily for eight years and then died of heart infarction. Joseph Murray later performed several other transplants between identical twins. However, most patients with incurable kidney damage had no twins, and it was therefore some time before such patients could become transplant candidates (7).

In its press release of October 8, 1990, The Karolinska Institute closed its statement, saying,

> Murray's and Thomas's discoveries are crucial for those tens of thousands of severely ill patients who either can be cured or be given a decent life when other treatment methods are without success.

Thoughtful reflections on each of these contributions by surgeons that led to their selection for the Nobel Prize again emphasize the significance of the quote by Edward B. Butler: "One man has enthusiasm for thirty minutes, another for thirty days, but it is the man who has it for thirty years that makes a success of his life." The discipline of surgery and all those who have made it possible owe a continuing debt to those master achievers whose scientific observations led to their worldwide recognition.

References

1. Wilhelm, P. *The Nobel Prize*. London: Springwood Books, 1983.
2. Nobelstiftelsen. *Nobel Lectures: Physiology or Medicine 1901–1921*. Stockholm: Elsevier Publishing Co., 1967.
3. Nobelstiftelsen. *Nobel Lectures: Physiology or Medicine 1922–1941*. Stockholm: Elsevier Publishing Co., 1965.
4. Nobelstiftelsen. *Nobel Lectures: Physiology or Medicine 1942–1962*. Stockholm: Elsevier Publishing Co., 1964.
5. Forssmann, W. Die Sondierung des rechten Herzens. *Klinische Wochenschrift 1929*; 8:2085–2087.
6. Nobelstiftelsen. *Nobel Lectures: Physiology or Medicine 1963–1970*. Stockholm: Elsevier Publishing Co., 1972.
7. Citation of Nobel Prize Presentation, 1990.

Chapter 9 &

Friedrich Trendelenburg

T hree-quarters of a century have passed since Friedrich Trendelenburg of Leipzig described his experimental observations in
the production and surgical management of pulmonary embolism.
This work was combined with one of the first reports of clinical pulmonary embolectomy and was presented at the 37th Congress of the
German Surgical Society in 1908 (1). It is astonishing to note the
scope and depth of the diagnostic, physiological, and therapeutic
aspects of pulmonary embolism recognized at such an early date by
this surgical master. For example, Trendelenburg opened his presentation with a description of the clinical manifestations of acute, massive
pulmonary embolism, stating quite succinctly:

> The face appears ashen; the lips are pale and slightly cyanotic, although the
> absence of color is more pronounced than the cyanosis. The jugular veins and
> the subcutaneous veins of the upper half of the chest appear abnormally dis-
> tended and show through the skin with bluish color. The patient's forehead
> is covered with cold sweat, the fear of death is reflected in his facial expres-
> sions, the extremities are pale and cool, his pulse is small and irregular. The
> pulse is often absent altogether for periods, and respirations are frequent and
> labored. The pupils are dilated and become fixed. The patient becomes less
> responsive with either transient or permanent loss of consciousness, and fi-
> nally death occurs after a few agonal respirations. (1)

Most would agree that this superb description can hardly be
improved upon by the most experienced of contemporary clinicians.

Of additional interest are the physiological features that Trendelenburg described primarily from his experimental observations of massive embolism:

The right ventricle is markedly dilated and packed full with blood. Finally, the heart arrests in diastole while a few agonal respirations follow. In general, the cerebral symptoms secondary to the lack of oxygen, namely, the loss of consciousness, the dilated and fixed pupils and even at times the emesis usually occur toward the end, although the attack may begin with the loss of consciousness....Systolic or systolic and diastolic murmurs are almost always present when the embolus hangs up in the right ventricle instead of in the pulmonary artery, although a second, previously broken off thrombus naturally could already be sitting in the pulmonary artery....In case the pulmonary artery is instantaneously and completely occluded, death occurs so quickly that it is instantaneous or comes after 1 or 2 minutes so that there is no time for an operation. (1)

It is fascinating that he also recognized the variability in the length of time between the onset of symptoms and death following massive pulmonary embolism:

In my experience, however, cases are more frequent in which the obstruction initially is only a partial one and death occurs after 15 minutes or later; sudden death is less common. Among the 9 cases of pulmonary embolism from the Leipzig Hospital, which we could observe more closely regarding the time passed between the onset of the attack and death, only 2 cases belong to the group experiencing sudden, immediate death. In the remaining 7 cases the time that passed between the beginning of the embolic attack and death was 10 minutes, 15 to 20 minutes, 30 minutes, 30 to 35 minutes, and approximately 40 minutes, and in 1 case even one hour. (1)

In specific comments about his experimental work on the calf, Trendelenburg stated:

In these experiments I have incised the right ventricular outflow tract after exposing the entire heart and through this incision have passed a wide cannula to the pulmonary artery and with the help of a suction syringe have removed emboli from the pulmonary artery. Even though this was repeatedly successful in animals, the procedure proved to be too uncertain and too traumatic. Further experiments showed that the same effect could be achieved more simply by incising the main pulmonary artery directly and extracting emboli using a polyp tong. Naturally, to do this one has to compress the pulmonary artery proximal to the incision. Sauerbruch has shown that one can occlude the vena cava for 10 minutes in animals, and one would expect that one could occlude the pulmonary artery for a similar length of time. However, this is not the case. On the average, after 45 seconds to 2 minutes in rabbits and after 45 seconds to a minute in sheep one observes gasping respirations and often convulsions that make it necessary to release the occlusion in order to avoid the risk of causing the animal's death....After complete occlusion of the pulmonary artery the blood pressure in the aorta drops to a third or a fourth of its normal pressure and after releasing the clamp within three-fourths of a minute the blood pressure rises rapidly, initially way above the normal level and then after 1 1/4 minutes following release of the clamp it returns to normal. The heart continues to work during the compression, both ventricles pump themselves full of blood, becoming markedly dilated, and the pulse wave disappears....These experiments indicate that after total compression of the pulmonary artery and the aorta one has approximately one-half to three-fourths of a minute to extract the emboli from the artery following an incision. (1)

In his first clinical attempt to treat a patient with acute, massive pulmonary embolism, Trendelenburg entered the left chest with a transverse incision beginning at the level of the second rib near the sternum and extending 10 cm laterally. A second perpendicular incision was made along the left sternal border from the manubrium at the level of the first rib to the level of the third cartilage. The two triangular skin flaps created by these incisions were dissected off the chest wall, and the second rib was divided laterally, bent medially, and removed. The third rib was divided through its cartilaginous portion and the pleura opened with the internal mammary vessels protected. The pericardium was then opened anterior to the phrenic nerve, exposing the pulmonary artery. Trendelenburg commented that this entire portion of the procedure could be accomplished easily within five minutes. Next, the retracting pulmonary artery and aorta had to be pulled into the wound to permit compression of the vessels. To accomplish this, a long, markedly curved probe with a button at the end was passed within the pericardium but behind and through the transverse sinus with a rotating movement from left to right behind the blood vessels so that the button of the probe appeared at the left sternal border. A thin rubber tube was then connected to the button of the probe with a small screw clamp and the probe was pulled back, thereby bringing the rubber tube as a loop behind the aorta and the pulmonary arteries.

Trendelenburg stated:

one stabs quickly into the pulmonary artery at the exposed site and dilates it in a longitudinal fashion toward the bifurcation of the vessel over a distance of about 0.75 cm. Then, the polyp clamp, which is blunted at the end so that it will not grab the arterial wall at the bifurcation of the artery, is passed first into the main pulmonary artery and then into its branches so that the emboli can be grasped and removed. (1)

It is also interesting that Trendelenburg used a partial occlusion clamp to control the pulmonary arteriotomy so that one could apply the clamp immediately with restoration of the circulation. Trendelenburg's first patient was a seventy-year-old woman with a fracture of the femoral neck. Six days following the fracture, about half an hour after turning in her bed, she suffered a sudden cardiovascular collapse with marked diaphoresis. Three minutes later she showed changes in consciousness and her pupils became dilated. Although her respirations continued, Trendelenburg stated, "One could not palpate a pulse anywhere in the periphery or hear any heart sounds." He further noted that at the time of the patient's acute attack he "was notified by telephone in my apartment, which is 8 minutes away from the hospital," so he immediately went to the hospital. He stated that "the operation lasted only 5 minutes, up to the time when the pulmonary artery was incised despite the fact that this was more difficult due to old adhesions of the lung and pleura." Trendelenburg regretted that he did not "use the pressure differential method in this case," since he surmised that "the pneumothorax that was created on the left side further worsened the condition of the patient." This comment was a reference to Sauerbruch's positive-pressure chamber. Trendelenburg then decried openly that in the first patient he elected to use an umbilical tape to pass beneath the pulmonary artery, instead of the smooth rubber tube he had used experimentally in the calf. The tape did not slide easily but rather was difficult to pull through the transverse sinus, causing a tear in the posterior wall of the pulmonary artery and producing "troublesome" and later fatal hemorrhage (2).

Trendelenburg closed his original communication on a more optimistic note:

The fact that the first attempt in man was unsuccessful does not disprove its feasibility, and I am now able to contrast this case with a complete success in an animal experiment. You see here the heart of a calf; I injected a 15 cm long strip of lung tissue into the animal's jugular vein on December 19, 1907, and then extracted it out of the left pulmonary artery. The animal was killed on March 21, 1908. One can see a small circumscribed area of thickening on the inside of the pulmonary artery at the site where the arteriotomy had been performed. The silk sutures were completely healed in and were not seen from the inside or the outside secondary to tissue overgrowth. Compared to the operation in man, the operation on the calf presents a much bigger challenge due to the shape of the thorax, the location of the pulmonary artery, and the communication of both pleural spaces. I would therefore hope that a successful attempt in man will soon follow this successful procedure in the experimental animal. (1)

In 1908, Trendelenburg published his observations of two additional patients on whom he performed pulmonary embolectomy with temporary occlusion of the pulmonary artery; these patients survived the immediate procedure. A translation of this report appeared shortly thereafter in the *Annals of Surgery* (3), in which it was stated that one of the two patients died of right heart failure sixteen hours following the procedure and the other thirty-seven hours postoperatively of hemorrhage from an internal mammary artery. Nevertheless, Trendelenburg had clearly demonstrated the procedure to be technically feasible, and in 1924 his student, Professor Martin Kirschner, performed a successful pulmonary embolectomy with temporary occlusion of the pulmonary artery (4). The operation was performed successfully in the United States by Steenburg and colleagues in 1957 at a time when only twelve other successful procedures had been reported in the world literature (5).

Although in contemporary practice, most authorities recommend the use of extracorporeal circulation in performing emergency pulmonary embolectomy, temporary occlusion of the inferior and superior venae cavae together with pulmonary arteriotomy, continues to be favored by some, and with acceptable results. For example, 42 patients who had massive pulmonary embolism were treated by emergency pulmonary embolectomy using normothermic venous inflow occlusion circulatory arrest. Among 26 patients without cardiac arrest before operation, 25 survived, although 7 eventually died of various causes. In contrast, there was only 1 survivor among 16 patients undergoing the procedure who had had preoperative cardiac arrest. In the entire series, 119 of the 42 patients (45 percent) operated on using the modified Trendelenburg procedure left the hospital alive. It was concluded in this recently reported series that "this simple and widely applicable technique has enabled an emergency pulmonary embolectomy service to be offered to all the hospitals in a metropolitan area" (6).

Once again, reexamination of a major contribution to the history of surgery provides a number of unexpected rewards, and serves as a continuing reminder of the importance of returning to the original literature.

References

1. Trendelenburg, F. Über die operative Behandlung der Embolie der Lungenarterie. Arch. Klin. Chir. 86: 686, 1908.
2. Johnson, S. L. *The History of Cardiac Surgery, 1896–1955.* Baltimore: Johns Hopkins Press, 1970.
3. Trendelenburg, F. General surgery, pathology and therapy: I. Operative interference in embolism of the pulmonary artery (abstract); translated by Pilcher J. T. ands Joerg W. *Ann. Surg.* 48: 772, 1908.
4. Alexander, J. Some dramatic thoracic operations. *J. Thorac. Surg.* 5: 1, 1935.
5. Teenburg, R. W., Warren, R., Wilson, R. E., and Rudolf, L. E. A new look at pulmonary embolectomy. *Surg. Gynecol. Obstet.* 107:214, 1958.
6. Clark, D. B. Pulmonary embolectomy re-evaluated. *Ann. R. Coll. Surg. Engl.* 63: 18, 1981.

Chapter 10 ☞

Allen O. Whipple, M.D.

*T*here are few in surgery whose honor is more appropriately remembered for surgical education than Allen O. Whipple. Both during his life and after his death, it can be stated with confidence that he was a heroic figure in surgery whose contributions as a teacher, investigator, and clinical surgeon were of extraordinary breadth. Born of missionary parents in Persia just south of Mount Ararat, where Noah is reputed to have landed the Ark, Dr. Whipple inherited from his New England ancestors a vigorous idealism combined with practicality. Graduating from Princeton in 1904, he received his medical degree from the Columbia College of Physicians and Surgeons in 1908. His house staff training in surgery was at the Roosevelt Hospital and following this, he was appointed to the faculty at Columbia. In 1911, he was made a member of the surgical staff of the Presbyterian Hospital. Ten years later the University decided to establish a full-time Chair in Surgery, to which Dr. Whipple was appointed.

Allen O. Whipple was one of those unusual scholars who achieved excellence in several fields. Not only did he accomplish brilliantly in surgery, but he was a student of music, painting, oriental culture, and medical history. As Wilder Penfield noted, he could write English that was pure and simple, like that found in the King James version of the Bible. As an example, Penfield quotes his description of the combined spleen clinic at Presbyterian Hospital: "The workers in these clinics, from whatever department they may be, speak the same language, see eye to eye, and there are no therapeutic miracles among friends. Here, as in no other clinic, pride and prejudice disappear and an honest integration of opinions and convictions results." It was from his association with his colleagues in this interdisciplinary clinic that his interest in portal hypertension began and subsequently led to the innovative contribution together with his colleague, Arthur Blakemore, in the development of the portacaval shunt. His contributions to surgery of the pancreas, especially the clinical description of islet cell tumors and of the radical pancreaticoduodenectomy for treatment of carcinoma of the pancreas, which bears his name, each originated in these formative years. His interest in surgery and surgical physiology was maintained until the end. In the year of his death, Dr. Whipple published his final work, a monograph entitled, "The Story of Wound Healing and Wound Repair."

Of especial interest regarding his contributions in surgical education, were Whipple's achievements in this area, and these bear emphasis today. He was a founding member of the American Board of Surgery, and he followed his long-time friend Evarts Graham as the second Chairman of the Board. The many fine residents "whom he trained as well as their subsequent contributions are a matter of record." He was a member of the Board of Trustees of the American University of Beirut, and after his retirement he was asked to reorganize the medical training program there. His alma mater, Princeton University, conferred upon him its Woodrow Wilson Award in 1958, given to the alumnus "best exemplifying Princeton in the nation's service." The recipient of honorary degrees from Columbia University, the University of Chicago, Washington University in St. Louis, and Princeton, he was also an officer of one of the leading surgical organizations in the United Kingdom, an Honorary Fellow of the Royal College of Surgeons of England.

Whipple's personal ideas concerning the importance of teachers and teaching are found in his own words: "Choose your teachers well, for their influence on you can be telling and lasting. I shall always be thankful for mine especially those in surgery here in New York..." and after a pause, Dr. Whipple added, "...and by adoption, Halsted." One of his closest associates, the late Fordyce B. St. John, said in this connection, "Of equal importance was his interest in Halsted and his championship of Halsted's principles of surgical technique and surgical training which have become the hallmark of the best in surgery today."

Perhaps one of the finest tributes paid Dr. Whipple is to be found in the minutes of the meeting of the Medical Board of the Presbyterian Hospital shortly after his death. There one finds the following statement:

> All of us here owe to him more than we know. With true humility, he disregarded his contributions and the honors they won him in the eager and continued search for new avenues of service. His stature rises, like a high mountain as we see it from a lengthening distance. Those of us who are privileged to be close to him, forget, with him, his many accomplishments and decorations, and remember him only with the filial respect of devoted professional children.

It is the high respect and stimulation for achievement that formed the basis of the founding of the Whipple Society. It is altogether appropriate that Dr. Whipple's memory be continued with constant reappraisal of major problems facing surgical education at all levels.

Chapter 11 &

Alfred Blalock

*A*s I reflect upon my own educational experience and the many teachers whom I have admired, there is one far more than any other who remains foremost. His breadth of vision, his concepts of teaching, his approach to clinical surgery, his emphasis upon original investigation, and his recognition of the importance of effective administration have remained since my first encounter with him as a second year medical student. With the passage of time, his shadow continues to lengthen, and a day seldom passes but that my thoughts return to him, usually with the simple question, "How would he have managed this?"

In reviewing the career of Alfred Blalock, I hope that his profile will especially interest the younger readers and cause them to reflect upon his careful planning of an outstanding career. Of equal importance is a clear recognition of the pleasure he obtained throughout his life, especially in his unique ability to help others. As one assesses his career and his achievements, it becomes indelibly clear that the entire span was carefully planned from the outset, and that he achieved in a stepwise and ever widening manner those goals which he had established many years earlier.

There is much to be learned from great people not only from a philosophic point of view, but more important from the practical aspects of those issues and problems of daily life. A glimpse of his early life, education, and training provides much insight into the remarkable contributions which were to follow. We learn from his cousin J. Dorsey Blalock that the first of the family to arrive from England was Patrick Blalock, whose name is listed in a colonial grant and who settled in Virginia in 1620. Further investigation shows that a number of his forebears served in the Revolution and in the War Between the

States, and in Georgia the name of Blalock is well known in a variety of endeavors, including law, business, agriculture, politics, and many other fields.

Alfred Blalock was born on April 5, 1899, in Culloden, a small town in mid-Georgia. His father owned a large cotton plantation and was a well-known merchant. Alfred was the oldest of five children and commented from time to time that his father was a strict disciplinarian. It is fortunate today that at one point he was asked to prepare a short biographical sketch of himself, and the insights obtained from reviewing it are penetrating.

Of his early life, he said, "I had a very pleasant environment at home....My father encouraged us to read worthwhile books...and he would help me with my studies." He attended the public schools in Culloden and then attended Georgia Military College, an academy recognized as being a preparatory school for the University of Georgia. As a result of academic success there, he was admitted to the University of Georgia as a sophomore in the fall of 1915, and of that time he was later to say, "My favorite study in college was zoology. Languages were fairly easy for me, but such was not the case with mathematics and physics." He continues his description of that period by saying:

> I received my Bachelor of Arts Degree at the University of Georgia in the spring of 1918, shortly having passed my nineteenth birthday. I had known for some several years that I wished to study medicine, and it was largely through the efforts of Dr. Campbell, Professor of Zoology, that I was accepted for admission to the Johns Hopkins School of Medicine.

While in medical school at Hopkins, his best work was in the surgical courses. For example, in his senior year, one finds in the class roll in the archives of the Welch Medical Library that he was awarded a grade of 9 out of a possible 10 as the final mark in the course. In fact, only four students of the eighty in the class outranked him. It is also interesting to note the number of outstanding students in the class of 1922, names later to become known for a wide variety of important contributions, including those of Arthur Blakemore, Robert Elman, Tinsley Harrison, Chester Scott Keefer, and Orthello Langworthy.

One of the most interesting letters to be found in the Blalock papers is one which he wrote to Dr. Halsted, while a senior medical student, in December 1921. It is interesting to note the similarity of his handwriting at that time with that which continued years later. In addition, his choice of words and expressions, even at that time, are characteristic and were often repeated in succeeding years.

Dear Dr. Halsted,

The writer of this letter is a member of the present fourth year class and it concerns an appointment in surgery for next year.

I would like very much to have the place in experimental surgery. My only work in this department has been in the third year elective course and a little work in which I assisted Dr. McLean. Despite the fact that I know little of the work I feel very interested in it and would like an opportunity to try it. If I should get an appointment and make good, I hope to work in a surgical clinic for a number of years, as I have no immediate desire to start practicing.

During my three years as a medical student, I have worked seven months in the summers in surgery, and I feel absolutely sure that I want to follow it. The past summer I substituted two months here in general surgery and I enjoyed it very much. As the greatest number of my patients were Dr. Dandy's, I think he could best give you an idea as to my work.

If my name is considered for the place, I would appreciate a personal interview. At any rate, I shall put in my application.

Yours sincerely,
Alfred Blalock

From this letter, it is apparent today that one can almost chart the course of Dr. Blalock's life since the code is clearly contained within it.

It is interesting to note the attention which Dr. Halsted gave to detail since, despite his duties as a busy and involved director of a department, he replied to this letter, stating:

Dear Mr. Blalock:

I am pleased to receive your letter of the first inst. and to know that you are an applicant for a position in the Hunterian

Laboratory. These positions will be reserved for men of high standing in the class, and I shall have to investigate your records before giving you a definite answer.

Very truly yours,
William S. Halsted

It is generally believed that Alfred Blalock was later greatly disappointed that he did not obtain one of the appointments for a position in Dr. Halsted's famed residency program. Nevertheless, it is a matter of record that he was always quite candid about the fact that he was not chosen to remain for the full program, and in his files are several references to this point. He once stated, "Following one year as an assistant resident on the surgical service, the competition became too keen and I sought a position elsewhere without success." He then turned to Dr. Samuel R. Crowe, Professor and Head of the Division of Otolaryngology, for assistance, and a letter to Dr. Harvey Cushing was forthcoming. Dr. Blalock continued, "Following Dr. Crowe's letter, I was offered a position at the Peter Bent Brigham Hospital under Dr. Cushing but later decided to go to Vanderbilt with Dr. Barney Brooks, who had been recommended to me by Dr. Halsted. After two years at Vanderbilt I became ill [with tuberculosis] and had to go to the Adirondacks."

As many know, the attack of pulmonary tuberculosis and his confinement at Trudeau Sanatarium were a very depressing experience. A small area of increased density of the left apex with mottling and scarring was noted in the chest film, and his sputum was positive for acid-fast organisms. After a year there he wrote:

> I requested that I be given pneumothorax treatments, but they refused. I then decided to go to Europe and on a visit to Berlin I became rather ill and sought the advice of Dr. Sauerbruch. He treated me rather miserably. Finally, he advised me to have a thoracoplasty, but I refused and returned to Saranac Lake.

Following the pneumothorax treatments, he returned to Nashville, but in spite of the fact that he remained under intensive treatment with pneumothorax for two years, he worked continuously and missed only one or two days' work during the entire time. This is a clear example of his perseverance, of his industry, and of his tenacity, each feature that was to characterize him throughout the remainder of his life.

Dr. Blalock's first paper was published in the *Journal of Ameican Medical Association* in 1924 while he was a resident in Baltimore and concerned a clinical study of biliary tract disease, concerning which he reviewed 735 patients with this disorder. The fact that it was a clinical paper is significant in that, despite his unconcealed love for the experimental laboratory, he always insisted that there be clear clinical implications in his laboratory investigation.

His first experimental paper appeared in the *Journal of Clinical Investigation* in 1925 and concerned the effects of changes in hydrogen concentration on the blood flow of morphinized dogs. It is interesting that at such an early date he and his colleagues employed exacting techniques for determination of pH with accuracies of 0.03, and performed concomitantly with determination of the amount of oxygen consumed and carbon dioxide released by the lungs.

His early work with Tinsley Harrison on circulatory problems led quite naturally to his becoming involved in studies relating to the pathogenesis of shock. He often referred to this period of his life and placed great emphasis upon spending considerable time in the experimental laboratory during the course of surgical training. He recognized clearly the importance of this phase of academic development, and this philosophy is reflected in his many hours of dedicated work in the laboratory.[1] Of particular significance in the development of his scientific career was the time spent in England at the Physiological Laboratories in Cambridge. In 1927 Blalock was introduced to painstaking and rigid physiological techniques. He referred to this period in later life, recalling that it was in that Cambridge laboratory he first learned the importance of meticulous attention to detail, particularly in the conduct and

---

1. From Blalock's emphasis on research experience during surgery training came Sabiston's emphasis on research time in the Duke Surgical Residency (see Chapters 5 and 14).

interpretation of experimental work. While in Cambridge, his work was on the subject of blood flow in skeletal muscle assessed by the anemometer. The principle involved was the employment of hot wire in the form of a spiral of platinum about twelve microns in diameter and mounted in a metal cylinder, a very involved technique for surgical investigators in that early day. The work entitled, "Observations upon the Blood Flow through Skeletal Muscle by the Use of the Hot Wire Anemometer," was published in the *American Journal of Physiology.* Another paper from that laboratory concerned the distribution of blood flow in the coronary circulation, and these studies represented his first work in cardiac physiology. It was entitled "The Distribution of the Blood in the Coronary Blood Vessels," and was published in the *British Journal of Physiology* in 1929. This experience at Cambridge, with a group of distinguished physiologists, provided a rigorous standard in the collection of experimental data which was to remain with him always.

In 1928, Dr. Blalock returned to Vanderbilt with a firm understanding of basic physiological principles and having mastered a number of important investigative techniques. These were rapidly put to work in the Surgical Research Laboratory in Nashville, and 1928 to 1941 was probably the most productive time of his life. Thus, he was to subsequently say, "My research problem was that of traumatic shock and my main clinical interest was thoracic surgery." During that period, the status of shock was in a state of total disarray, with many conflicting views concerning its pathogenesis. As was characteristic of all his undertakings, he insisted that simple questions be answered first and therefore designed an experiment which was to remain a classic. In an anesthetized animal, the thigh was injured by blunt trauma and some hours later its weight was compared with that of the control limb following exacting dissection. In the traumatized limb, the increased weight was shown to account for 66 percent of the circulating blood volume, thus explaining the loss of intravascular volume into the tissues and accounting for the hypotensive state. In this simple, but brilliant, experiment, he was able to show that shock is due primarily to the loss of circulating blood and plasma from the vascular compartment, either externally or into the tissues.

These early studies were noted widely, and at the young age of thirty-four he was elected a member of the American Surgical Association. In 1933 he was invited to give the Arthur Dean Bevan Lecture in Chicago, almost certainly the youngest ever to deliver this distinguished lectureship. He reviewed his important contributions under the title of "Acute Circulatory Failure as Exemplified by Shock and Haemorrhage."

His work on experimental and clinical shock was summarized in a well-known monograph entitled, "Principles of Surgical Care, Shock and Other Problems," and his warm interest in people and his appreciation of their assistance were typified when he said in the introduction: "My excellent technician, Vivien Thomas, has been responsible for the execution of many of the experiments." Dr. Blalock spent many hours with him and he became an outstanding assistant who was to have a major role in subsequent years. While in Nashville, Dr. Blalock met and married Mary O'Brien, a Nashville native who was known for her charm and beauty, and the wedding was widely reported in the newspapers of the day. All their friends recognized the great support which she provided him and their three fine children, Bill, Betty, and Dandy Blalock.

It was also at Vanderbilt that Dr. Blalock's pioneering work on myasthenia gravis and its relationship with the thymus was performed. Of this period he was to say: "I remained at Vanderbilt for 16 years advancing from Instructor in Surgery to full Professor in the Department directed by Dr. Brooks." It is appropriate to emphasize that he had already made a number of important scientific contributions and was clearly a national figure. He was respected not only by clinical surgeons but by physiologists, biochemists, and others in basic science alike. In subsequent years, his general insistence upon having achieved a rather solid scientific background before assuming major administrative duties was a principle that he frequently emphasized. Certainly it was clear in his situation that the strong background in teaching at Vanderbilt, the fact that he was a pioneer in clinical thoracic surgery, particularly in diseases of the thymus and pericardium, and his brilliant research combined to make him an ideal choice for a prominent chair in surgery.

In 1940, there was considerable controversy in Baltimore concerning the choice of a successor to Dr. Dean Lewis as Professor of Surgery at Johns Hopkins. The first letter in the Blalock files referring to this issue is one from his close friend Samuel Crowe, who wrote:

Dear Al:

Thank you for sending me a copy of your book. I am just leaving for a few weeks rest in some cool spot and will there read your book with a great deal of interest and pride. We need you here and I wish I had the authority to make the appointment.

As ever yours,
Samuel J. Crowe

The Surgical Search Committee recommended as its first choice a former resident of Halsted, Dr. Mont Reid, Professor of Surgery at the University of Cincinnati. However, he chose to remain in Cincinnati, and Evarts A. Graham was next offered the post. In declining the position, he took the opportunity to recommend to President Bowman the name of Alfred Blalock. During a visit shortly thereafter, it became obvious that President Bowman was greatly impressed by the forty-one-year-old Blalock and was quite influential in the Committee's decision to make him the offer, an offer which was accepted.

One of the recurring features of much significance is the admiration which those in other disciplines had for his clinical and investigative work. For example, the late Edward A. Park, regarded by some as the most outstanding pediatrician thus far in this century, wrote him several months after his arrival in Baltimore, saying:

Before starting in work tonight, I wish to state again my admiration at the moves you are planning for your Department. You will have soon a unique Department of Surgery which will stand above and set an example to all other Departments in the country. I feel like giving three cheers that you are thinking of surgeons in terms of physiology as well as surgery.

While in Baltimore, the Friday Noon Clinics, which had been begun by Halsted, were always exceptional and attended by students, residents, and faculty alike. On the investigative side, Dr. Blalock's early work was a continuation of studies on shock, but shortly thereafter his major attention turned toward the heart. At that time, Dr. Helen Taussig was Head of the Congenital Heart Disease Clinic in the Department of Pediatrics and was involved in the care of cyanotic and desperately ill children with the tetralogy of Fallot. She presented the problem of inadequate pulmonary blood flow in these patients and asked Dr. Blalock if there might not be a way to increase this flow by a surgical approach. He recalled that six years earlier, in an effort to produce experimental pulmonary hypertension, he had joined the systemic and pulmonary circulations by direct anastomosis with marked augmentation of pulmonary blood flow. Although the laboratory experience had been negative from the point of view of producing pulmonary hypertension, he nevertheless remembered the technique and particularly the fact that in long-term follow-up there were no adverse changes to be found in the pulmonary microcirculation. In fact, the animals tolerated the subclavian artery to pulmonary artery anastomosis amazingly well and without ill effect, work that was published in 1939. Nevertheless, he wished to be certain that the polycythemia and cyanosis, which occurred in patients with pulmonary stenosis and atresia, could be reversed by a systemic pulmonary shunt. For these studies, he developed a rather complex but appropriate experimental model by a combination of pulmonary resection and arteriovenous shunts in the remaining lung. Following these studies in the laboratory, he was convinced that a systemic pulmonary shunt would not only reduce the cyanosis but also decrease the high hematocrits in patients with tetralogy of Fallot.

On November 29, 1944, he operated upon a severely cyanotic infant who had spent a prolonged period in oxygen and created the first pulmonary systemic shunt. Fortunately, the child obtained an excellent response, and the procedure was repeated shortly thereafter in several additional patients with equal success. Within a short period, a new and historic surgical procedure became established, and news of this rapidly spread throughout the nation and around the world. This work was published in the *Journal of the American Medical Association,* and in a short time, patients were referred in large numbers from both this country and abroad. A new era had opened in the life of Alfred Blalock and for the entire field of cardiac surgery. In 1948, Dr. Blalock was invited to give the first Rudolph Matas Lecture at Tulane, which was on the topic of "Surgical Procedures Employed in Anatomical Variations Encountered in the Treatment of Congenital Pulmonic Stenosis." This paper was to become one of the most frequently quoted of all his publications and contained the beautiful illustrations of the anatomic variations and stepwise surgical procedures by the well-known medical artist Leon Schlossberg. Matas was very impressed with this lecture and was to wire Dr. Blalock:

> TIS MIDNIGHT AND ONLY ONE HOUR SINCE I HAVE MY FIRST GLIMPSE AT OCTOBER NUMBER SO I COULD NOT FINISH READING YOUR MONUMENTAL NU SIGMA NU LECTURE WITHOUT RUSHING TO THE PHONE TO TELL YOU THAT MY PRIDE AND VANITY HAVE BEEN SO DEEPLY STIRRED BY YOUR DEDICATION AND MELODY OF YOUR PRAISE HAVE STARTED A FLUTTER IN MY HEART-STRINGS THAT WILL KEEP ME FROM SLEEPING TONIGHT BUT I FORGIVE YOU CORDIALLY NONE THE LESS.
>
>   R MATAS

Today, the Blalock operation continues to be used, primarily in severely ill infants with tetralogy of Fallot, and one recently published paper stated that this operation was the procedure of choice in infants requiring an operation in the first year of life.

There is also a very interesting episode which Dr. Blalock had with Yousuf Karsh, the noted Canadian portrait photographer. Karsh said:

> In 1950, as he was about to perform his thousandth blue baby operation, his colleagues commissioned me to commemorate the event, but the surgeon, I was told, "would take a great deal of persuading." As one of his associates explained to me, he could be enticed before my camera only with an innocent subterfuge. I was to tell him in the interest of his profession he must be included in my gallery of scientists. We spent a lively evening together. At dinner, by way of discovering his personality, I talked freely about doctors and remarked rather brashly that in the main they were very vain creatures. He took this in good part and suggested that, if I were interested in his profession, I had better see a blue baby operation for myself.

Accordingly, I was amazed and not a little nervous to find myself in an operating room next morning wearing a mask and gown and standing at the left hand of the surgeon. Then for two hours he applied the magic of his mind and fingers to the body of a child seven years old. I was awed by Dr. Blalock's dexterity and more by his calm. He proceeded easily and naturally, often talked to me with no sign of tension, explained his methods to visiting doctors from many parts of the world who sat in the operating amphitheater. As time wore on I lost my awe and two hours stretched into eternity. Nothing disturbed Dr. Blalock. He finished his incredible task on schedule, ordered the patient wheeled out of the operating room, and removed his gloves like a man who had done an ordinary morning's work. But his single thought was for the mother of the child. Before he had even removed his gown, he went to telephone and assured this anxious woman that the operation was successful. His telephone conversion, more than his skill, told me what sort of man I was going to photograph. And I hastened to say to him, "Dr. Blalock, I take back everything I said last night about the vanity of doctors. If you have such a thing, which I doubt, you are more than entitled to it."

Karsh was to subsequently publish an album of his portraits of the world's greats, and it is rather poignant that there are five physicians included in this album entitled *Portraits of Greatness*, Charles H. Best, Sir Alexander Fleming, Wilder Penfield, each of whom is a Nobel laureate, and, in addition, Jonas Salk and Alfred Blalock.

In April 1945, Dr. Blalock was elected a member of the National Academy of Sciences, the highest scientific and academic honor. He received a large number of commendations from scientists throughout the country. Representative ones include that from Donald D. Van Slyke of the Rockefeller Institute, who said, "It was a great pleasure to learn that the Academy had honored itself by electing you." And another from Vincent Du Vigneaud, who said, "Just a little note to extend to you my most hearty congratulations on your election to the National Academy of Sciences. This recognition of you and your work is richly deserved." And from Charles Huggins:

Dear Al:

I have just read in *Science* the good news of your election to the National Academy of Sciences. The wisdom of the electors is apparent and has made us feel very happy. I wish to extend my very best congratulations to you on this well deserved recognition of your brilliant scientific accomplishments.

With his usual humility, Dr. Blalock replied:

Dear Charlie:

It was exceedingly thoughtful of you to write to me regarding my election to the National Academy of Sciences. It was a great surprise to me and I hope that those responsible have not made too bad a mistake.

To Dr. Blalock came many national honors, including the Presidency of the American Association of Thoracic Surgery in 1951. In 1954 he was President Elect of the American College of Surgeons, and a number of the members of the College traveled jointly to Scotland, England, and France during April for combined meetings with surgical organizations in those countries. At Harrogate, near Leeds, the American College met jointly with the Association of Surgeons of Great Britain and Ireland. The author had the privilege of accompanying Dr. Blalock on that month's tour, and it was an extraordinary experience. While at Harrogate, Professor Allison was our host in his beautiful home in nearby Leeds, which had extensive gardens and a cricket field (see photograph, page 128). The close friendship which was to subsequently develop between Alfred Blalock and Philip Allison began during that week and continued throughout Blalock's life.

In his Presidential Address to the College, Dr. Blalock showed a deep insight into current problems as well as the future. He stated: "Our system of medical education, undergraduate teaching, and residency training is in serious danger." He proceeded to emphasize that tuition had been greatly increased, but that still such fees accounted for only a small part of the actual cost of medical education, stating further:

"Worthwhile candidates who simply cannot afford to go to medical school are eliminated from the profession." He further feared the fact that private endowments were not likely to increase significantly under the present tax structure and he hoped that more aid would he available "without strings" for medical schools in the future. It is striking to recognize the current significance of this farsighted address delivered more than twenty years ago.

In 1956, when Alfred Blalock was President of the American Surgical Association and presented his address on the topic "The Nature of Discovery," he stated:

> For many years I have been interested in the background or the nature of discoveries in medicine and this is the subject of my address. Discovery may be defined as the act of finding out what was unknown, such as Harvey's discovery of the circulation of the blood. One discovers what already exists but was unknown previously, such as the applicability of steam to the purposes of locomotion.... It must be admitted, however, that the distinction is often a close and debatable one. Whereas we usually give the name "discovery" to the recognition of a new fact, Claude Bernard maintained that the idea is what really constitutes the discovery. He said, "The idea is the seed; the method is the earth furnishing the conditions in which it may develop, flourish and give the best of the fruit according to its nature. But as only what has been sown in the ground will ever grow in it, so nothing will be developed by the experimental method except the ideas submitted to it."
>
> What are the methods by which discoveries are made? We may distinguish roughly four general categories: (1) Some are made by chance or accident; (2) some are made by intention or design; (3) some are made by intuition or imagination or hunch; and (4) some are made by combinations of two or all of the above methods. The mode of discovery is not always clearcut. It has been my experience, and I am sure yours, that one cannot always recall exactly how one spotted the clue that allowed him to solve the problem.

In this remarkable address, he reviewed accounts of the background of a number of major contributions in medicine. For example, Blalock chose to cite Claude Bernard's maxim, which all of those who worked with him knew he fully endorsed: "When we meet a fact which contradicts a prevailing theory, we must accept the fact and abandon the theory, even when the theory is supported by great names and generally accepted."

During these remarks, his abiding dedication to hard work was brought into focus when Blalock said:

I would place first among the requisites of an investigator the willingness and the desire to work. No amount of brilliance or good fortune relieves one of the necessity of hard work. Even the brilliant accidental observation has to pass rigorous tests before it is proved and accepted.... No satisfaction is quite like that which accompanies productive investigation, particularly if it leads to better treatment of the sick. The important discoveries in medicine are generally simple and one is apt to wonder why they were not made earlier. I believe that they are made usually by a dedicated person who is willing to work and to cultivate his power of observation rather than by the so-called intellectual genius. Discoveries may be made by the individual worker as opposed to the current practice of a large team research. Simple apparatus may suffice: all the analyses need not be performed by technicians; large sums of money are not always necessary. Important basic ideas will probably continue to come from the individual. Whether by accident, design or hunch, the diligent investigator has a fair chance of making an important discovery. If he is unwilling to take this chance, he should avoid this type of work.

In 1960, Henry Bahnson, Mark Ravitch, Glenn Morrow, and the author arranged a dinner in Blalock's honor. On that occasion a large number of friends from around the world met in Baltimore to honor him. The *Baltimore Sun* made the event a special feature, stating in part:

Medical men from various parts of the western hemisphere and Europe gathered at the Southern Hotel last night for a dinner honoring Dr. Alfred Blalock, Professor of Surgery at the Johns Hopkins Hospital. The guest list totaled nearly 500 persons and a number of those present were surgeons trained by the soft spoken, Georgia born Dr. Blalock. The dinner was arranged by a Hopkins group and preparations were made without the knowledge of the man being honored.

The tributes that evening were superb and brought obvious joy to the professor. The distinguished physiologist Philip Bard, who was for many years Professor and Director of the Department of Physiology at Hopkins and later Dean of the School of Medicine, said:

I have known Al personally for 20 years. Before that I knew him through those of his published papers which every respectable physiologist interested in the cardiovascular system had to read if he were to keep abreast of the subject.... To a physiologist, his studies were of the utmost importance. After World War I, physiologists lost all interest in somatic and other kinds of shock and the surgeons took over, led by Al. This was a classic, and the work during World War II confirmed it, and I merely want to state as a physiologist how indebted we are to him.

Dr. Blalock's talents in administration were underscored by Philip Bard when he said:

During my term of service as Dean of the Medical Faculty, administrative duties gave me an insight into the difficulties he had in directing a huge Department filled with personalities and individualities that cover a broad spectrum of human nature. During that period, I also felt the impact of his resourcefulness as the Head of the Department in obtaining what he deemed necessary for the Department and its staff, particularly the younger members.

Philip Bard concluded his remarks by quoting from Samuel Crowe's biography, *Halsted of Johns Hopkins—The Man and His Men*: "Halsted was the founder of a school, the disciples of which have perpetuated his influence and prestige as one of the great creators of scientific surgery." Moreover, Crowe said, "The spirit of Halsted has been reincarnated in his successor. Alfred Blalock."

Joseph Beard,[2] who worked with Dr. Blalock in the experimental laboratory early in his career and was to become a virologist of worldwide renown, receiving both the Borden Award and the Crowes Cancer Award, said of Dr. Blalock that evening:

I don't know how well you all really know Dr. Blalock but you know as you look at him here he looks so calm, self-possessed, composed, kind, and all that sort of thing, but you never really did work for that fellow. The trouble with him, so far as I was concerned...a 24 hour day was just nothing at all. He would come in the laboratory and start about 7:30 or 8:00 in the morning and about 1:00 a.m. he'd leave me holding the sack until the next morning just before 7:30 a.m....But this I can tell you, Dr. Blalock is a friend of enduring and lasting capacity. All through the years that I have known him he has never forgotten the fact that once upon a time I worked for him and he has never forgotten the obligation of a teacher to aid and to sympathize with the advance of one of his students.

---

2. Joseph Beard was a professor of Experimental Surgery at Duke who developed the equine infectious anemia virus vaccine.

His coworker, Helen Taussig, said: "It is with the greatest of pleasure that I salute you tonight.... It was in 1942 that Dr. Blalock first proved to everyone at Hopkins that he was a great thoracic surgeon with our first successful ligation of a patent ductus arteriosus." Regarding the work on the tetralogy of Fallot, she said: "Al, the true scientist, took the problem to the laboratory where he performed the many tests to establish the fact"...and to develop a technique which made the operation so successful."

The Professor of Surgery at the University of Turin, A. Mario Dogliotti, cited the fact that the largest cardiovascular surgical center in Europe at that time was the Blalock Center—at the University of Turin. He concluded, saying, "From your lips and through your eyes tell the happiness of everybody who knows you, and loves you."

The late Isidor Ravdin paid him a remarkable tribute when he said: "Alfred Blalock's work in shock was monumental in concept and in analysis. It was he who demonstrated firmly the effects of trauma and blood loss. Alfred Blalock represents the finest of the physiologically minded surgeons who followed after the death of Dr. Halsted."

His close friend from Oxford, Philip Allison, said, "You, Alfred Blalock, by your continuing scholarship, integrity, and insatiable curiosity have grown to immense proportions for these men and many more throughout the world."

Mark Ravitch, speaking for the residents, said:

> It didn't take us long to find out that what we had formerly thought was superb clinical performance, that is, working 24 hours a day...was merely expected and accepted. It was really infuriating, but it was a fact of life. Even more work, more detailed attention to the students, to experimental work in the Hunterian Laboratory, in the Library, in the operating rooms, all became the order of the day for all of us after his arrival at Hopkins.

His close friend and coinvestigator of many years, Tinsley Harrison, the distinguished Professor of Medicine and Editor of the well-known *Textbook of Medicine,* said:

> A teacher is an individual who has the capacity to influence the horizons of his pupils. Al has had that capacity all of his life. And there is another part of the story, one to which many individuals can testify, and perhaps no one quite

as much as I, having been his intimate friend for more than 40 years. The story is that none of us who have ever touched him have been left without the impact of a broader and better educational influence and a greater and stronger inspiration.

His fellow classmate and longtime friend, Arthur Blakemore, commented on his remarkable productivity and ended by proposing a toast to the more than 500 present when he said, "A toast to this man, the finest house officer Johns Hopkins ever had."

At the table with him that evening was Alice, his second wife, who had been a close friend of Mary Balock before her death and who brought him much happiness in the remaining years. It was apparent to all present at the dinner that Dr. Blalock had been deeply moved by the many tributes paid him, and in closing said:

> With the exception of my family, and personal friends of my own vintage, many of whom are here tonight, my greatest pleasure in life has come from the house staff here, and at Vanderbilt. At Hopkins we have had 37 senior residents in the past 19 years. Most of them are here tonight, much to my delight. All of these 37 are successful. A number of them are known nationally and internationally. All are fine gentlemen and superb friends. At the dedication of the Brady Urological Institute some years ago, Diamond Jim Brady simply said, "The sky was never so blue and the grass was never so green as they are this day for me." These are my sentiments tonight, thanks to you.

There is little doubt among those who knew him well that his last public appearance and the address that evening provided his listeners with an insight into his philosophy and into the deepest recesses of his mind. He had been invited to deliver the keynote address of the seventy-fifth anniversary of the opening of the Johns Hopkins Hospital on May 14, 1964, this being only a few months before his death. Although at the time his diagnosis was not known, and there was little reason to suspect what was to happen shortly thereafter, nevertheless, the author and many others had a sense of the impending event and indeed that he himself was aware of it. He had recently undergone a fusion of the lumbar spine for what was thought to have been a herniated vertebral disc but was later proven to be metastatic carcinoma to the vertebrae. He had lost considerable weight, was in continuous pain, and was deeply worried about a group of recent administrative problems and decisions at Hopkins. Despite this combination of concerns, his tenacity and loyalty to the institution made him determined to deliver the address to which he had previously committed himself.

A special chair and support system were placed behind the lectern, and he then began the most poignant and certainly the most deeply felt address of his entire life. His opening remarks had a touch of humor, probably included more than anything else to help place the audience at ease, since all were aware of his recent operation and continuing pain. He greeted the mayor of the city, who was in attendance that evening, and who had also recently been a patient at Hopkins for treatment of asthma. Dr. Blalock began his remarks by saying, "Unlike Mayor McKeldin, I fell into the hands of surgeons, and I hope the next time I am in the hospital I will have asthma." From that point, he then reflected upon the proceedings of the twenty-fifth anniversary of the Hospital, and of that era he quoted Osler who said:

> And binding us all together there came as a sweet influence a spirit of the place; whence we knew not but teacher and taught alike felt the presence and subtle domination. Comradeship, sympathy one with another, devotion to work were its fruits and its guidance drove from each heart hatred and malice and all uncharitableness.

At this point, he began a review of the many problems which then faced the Medical School and the Hospital. In fact, a number of these same problems continue in some of our institutions today. I think it is useful for all of us, and for many reasons, to emphasize the practical advice and admonitions he stressed at that time. He said:

> Quality is more important than quantity, and too great a size may mean unwieldiness. Next, excellent patient care and teaching and clinical research should be accorded a status of dignity equal to that of the so-called laboratory research.

He further emphasized: "The full time members of the hospital staff should consist, with few exceptions, of clinicians who have great interest in patient care and teaching." He concluded that while he admired tradition greatly he recognized that it should serve only as a stimulus and not as a wall behind which to retreat. These were his last public remarks.

During the next several months, as his physical condition rapidly weakened and he was in constant pain with multiple bony metastases, the author had the privilege of sitting with him for many hours. His primary pleasures at that time were reminiscences about his residents and reflections upon his, and their, earlier work. He was especially close to Bill Longmire and spoke of his good fortune in having him as first assistant during the first tetralogy operation in 1944. He recalled the work with Rollins Hanlon in developing the Blalock-Hanlon operation during many hours in the Hunterian Laboratory. He was also pleased that H. William Scott had succeeded his former chief, Dr. Barney Brooks, particularly in that happy and productive environment he recalled so clearly.

He spoke of the visit he and Henry Bahnson made to England and France in 1947 where they introduced the Blalock operation in Europe.

Another of those with whom he was particularly close was William N. Muller, Jr. The last meeting of the Blalock residents was held at his department at the University of Virginia in March 1964, and at that time Dr. Blalock was presented a silver tray upon which were the engraved signatures of the Hopkins residents whom he had trained.

Dr. Blalock's influence in creating clinical surgeons, teachers, investigators, and department chairmen had been similar to that of Halsted, and as he reviewed it all in perspective, he was warmly grateful that he had had such an opportunity. Longmire headed the department at the University of California at Los Angeles, Hanlon at St. Louis University, Scott at Vanderbilt, Muller at the University of Virginia, Bahnson at Pittsburgh, and the author at Duke. Others were chiefs of divisions, including Sloan at the University of Michigan, Pickrell at Duke, Morrow at the National Heart Institute, Cooley at Baylor. Maloney at the University of California at Los Angeles, Hailer at Hopkins, Hatcher at Emory, Weldon at Washington University, Kay at the University of Southern California, and Jude at the University of Miami. Subsequently, Rainey Williams was to succeed in the chair at the University of Oklahoma, Lazar Greenfield at the Medical College of Virginia, and Paul Ebert at Cornell and later at the University of California at San Francisco. Among the remainder of the residents, six were in the private practice of surgery and seventeen held academic appointments.

A special cabinet was presented to him for appropriate placement of his many medals and honors, including the Passano Award, the Rene Leriche Award, the AMA Distinguished Service Award, the Lasker Award, the Roswell Park Medal, the Gairdner Award, the Bigelow Medal, and the Chevalier de la Republique Francaise Nationale de la Legion de Honneur.

As the remaining days passed, he recalled each resident with much fondness and warm reflection. As Mark Ravitch was to write later in his *Collected Works of Alfred Blalock*,

> His intermittent stupor mercifully lightened two days before his death when one by one his old residents—Longmire, Scott, Hanlon, Muller, Bahnson, Sabiston—now away in chairs of their own, came in to see him. These last visits made deep impressions upon us for, despite his illness and pain, he continued to maintain his gracious attitude, his appreciation, and his loyalty to all of us.

As the candle grew dim, and when on September 15 the final day came, all knew that his life had been fully complete, touching a vast number of grateful patients, many admiring students, a group of loyal residents, and a host of warm friends everywhere. His productive life, characterized as it was by many original ideas and achievements, fulfilled in all dimensions the criteria of the noted medical historian, Henry F. Sigerist, when he said:

> Posterity weaves garlands for those alone whose work has been creative. No doctors live on in the memory save the exceptional beings who enriched the healing art with new outlooks, who forged new weapons for the fight against disease, whose activities were vital to the development of medicine, to those who incorporated a trend, founded a school or represented an era. We remember those choice spirits who, becoming aware of divine thoughts that were still inchoate, were able, by strenuous labor, to make them generally known and practically applicable. It is only of such great doctors that I can write.

Finally, the statement of Henry Brooks Adams penetrates directly to the mark when he said, "A teacher affects eternity, he can never tell where his influence stops"—surely, this can he said of Alfred Blalock.

Chapter 12 ☙

Henry T. Bahnson

H enry T. Bahnson was a native of Winston-Salem, North Carolina, and a summa cum laude graduate of Davidson College (B.S. 1941). He was elected to Phi Beta Kappa and Omicron Delta Kappa during his junior year and served as president of the student body. In addition, he was president of his fraternity, a member of the varsity football team, and he graduated third in his class scholastically. He was later elected permanent President of the Class of 1941.

Following graduation he entered Harvard Medical School, where he was a thoroughly outstanding student and graduated cum laude (M.D. 1944). While in his second year at Harvard, he performed research on blood coagulation at the Thorndike Laboratory at Boston City Hospital under Dr. George Maynard and Dr. Charles Davidson, and in his senior year he worked with Dr. Lewis Dexter at the Peter Bent Brigham Hospital. He was one of six third-year students elected to Alpha Omega Alpha and one of three to be awarded a John Harvard Fellowship. He was also the student head of the Boyleston Medical Society.

Dr. Bahnson spent the summer following his second year in medical school working with Dr. Tinsley R. Harrison, the noted professor of medicine and editor of the well-known text *Principles of Internal Medicine*. In October of 1943, Dr. Harrison wrote to Dr. Alfred Blalock, Professor and Director of the Department of Surgery at Johns Hopkins, a letter recommending Dr. Hahnson for internship, in which he said,

> The purpose of my letter is to tell you something about Mr. Henry T. Bahnson who is a third year student at Harvard, and writes me that he is going to apply to you for an internship. Last summer when he was on his vacation from

Harvard, he bobbed up in the labs here the day he got home and said he wanted to do some research. I laughed at him when he told me he had only three weeks vacation and told him to go and have a good time. His answer was that he could have a good time and do research, too.... When the three weeks were up, the boy came and brought me some beautiful data which demonstrated quite conclusively that removal of the kidneys made the rats more susceptible to hemorrhage.... It was the best research performance I have ever seen in a lad who has had only two years of medical school.

This work was published in the *American Journal of Physiology,* and following that experience Henry Bahnson began a remarkable career in scientific surgery and was to make many basic and clinical contributions in the years ahead.

After entering the Surgical Residency Training Program at Johns Hopkins under the direction of Alfred Blalock, he rapidly recognized his mentor's many outstanding traits and especially his dedication to research and teaching. Stimulated by these factors, he decided to do basic work on the pulmonary circulation and arranged to spend a year at the University of Rochester in the laboratory of two great pulmonary physiologists, Dr. Wallace O. Fenn and Dr. Herman Rahn. While there he held a National Science Foundation Fellowship and made funndamental observations on the effect of unilateral hypoxia on gas exchange and calculated pulmonary blood flow in each lung. In addition, he studied adaptation to high altitudes including changes in breath-holding time and a study on blood and tissue cases of animals exposed to one and seven atmospheres of oxygen or air. These observations were also published in the *American Journal of Physiology.* After Henry Bahnson returned to continue surgical training at Johns Hopkins, Dr. Fenn wrote Dr. Blalock, stating,

I want to tell you how much we appreciated having Dr. Henry Bahnson this year. We all became very much attached to him personally, and we also valued his professional ability and industry very highly indeed. I am sure that we shall hear from him in the years to come. His surgical skill was a very great asset to our group and he gave a big boost to the work of the laboratory. We consider it a great privilege to have had him here for a year and we want you to know what a fine impression he left upon us.

While Henry Bahnson was in residency training, Dr. Blalock became very impressed with his brilliance and hard work. Together they exchanged ideas and performed studies which led to the publication of a number of outstanding papers. By the time he finished the residency program, Bahnson had published works on angiocardiography in congenital heart disease, coarctation of the aorta at unusual sites, causes of death following operation for congenital heart disease of the cyanotic type, aorta vascular rings encountered in the surgical treatment of congenital pulmonic stenosis, observations on tricuspid stenosis or atresia with hypoplasia of the right ventricle, and evidence for a renal factor in the hypertension of experimental coarctation of the aorta.

In retrospect it is clear Dr. Blalock recognized very early on that Bahnson was quite exceptional. In fact, while he was a junior resident he wrote Admiral Lamont Pugh saying, "Bahnson is a very outstanding young man who will go far in academic work. I have never known a young man with more ability along these lines!" It soon became recognized nationwide that Alfred Blalock had a unique ability to select individuals who were destined to have successful careers in the field for his training program.

In a letter nominating Henry Bahnson for a Markle Scholarship, Dr. Blalock said, "Probably the most significant statement is that he is an excellent clinical surgeon, having performed a great variety of major operations successfully, that he is a successful teacher, and he still finds time to carry on problems in the laboratory. It is of interest that he performed the first successful closure of a patent ductus arteriosus in France while visiting the Hospital Broussais in Paris in 1947 (while still a young resident)." He then proceeded to laud his fundamental studies on the pulmonary circulation, on oxygen poisoning with special reference to pulmonary edema, climatic studies at an altitude of 14,000 feet, the role of the kidney in hypertension associated with coarctation of the aorta, and his commitment to academic surgery. Latter, Dr. Blalock emphasized his pioneering role in the excision of thoracic aortic aneurysms, and he cited his first pioneering procedure, performed in 1952, as a milestone in the surgical treatment of this condition.

In 1957, Henry Bahnson and Frank Spencer were invited to Australia to initiate open heart surgery at the Royal Prince Albert Hospital in Sydney. Following that visit, Sir Herbert Schlink wrote to Dr. Blalock, "Dr. Henry T. Bahnson left the hospital yesterday to return home. He has been with us for the past month and l am writing to tell you how much we have enjoyed having him with us. Dr. Bahnson has proven himself to be a most competent surgeon, a congenial and inspiring colleague and a worthy ambassador of your great Country. All patients operated on have done well and his advice and practical example has been of immense help in initiating open heart surgery in this Country." The noted Australian cardiac surgeon, Rowan Nicks, wrote, saying, "We have had a most stirring visit from Henry Bahnson and Frank Spencer. The results of their work here had a profound effect on Australian Surgery. We found them both fine companions who took us up, cemented us together to their own world, and left us with their 'Know how' and their stamp to carry on with some confidence. Myself, I think that this gesture of theirs, in coming on such an assignment revealed great depths of moral courage."

On the faculty at Johns Hopkins, Henry Bahnson was very creative and established the open heart program, training a number of residents in this field, including the author who remains deeply indebted to him. He was also devoted to the experimental laboratory, and he and his co-workers continued outstanding research. In 1961 he was promoted to the rank of Professor of Surgery and the following year was invited to spend three months at the University of Vienna to assist Professor Fritz Helmer in establishing a new cardiovascular surgical service. On return from Vienna he was appointed the George V. Foster Professor of Surgery and Chairman of the Department of Surgery at the University of Pittsburgh. There he built an unusually strong surgical residency training program combined with basic surgical research. He initiated a highly successful cardiac transplantation program which was further extended to other organs, especially the liver, when he successfully attracted the brilliant and exceedingly productive pioneering academic surgeon, Thomas E. Starzl, to lead this effort. In a short time Pittsburgh became and has remained the leading transplant center in the world (1).

A remarkable contributor across the broad field of clinical and investigative surgery, Henry T. Bahnson's achievements have been of monumental proportions, and he has clearly achieved a well-deserved place in the history of surgery.

Reference

1. A note about the surgeon. In *Surgical Procedures: The Pictorial Preview of Significant Developments in Surgery. Warner-Chilcott Laboratories* 2:7, Morris Hill, N.J. (1965).

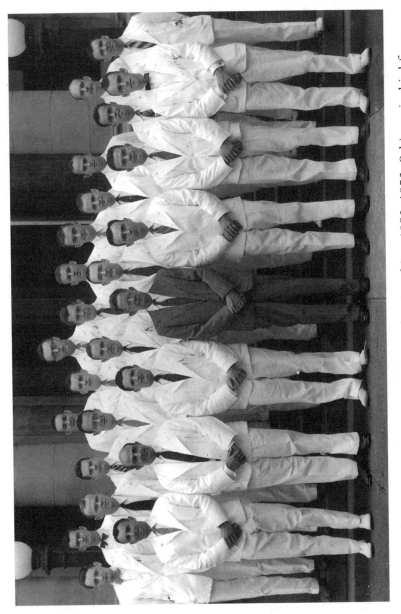

David C. Sabiston's Chief residency year at Johns Hopkins, 1952–1953. Sabiston is third from left, front row. Alfred Blalock is to his left.

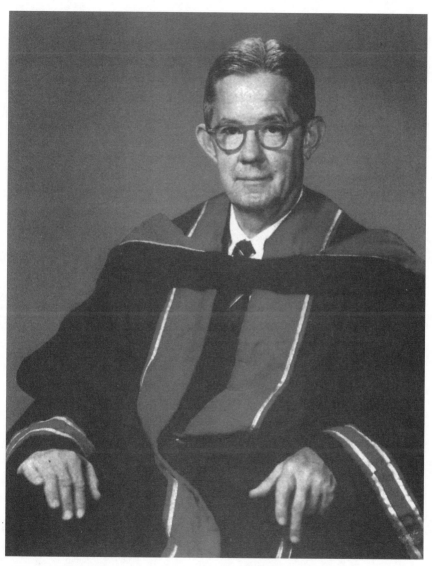

Alfred Blalock, Chief of Surgery at Johns Hopkins Hospital, 1941 to 1964.

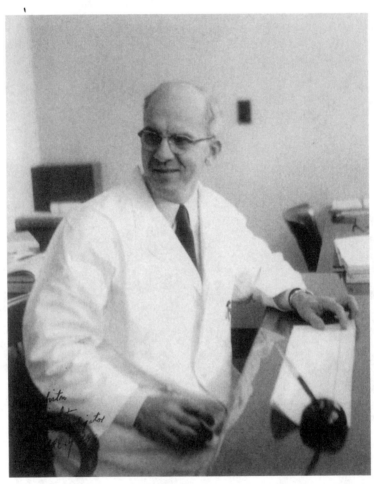

Dr. Donald Gregg, Chief of Cardiorespiratory at the Army Institute of Research in Washington, D.C.

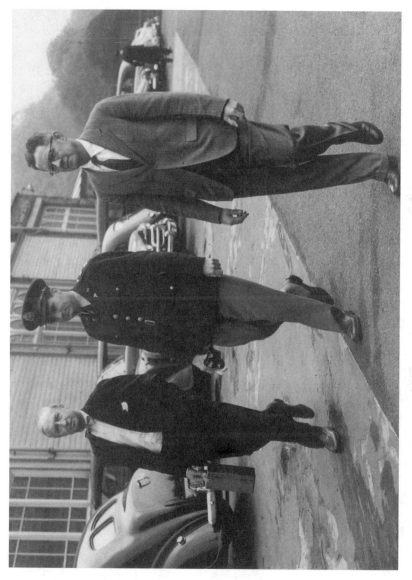

Sabiston in Oxford in 1954, walking between Philip Allison, Chairman of Surgery at John Radcliff Hospital (left), and Alfred Blalock (right).

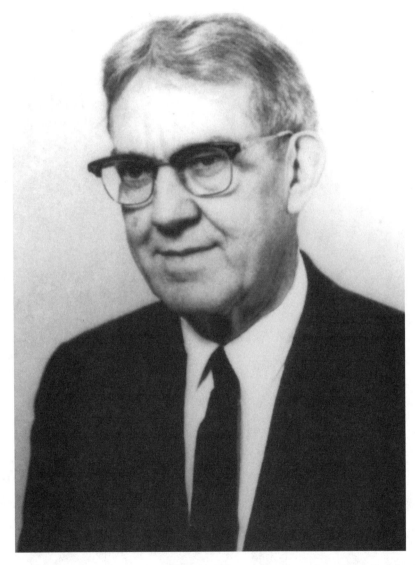

Dr. Deryl Hart, Founder and first Chair of Surgery at Duke School of Medicine, 1929 to 1960, and President of Duke University, 1960 to 1963.

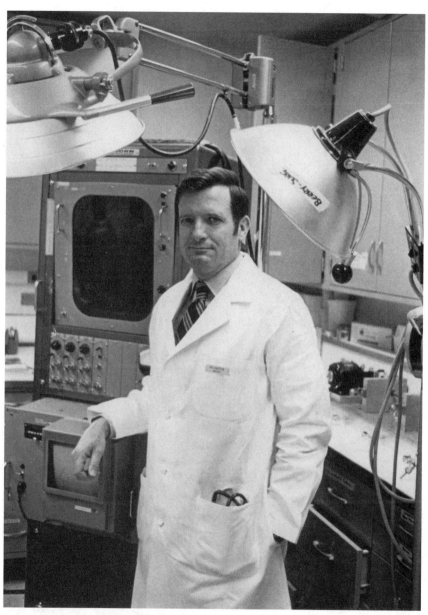

David Sabiston in the Animal Surgical Laboratory at Duke where he taught medical students and young surgeons the science of surgical research.

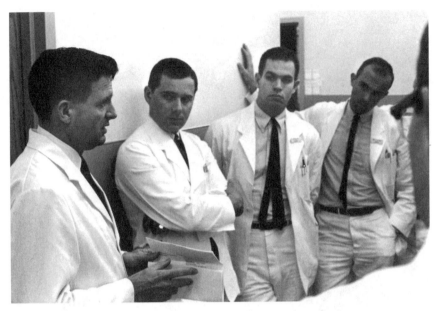

David Sabiston teaching on the wards in Duke Hospital.

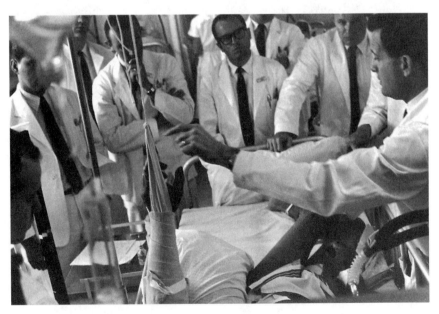

David Sabiston teaching at the bedside in Duke Hospital.

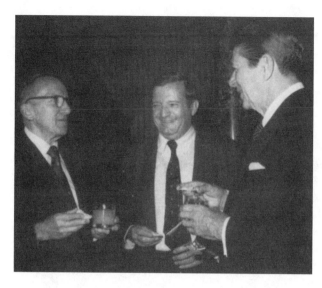

Dr. Rollin Hanlon of the American College of Surgeons (ACS) (left) and Sabiston (center) chat with President Ronald Reagan at the headquarters of the ACS in 1983. (Photograph courtesy of the American College of Surgeons.)

David Sabiston with his wife, Aggie Sabiston, after receiving an award for Surgical Excellence from the Spanish Surgical Society.

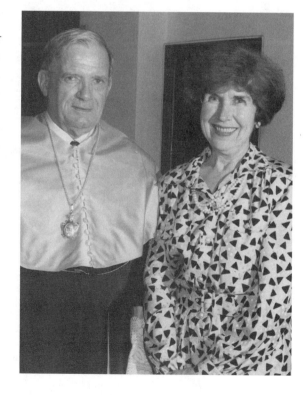

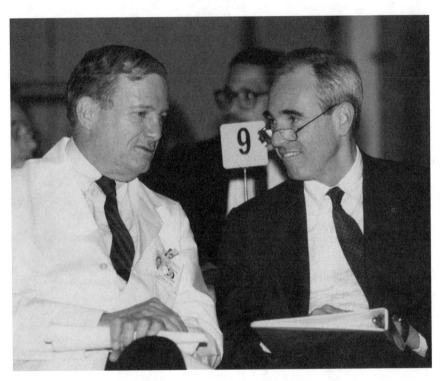

Sabiston with H. Keith H. Brodie (right), President of Duke University from 1985 to 1993.

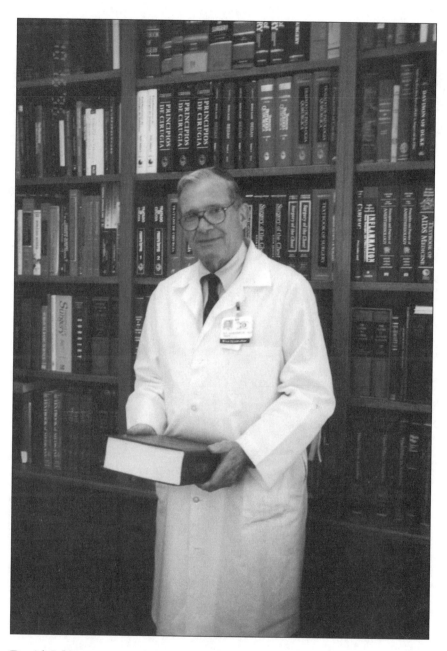

David Sabiston at age 72 with his classic textbook, *Sabiston's Textbook of Surgery.*

IV

Surgical Education

*I*n our program at Duke through the years, residents take at least two years of basic research, not just going to their laboratory and doing experimental operations, but doing basic research and recording their data. Nowadays, it has gone even a step further; they are not only physiologists, biochemists, and bacteriologists, but they also have to be molecular biologists.

Chapter 13 ☙

Medicine as a Career

O f the many decisions which confront the college student today, the choice of a career is one which demands much incisive thought and firm conviction. Experience has shown that the selection of one's life work should be determined by a combination of individual qualifications, personal interests, and ultimate goals. The complexity of modern society has placed an additional demand on the contemporary student in that it has become apparent that the early choice of career is often associated with definite advantages. The current requirements for preliminary preparation in depth has focused attention on the selection of a career, and it is fortunate that the ability of students today is superior to that of previous years, a fact which makes this responsibility both realistic and justifiable.

The origin of the word career has an interesting background. Derived from the Latin *carraria* (meaning a "carriage-road"), it was later broadened in the Italian *carraria* to include "a horse at full gallop, at full speed;...or as a walk in life...such as a career officer." The French accepted this version in their *carriere* but introduced more depth with an added meaning, "to give free scope to one's imagination ...to throw off all restraint." The current Oxford English Dictionary defines career as "a person's course or progress through life....to move at full speed." It becomes apparent that the term had its origin in a concept of both action and maximal effort. Furthermore, its definition places emphasis on the vital element of the imaginative mind, the key to original contribution.

Of the many careers available to the present generation, medicine ranks among the oldest. The history of medicine is a fascinating one, being marked by both superstition and mistake as well as progressive advancement. Since its earliest documentation as found in the figurative drawings of the caveman, it has evolved through successive periods of ancient Egypt to the Grecian advances of the fourth century B.C. This was the era of Hippocrates, upon whom historians have bestowed the title of "Father of Medicine," and who his countrymen were confident was descended from Aesculapius, the God of Healing. It has become apparent that a remarkable power of observation was Hippocrates' most significant characteristic, a quality which has since remained of great importance in medicine. He shifted the basis of medicine from the spiritual concept to the introduction of rational bedside observation with stress upon the patient, the symptoms, and an explanation of disease on the basis of organ malfunction. Even today, his descriptions of numerous diseases are unsurpassed for their accuracy. During the two thousand years that followed Hippocrates, medicine advanced slowly through phases of ill-directed spiritual domination, inadequate professional training, witchcraft, and the barber surgeon to the introduction of the concept of physiology in the seventeenth century. It was at this time that William Harvey, a physician himself, discovered the circulation of the blood. Rapid advances then followed, with the establishment of the germ theory of disease by Pasteur, the specific identification of disease by microscopic study of tissues and organs by Virchow, the introduction of the antiseptic technic in surgery by Lister, and the general application of physiology and biochemistry to the study of human disease. It is the summation of these advances that has led to the current era of modern medicine, and it is this present profession upon which the student is to pass thoughtful judgment today.

In the selection of a career, students necessarily choose the discipline toward which their further training and subsequent learning experiences are directed. In this sense, they are placing emphasis on their role as individuals rather than upon previous experiences as a part of a group. Thus, they may examine the fields of business, law, engineering, education, medicine, or a variety of other professional paths. Most young men and women have an image of medicine in its contemporary sense, although the depth and background of this information may vary considerably.

Medicine appeals to a wide variety of young students with varying outlooks and for diverse reasons. The explanation for this circumstance can be found in the scope of modern medicine, since in contemporary terms it is a profession comprised of what is actually a wide spectrum of careers. In broadest terms, physicians may devote themselves to lives solely engaged in clinical practice, or to a combination, including clinical work, research, and teaching, or to the single pursuit of research in the laboratory. Furthermore graduating physicians have the opportunity to choose a general career embracing the entire field of medicine, or if they wish they may limit their scope of interest in practice by choosing a specialty such as pediatrics, obstetrics, psychiatry, or surgery. With the increasing complexity of current socioeconomic structure, medicine is also asked to supply a number of medical administrators. This group has become an ever important one in the planning and direction of medical activities and is yet another vital front in the broad field of medicine.

Despite the individual differences that tend to subdivide the medical profession, the fact remains that there are a number of basic similarities that bind each of its branches. Fortunately, all who enter the field are required to obtain a degree of Doctor of Medicine, a factor responsible for the broad primary training necessary in this discipline. Although the training program leading to the M.D. degree is now quite similar for all students, there is increasing recognition of a need for individually selected programs more closely related to the needs and interests of each specific student. Duke University will inaugurate a program next fall that embraces this concept by providing a curriculum individually suited for each student's future needs. Furthermore, the student will be introduced rapidly to clinical experiences with assignment in the latter part of the first year in medical school. The second year will be devoted entirely to clinical medicine, while the third year is designed as a return to the basic sciences permitting independent research. The last two years of the course will be highly individualized, permitting the student considerable flexibility in the curriculum. The faculty of the School of Medicine has carefully studied the many aspects and implications of this change over a period of several years, and it is enthusiastic about the future of the program.

In choosing medicine as a career, the student is apt to recognize certain characteristics frequently regarded as important in its selection.

In its broadest sense, a career should provide personal happiness as well as a reasonable likelihood of success. Medicine offers many challenges and individual rewards, while at the same time it is clearly a demanding profession. It offers excitement in that no day spent in its endeavor is like another. New problems, different people, and changing concepts emphasize the point that the follower of this profession must be amenable to change. Of particular meaning to those in medicine is the admonition of Douglas Maitland Knight, President of Duke University, in the baccalaureate address of 1965 in which he said: "Accept change...and use it as your servant." Physicians must continually bear this in mind if they are to be effective members of the profession.

Traditionally, the physician has been recognized as one who holds not only a like but a love for people. An understanding of human behavior with its attendant frailties is an integral part of the doctor's life. Despite the numerous contributions of modern science, the fact remains, as Galen stated centuries ago, "He cures most successfully in whom the people have the greatest confidence." This long recognized truth places emphasis on this quality of the physician as a healer, as well as on the importance of scientific knowledge and skill. While a medical career brings numerous satisfactions, by its very nature, the physician must realize that disappointment is also a recurring component. Fatal illness is encountered for which cure is not currently known, yet experience has taught that future discovery will likely provide the solution. Such disappointment frequently acts as a stimulus for continued research and advance, and reflection upon a number of fatal illnesses of the past provides adequate evidence of discoveries which led to their conquest. The discovery of insulin in the treatment of diabetes is a widely known example, and the introduction of penicillin by Fleming and Florey has prevented the death of thousands from previously fatal infections. The use of liver extract and more recently of vitamin B_{12} cures the once fatal pernicious anemia. The condition of the infant born with a severely malformed heart can now be completely corrected with expectation of a normal life, a result of advances in cardiac surgery. These examples are but a few of those which comprise modern medicine, facts that make medicine the stimulating field so many have found it to be in the past.

Although awarding of the M.D. degree was once considered the end of one's professional training, this concept is now completely outdated. Medicine requires that its followers be continuous and lifelong students. The rapid advances in scientific knowledge today far exceed those of any other previous period in the history of civilization. These facts have emphasized the necessity for utilization of the basic sciences in the daily advances of clinical medicine. With this concept in mind, the demand for continuing education in medicine becomes apparent.

An additional point that bears emphasis is that students are sometimes led to exaggerate the long period of training required for an adequate medical education. While it is certainly true, one should nevertheless consider the rewards medicine offers as well as the modern aids which make its objectives more easily accomplished. Increasing numbers of medical scholarships, an awareness by the government of its responsibility to train and provide adequate numbers of physicians, and higher salaries offered by hospitals during intern and residency programs have made these problems considerably fewer today than were a decade ago. In fact, all indications point toward increased relief of financial burdens for students of medicine in attaining the education required for a complete career. Such a trend is a welcome one, since it will allow a more equitable entry of those interested in the field and should greatly reduce the burden of financial worry. Furthermore, the increasing interest of Congress and the National Institutes of Health in medical research is one of the most outstanding aspects of medical education and research of the last decade.

Of the many stimulating aspects of medicine, none is more exciting than its future. The many advances made possible by the application of basic research to clinical problems is increasing at the greatest rate in history, and every indicator points toward further acceleration in the years ahead. There are numerous examples, including the treatment of infectious disease by antibiotics, the advent of the heart-lung machine, and the development of plastic arteries and valves for extension of the ability to treat and cure heart and blood vessel disease. The recent advances in transplantation of tissues and organs, such as a kidney, are now associated with the likely prospect of immunological matching for selection of donors and recipients, just as blood is typed and chosen for transfusion. The application of genetics to the origin and understanding of numerous heritable diseases is yet another of the rapidly expanding fields of medicine which are now of benefit to the individual patient. To this list should be added the utilization of nuclear physics and radioisotopes in the diagnosis and treatment of a number of human ills, a field that represents a prime example of the development and application of basic science to clinical medicine. With these advances now a matter of record, the future of medicine can be predicted to become even more closely associated with the basic sciences, and this combination can be confidently forecast to insure widely increased horizons of medical discovery.

While the field of medicine offers unlimited scientific opportunities and much individual satisfaction, it is clearly not an easy way of life. The responsibility which its members accept is great, and the efforts necessary to obtain adequate training are not exceeded by any other profession. Nevertheless, for those who enter after thorough consideration, its rewards are unmatched. First among its requisites is conscientious and vigorous pursuit. It is closely allied to the master word *work*, of which Sir William Osler, the noted Regius Professor of Medicine at Oxford, said, "It is the open sesame to every portal, the great equalizer in the world, the true philosopher's stone, which transmutes all the base metal of humanity into gold. The stupid among you, it will make bright, the bright man brilliant, and the brilliant student steady. With the magic work in your heart, all things are possible, and without it, all study is vanity and vexation."

There is little doubt that Osler's description of work is a meaningful solution to a number of daily problems and certainly to many that pertain to medicine. Lest the student be overwhelmed and place undue emphasis on the amount of effort necessary to enter the field, one should recall the statement of John Shaw Billings, the great educator, statesman, and medical bibliographer, who replied to a query regarding the secret of his success by saying, "There's really nothing difficult if you only begin. Some people contemplate a task until it looms so big, it seems impossible, but I just begin and it gets done somehow. *There would be no coral islands if the first bug sat down and began to wonder how the job was to be done.*" This is an answer to a number of questions that contemporary students ask about medicine.

Chapter 14 &

A Continuum in Surgical Education

Recently, much unrest has become manifest on college and university campuses both in this country and abroad. A major portion of the apprehension has been related to student and faculty concern with socioeconomic problems and especially to the solutions proposed to meet these crises. Of additional importance have been overt expressions of dissatisfaction with existing educational patterns and particularly with the structure of the curriculum. In response to these and other pressures, pronounced changes have been either recommended or actually accomplished, and these changes have posed both problems and opportunities for all aspects of higher education. Ferment in education has clearly become widespread, and critical appraisal by both students and educators is in the forefront of current academic life.

Despite the increasing emphasis being placed upon curricular structure at all levels of education, the present trends are for the most part neither new nor original. Rather, the concepts constitute basic features of educational philosophy and are being reintroduced to meet critical needs. Moreover, it should be emphasized that innovative changes are being made and successfully accomplished in a number of centers. Recent examples of such changes in graduate surgical programs have stimulated renewed interest in solutions for numerous pressing problems. In this chapter, I have elected to present innovations from Duke University, primarily because the experience and specific data involved are personally familiar. It is recognized and fully appreciated that other groups have faced similar problems and are providing necessary solutions (9). In fact, the fundamental basis of the plans to be presented in the following discussion is best expressed in a quote from the last century by Thomas Huxley, who said, "The great aim should be to teach only so much science as can be taught thoroughly, and to ground in principles and methods rather than to attempt to cover a large surface of details."

The undergraduate curriculum at Duke University has remained essentially the same since 1924. The Baccalaureate Course is comprised of four academic years totaling 124 semester hours. Of these, more than 100 are listed in the Uniform Course Requirements, with less than 20 percent of time available for genuine electives. As in other universities, unrest became apparent, especially among the more scholarly students, and complaints were voiced that many of the courses demonstrated a "lack of intellectual climate." Primary criticism was directed toward the large class exercise in which the student seldom has an opportunity to communicate or adequately know his teachers. After a careful survey involving much thought and tedious work, a select faculty committee recommended changes which promise to alter the university undergraduate curriculum. The basic innovations in this curriculum include a significant reduction in required courses, the introduction of preceptorials, seminars, and tutorials on an individual basis, beginning in the first year and extending through the senior year. The basic philosophy of these changes is perhaps best expressed in a statement from the committee's report: "If every student must take some classes in which the format, size, and instructor all compel him to take a position, and defend it orally, and in which they encourage him to consider the positions of his fellow students and professors, he should develop a skill, assurance, and mental agility to speak under stress" (9). It is upon this foundation that the basic changes in the structure of the undergraduate courses have been proposed and will become effective in the autumn of 1969. In the new curriculum, a student with a committed interest may choose a highly individualized program as designed in conjunction with any department in the university. In emphasizing the primary objective, Dr. Robert Krueger, the Director of Review, stated pointedly that under the new curriculum "the university is guaranteed that no student can idly pass through on the back row, an anonymous and shady figure appearing only in a grade book" (9).

Upon completion of college, the student may elect to enter graduate school. In most circumstances he immediately finds much emphasis placed upon individualization for the three or four years leading to the Ph.D. degree. Considerable flexibility is offered with an opportunity through the thesis to pursue in depth a clearly defined subject. In this format, the student is permitted to develop as a true scholar. He is a graduate student in the most meaningful definition and with appropriate guidance becomes an investigator with attention directed toward the making of original observations.

The student who selects medicine as a career has in the past been apt to enter a highly structured four-year curriculum with minimal opportunity for career planning. It is recognized that since the Flexner Report, elective courses have been a part of the curriculum of many schools. Nevertheless, in many instances there has been a lack of evidence that either sufficient time or appropriate format has permitted electives to represent individualized programs for the student. In the recent past, considerable thought and effort have been directed by several medical faculties to this important problem with development of innovative plans.

In 1960 the Medical Faculty at Duke began serious consideration of a far-reaching plan for the medical curriculum. The concept originated in the thoughts of several imaginative teachers and investigators, especially Drs. Eugene A. Stead[1] and Philip Handler.[2] A six-year period ensued during which much discussion, planning, and research were directed toward the structure of a new and innovative program which drastically altered the medical curriculum. Control data from the classes immediately prior to entry into the new curriculum were obtained during this period for later comparison. Although predictable opposition to change developed among some members of the faculty, the opponents were gradually converted during the six-year period of extended planning. The New Curriculum was ultimately adopted by a large majority of the Faculty and made effective in September 1966 (15).

The primary objectives of the Duke curriculum are: (1) to provide relief from the "overload" of information to which the student is subjected, (2) to emphasize the understanding of biologic principles and

---

1. Chair of Medicine at Duke University, 1947–1967.
2. Chair of Biochemistry at Duke University, 1949–1969.

experimental methods, adding factual material in sufficient quantity to enable the principles to be understood, (3) to foster the development of an attitude of scholarship and learning constructed to continue throughout professional career, and (4) to provide an objective basis for the student to make an early career choice. This curriculum radically changes instruction such that all the *required* courses in the basic sciences are given in the first year. These courses are termed "core courses" and include anatomy, biochemistry, pathology, pharmacology, physiology, and microbiology. The student is introduced to the principles of these disciplines with emphasis placed upon a maximal opportunity for discussion. In Year II, the five major clinical subjects (medicine, surgery, obstetrics and gynecology, pediatrics, and psychiatry) are each presented in separate terms. Again, the principal concepts of these disciplines are presented, and the student is taught the basic approaches to problem-solving as well as diagnosis and management of disease. It is apparent that appreciable modifications have been required in all courses. In the clinical experiences these changes have been accomplished by utilization of two primary principles: (1) the assignment of students in small groups working with patients in close association with the faculty and resident staff, and (2) the organization of informal seminars for the establishment of a dialogue between instructor and student. In surgery, primary emphasis is given the subjects of wound healing, inflammation, fluid and electrolyte balance, the metabolic response to trauma, shock, blood coagulation and thrombosis, gastrointestinal physiology, as well as tumor and homotransplantation biology (1). It can be recognized that these subjects are fundamental and apply broadly to all aspects of medicine.

The third and fourth years of the Duke curriculum are entirely *elective.* This aspect of the program is of the greatest importance, since clearly it permits students to make a choice, that is, to develop their interest in depth in the true sense of a graduate student. The third year is primarily designed for electives in the basic sciences, while in the fourth year the electives are chosen primarily in the clinical sciences. The student may select, with the advice and consent of a faculty advisor, from more than 250 courses among the various departments. In the Department of Surgery, 43 electives are currently offered. Of perhaps greater significance is the fact that a selected area of endeavor can be chosen for one or both the elective years. A student may elect a correlated system of study in both the basic and clinical sciences in a unified subject such as (1) cardiac-renal-vascular disease, (2) the neural sciences, (3) the endocrine system, (4) psychobiology, or (5) a research training program. The last is a year in which the background and fundamental techniques of modern investigation are presented. These five programs are developed by a faculty group representing all departments bearing an interest in the particular program. Additional electives of this type are planned for the future.

By placing the required courses in the first two years, provision is assured for maximal individualization in the last two years. Moreover, with a consecutive two-year block of elective time, students have an opportunity to plan a meaningful study and relate it to their future career. It should be emphasized that students need not necessarily select a specialized area. They may choose a more general program for any elective courses offered and which they consider the most suitable for their career. Thus, students interested in a career in academic pathology, medicine, or surgery would be apt to select quite a different program for Years III and IV than would students interested in community practice. Nevertheless, the curriculum is sufficiently broad to embrace virtually all possibilities, and our experience indicates that a majority of students have indeed selected their career choices by the senior year. In a recent study of our medical students, Preiss and Long (4) found that by the end of the third year, 25 percent of the students had decided upon a career in surgery, which represents the great majority of the 32 percent who ultimately entered surgery.

While it is admittedly too early for a full assessment of this curriculum, nevertheless a progress report can he made. Both the students and faculty have demonstrated a clear enthusiasm which can be appreciated throughout the medical school. Comparative data between the classes immediately preceding the curricular change and those since the autumn of 1966 are quite encouraging. The evidence from examinations prepared by authorities unassociated with the university and given both groups indicates that the data presented during the course of a single academic year in the basic sciences can be mastered by the students with a similar competence as formerly accomplished in the traditional two-year period.

It should be emphasized that this experiment in medical education requires dedicated student and faculty cooperation, and a strong and committed administration is essential for its support. Under the vigorous and thoughtful leadership of our dean and associate provost, William G. Anlyan, these have been attained effectively, and currently both students and faculty exhibit much confidence. Moreover, with such freedom available during the final two years of medical school, it becomes apparent to those responsible for postgraduate amid residency training programs that these students are not likely to view entry into highly structured residency programs with favor. Having benefited from individualized training and an opportunity for personal choices, continuation of this concept at the graduate level is justifiable on the part of the student. Thus, several years ago, we began to direct attention toward this important problem. Furthermore, the motivation was due not only to the newly adopted curriculum, but also, more importantly, to a conviction that such a change was in itself imperative.

It is the fortunate responsibility of surgery, defined in its broadest sense, to be comprised of a number of distinct disciplines. Beginning with the field of general and thoracic surgery, the branches of neurosurgery, orthopedics, plastic surgery, otolaryngology, urology, and others have since developed. The trend during the past several decades has been toward a sharper differentiation between these specialties and, as a result, much specific progress has been made in each of these disciplines. More recently, emphasis is being placed upon a form of reunification with the concept that the first portion of graduate surgical education should be devoted to a "core" education in the basic principles of surgery. There should be a period of perhaps two years devoted to the management of all types of surgical problems during which those subjects relative to the management of such patients are taught. It is fortunate that the representatives of the Surgical Specialty Boards (17) have initiated efforts in this direction, and the concept offers considerable promise of consolidating our joint educational objectives. As a means of evaluating attainment of these goals, a primary examination designed to cover this "core" material has been proposed for trainees in all aspects of surgery and appears very likely of adoption.

There is no longer doubt that change in graduate education is overdue (6). The Coggeshall Report (5) candidly states, "Perhaps most important there is a growing need for the university to assume responsibility for education for health and medical services." The Millis Commission (11) also made strong recommendations that residency training programs be drastically restructured and advised a shift of responsibility from a hospital base to the university. Few, if any, programs in medical education have been more pervaded by a concept of uniformity and conservatism than have those of surgery.

During the past several years, the Surgery Residency Training Program at Duke has been substantially revised. At present 18 interns are chosen, of whom 10 have already decided upon a specific surgical specialty. These candidates are selected in consultation and with the approval of the chiefs of the Divisions of Surgery. These interns continue their residency programs in the various specialty areas of the department. Eight interns are selected for the General and Thoracic Program, and included among these are any applicants for internship who are "undecided" concerning their future career. No attempt is made to insist that every student make a career choice at this time. Thus, there is a group of four or five who, after two years of basic training, become committed to a career in general and thoracic surgery. Appointments are available for each of these in the Senior Program and each can finish with a Chief Residency. The period of training can vary from five to eight years, depending upon the goals and wishes of each resident. Moreover, a similar situation exists for each of the interns selecting a specialty career. By specific design the residency program is in one sense pyramidal, since it has a broad base for the first two years, but later progresses as a rectangular pattern in that virtually all candidates who enter the internship are able to complete a Chief Residency in the field of choice. The only requirement for advancement is that performance must meet the standards of the director of the specific program. Thus, appointment to successive positions on an annual basis is possible for all qualified residents, since the positions are available and mandatory elimination of able candidates is avoided.

The recent trends in collegiate education have convinced students that the choosing of a career early is advantageous, since the ability to select appropriate programs strengthens their development considerably. Similarly, the majority of our medical students plan career goals early. In most instances these students choose a field during medical school and rapidly gain a firm conviction about their future plans. It is in this setting that the Department of Surgery has made available to all its residents a completely flexible and individualized program. It is the aim of this program to produce first a surgeon who is broadly based in those elements which constitute general surgery and especially to provide an adequate operative experience. Second, the resident has the opportunity to select a particular area of general surgery which he wishes to pursue in depth. Thus a resident may preferentially select clinical rotations of interest along with the core standard assignments. Examples of such special interests currently being followed include transplantation biology, vascular surgery, pediatric surgery, cardiac surgery, tumor biology, shock and metabolism, thoracic surgery, endocrine disorders, gastrointestinal surgery, computer science, and biomedical engineering. The clinical area selected is made meaningful by preferential and flexible assignment of patients with these disorders to the particular resident throughout the training program in addition to and concomitant with his registrar rotations. The special clinical interest is supported fully by one or, more often, two years in basic investigation. The former "year in the dog lab" has been abandoned and replaced by research appointments with selected basic scientists in physiology, biochemistry, pharmacology, immunology, nuclear medicine, and biomedical engineering.

One's strongest convictions are often the result of personal experience, and the author is convinced that all extended association with a basic scientist is invaluable in preparation for clinical investigation. It is for this reason that much appreciation is due and fully accorded Dr. Donald E. Gregg,[3] a most exemplary physiologist, with whom the writer spent two years studying basic aspects of the coronary circulation. To the young resident surgeon, a committed association with an investigator in basic science provides bountiful rewards. The stimulation, objectivity, critical manner of thinking, adoption of precise methodology, and the accurate interpretation of results are each essential components which lead to successful clinical investigation. For our

---

3. Donald E. Gregg played a major role in training David Sabiston as a scientist (see Chapter 1).

residents, such an experience may be taken either locally or in another institution. Currently, one of the senior residents interested in transplantation biology is obtaining a doctorate under Dr. D. Bernard Amos.[4] He is remaining for most of the senior year of the program that is termed the "Teaching Scholar," an appointment that follows the Chief Residency and during which selected operative procedures of his choice are performed. In addition, this trainee has teaching responsibilities and continues basic laboratory investigation. This appointment is especially suitable for those interested in an academic career with a strong commitment to basic investigation. Another one of our trainees has recently returned from the Karolinska Institute in Stockholm after spending a year with George Klein studying basic tumor biology which he plans to follow in a clinical and investigative career. Another resident, who has a basic interest in pulmonary surgery, has just returned from a year with Dr. Julius Comroe, working in basic pulmonary physiology — at the Cardiovascular Research Institute of the University of California. Two others have had investigative experiences at the National Institutes of Health, one of whom will become the Teaching Scholar next year with a commitment to cardiac surgery; the other is spending a year in the Department of Physiology, studying cardiac metabolism.

Planning for a surgical career optimally begins during the last two years of medical school, during which time all courses are elective. A current example is a medical student whose goals are a doctorate in biomedical engineering as well as a complete residency training in cardiothoracic surgery. His curriculum is being planned jointly between the School of Engineering and the Department of Surgery. It is apparent that these scholars, who have accumulated both unique abilities and imaginative minds, should be provided with the most suitable facilities to pursue their interests. Toward this end, the faculty is constructing a research unit to be attached as a wing of the new Basic Sciences Building. Here, these surgical scholars will be provided laboratories immediately adjacent to those in biochemistry, physiology, and

4. Randy Bollinger, M.D., Ph.D., former Chief of Transplantation Services at Duke, received the Ph.D. while studying with the great Duke transplantation immunologist, D. Bernard Amos. Dr. Amos was Chair of Duke Section of Immunology, 1962 to 1990.

anatomy to allow maximal contact and interchange. We have termed these investigators the "third faculty," whose role will be a liaison and a continual bridge between the activities of the basic science faculty and those of clinical medicine. The goal of this special environment is the establishment of objectivity in research as applied to clinical problems. This concept has been most adequately expressed by the famed Scottish physicist, Lord Kelvin, who said: "I often say that when you can measure what you are speaking about, and express it in numbers, you know something about it; but when you cannot measure it, when you cannot express it in numbers, your knowledge is of an unsatisfactory —kind; it may be the beginning of knowledge, but you have scarcely, in your thoughts, advanced to the stage of science, whatever the matter may be." Insistence upon this philosophy bears repeated emphasis as the principle is the foundation upon which all important contributions rest.

An initial response to this surgical training program may draw the immediate criticism that it tends to produce highly specialized products at the expense of a broader education. It must be emphatically stated that this is neither the intent nor the result. The particular area of interest that is pursued in depth is attained in addition to a firm background in general surgery. While controversy remains concerning time necessity for the accumulation of significant numbers of actual operative cases performed by the resident, we hold the view that this aspect is both a strong and critical part of the program. There are few aspects of surgery more distressing than the surgeon who does not possess surgical confidence. The uncertain and timid operator is most often the result of an inadequate clinical training experience. Thus, we emphasize a continuing belief that an extensive and properly supervised operative experience forms the basis of superior surgical training.

Not only is an in-depth experience in a particular aspect of surgery an ideologic objective in the training of surgeons, but it becomes apparent that it has a highly practical meaning in preparation for academic positions. With adequate planning in the elective years of medical school and progression to an individualized residency program, the surgeon produced most resembles a second- or third-year member of the junior faculty. In other words, such a resident has accumulated a thorough familiarity with a specific field in surgery that has been documented both by clinical experience and investigative accomplishment.

It is apparent that a program providing individualization in graduate surgical training requires considerable fiscal support. One of the most significant of the recent advances in surgical education has been the creation of the Surgery Training Committee of the National Institute of General Medical Sciences of the National Institutes of Health.

The general program was initiated in July 1966, and 28 programs with 115 trainees have been established. This effort is currently being financed by an annual appropriation of $2,450,000. There can be no doubt of the importance of this program and the stimulus it is providing surgical residents currently in training. The emphasis placed on basic science and the relationship to clinical surgery has already had a strong impact, and the future careers of these trainees are predictably to be filled with excitement and accomplishment. Surgery owes much to the foresight of those who made this program a reality.

At a recent meeting of the Directors of the Surgical Training Programs, an interim progress report was presented. Among the more important aspects was a survey made by Marshall Orloff concerning the need for academically trained surgeons as evidenced by current and future openings in departments of surgery throughout the United States and Canada. In this study it was shown that some 2,352 additional academic surgeons will be needed by 1975, a figure approximately twice the number of current appointments.

Much recognition is also due the American Board of Surgery for its vital role in improving and strengthening surgical training in the United States and Canada. Since its inception in 1937, it has qualified 15,908 candidates (as of November 1, 1968). The principles upon which the Board was founded and the diligence with which the members have performed their function are both noteworthy. Fortunately, the American Board of Surgery recognizes the importance of its leadership in meeting the challenges of the changing needs of surgical education. At its recent midwinter meeting, a subcommittee of the Board recommended a plan permitting liberalization and selected experimentation in residency training programs. It is predicted that this measure will be adopted and thus allow directors of training programs more experimentation and individualization.

This is a most important and highly significant move and represents an opportunity to improve many aspects of postgraduate surgical education.

It is recognized that significant changes in training programs are not developed solely in the thoughts of a single individual or of a group, but clearly the major advances and most meaningful ones are the result of continuous exchange between program directors, the faculty, and major organizations such as the Society of University Surgeons. Programs such as that advocated require an appropriate environment. In our own program, appointments of trainees are made primarily to Duke University Medical Center but include four other hospitals, each of which provides one or more special opportunities in the total training experience, but all of which are closely integrated in the teaching structure. The characteristics of each plan depend upon the qualifications and goals of the trainees in harmony with the interests and commitment of the faculty together with the physical resources available. It is doubtful that any single plan is suitable for general adoption, and the ideas presented in this program are feasible only insofar as they fit an appropriate environment. Thus, a spectrum of programs is not only desirable but mandatory.

Finally, the continuum of surgical education as reviewed here, or in fact any program yet devised, contains controversial elements. Some of the thoughtful observers in surgical education hold the view that structure and format are actually unimportant and do not deserve the attention which they have been given. While such may be true, it is likely that all will agree that a particular and special ingredient is necessary to accomplish successfully the goals of any training program.

The attainment of success has been the subject of much discussion and learned writing. It has been my own experience from the observation of others that the single most important factor in this quest is in fact a very simple one. Moreover, it is available to all. My own Chief, Alfred Blalock, discreetly called it to the attention of his trainees as frequently as the occasion presented. Certainly, he was a prime and daily example of this basic characteristic. Dr. Blalock (3) expressed his view in the following statement:

> No satisfaction is quite like that which accompanies productive investigation, particularly if it leads to better treatment of the sick. The important discov-

eries in medicine are generally simple and one is apt to wonder why they were not made earlier. I believe that they are made usually by a dedicated person who is willing to work and cultivate his power of observation rather than by the so-called genius.

Many have attempted to express this concept with both clarity and precision. None has succeeded so well as Sir William Osler, who in his talk before the medical students at Yale said succinctly:

> It seems a bounden duty on such an occasion to be honest and frank, so I propose to tell you the secret of life as I have seen the game played, and as I have tried to play it myself.... This I propose to give you in the hope, yes, in the full assurance that some of you at least will lay hold upon it to your profit. Though a little one, the master-word looms large in meaning, WORK. It is the open sesame to every portal, the great equalizer in the world, the true philosopher's stone, which transmutes all the base metal of humanity into gold. The stupid man among you it will make bright, the bright snail brilliant, and the brilliant student steady. With the magic word in your heart all things are possible, and without it all study is vanity and vexation. The miracles of life are with it.... To the youth it brings hope, to the middle-aged confidence, to the aged repose. It is directly responsible for all advances in medicine during the past twenty-five centuries.

It is very likely, in fact certain, that the present continues to be governed by the same principles that Osler emphasized. Work remains the master-word, and substitutes are destined to failure. As surgical teachers entrusted with the training of those who are to create the surgical future, it is suggested that Osler's admonition deserves our repeated recognition. With continuous emphasis on work, all efforts become simpler and progress in any reasonable plan of graduate surgical education becomes assured.

References

1. Anlyan, W. G., and Sabiston, D. C., Jr. A new approach to medial education, *Surgery* 62: 134, 1967.
2. Blalock, A. Problems in the training of the surgeon, *Ann. Surg.* 131: 609, 1950.
3. Blalock, A. The nature of discovery, *Ann. Surg.* 144: 289, 1956.
4. Carter, B. N. The fruition of Halsted's concept of surgical training, *Surgery* 32: 518, 1952.

5. Coggeshall, L. T. Planning for medial progress through education, Evanston, Ill., 1965, Association of American Medical Colleges.

6. Funkenstein, D. H. Our obsolete residencies, *Arch. Int. Med.* 122: 279, 1968.

7. Garrison, F. H. *History of Medicine.* Philadelphia: W.B. Saunders Company, 1929.

7a. Gloyne, S. R. *John Hunter.* Edinburgh: E.&S. Livingstone, Ltd., 1950, p. 60.

8. Halsted, W. S. The training of the surgeon, in *Surgical Papers by William Stewart Halsted.* Vol. II. Baltimore: The Johns Hopkins Press, 1924, pp. 512–531.

9. Krueger, R. The new curriculum, *Duke Alumni Register* 54:1, 1968.

10. Lee, P. V. Medical schools and the changing times: Nine case reports on experimentation in medical education, 1959–1960, Evanston, Ill., 1962, Association of American Medical Colleges.

11. Millis, J. S. The graduate education of physicians, Report of the Citizens Commission on Graduate Medical Education, 1966, American Medical Association.

12. Orloff, M. J. Faculty positions for surgeons completing the academic surgery training programs, talk delivered to meeting of Surgical Training Committee Chairmen, Boston, Mass., April 20, 1968.

13. Osler, W. *Aequanimitas with Other Addresses.* Philadelphia: P. Blakiston's Son & Company, Inc., 1932.

14. Preiss, J. J., and Long, E.C. Personal communication.

15. Sieker, H.O. A new curriculum for medical education, *Clin. Res.* 13: 3, 1965.

16. Zuidema, G.D. Society and surgical education, *The Pharos* 31: 2, 1968.

17. Association of American Medical Colleges, Council of Academic Societies: Workshop on the role of the university in graduate medical education, Washington, D.C., 1968.

Chapter 15

The Training of Academic Surgeons for the Future: The Challenge and the Dilemma

*J*ulius Comroe[1] has had a tremendous influence both in the individual stimulation of young investigators and in science generally, both nationally and internationally, and he states the challenge forthrightly: "I have always believed that a main responsibility of a faculty member is to be a talent scout—to determine the special abilities of medical students in clinical care, in teaching, or in research and then to encourage them to do the very best they can in their field of unusual competence. One field, of course, is research. I see no way for faculty to determine this special talent of their students unless students have contact with research while they are still in medical school" (1). That statement can be supported by the achievements that match this definition in the history of medical science.

To pursue Comroe's admonition that we should stimulate students to enter research while they are still in medical school, I will cite several specific examples from the past. Andreas Vesalius is an excellent example, since the day following his graduation in medicine at the University of Padua, he published his scholarly work on human anatomy and was made a full professor at the age of thirty-one, largely on the basis of his original work. Today, medical historians and anatomists alike agree that Vesalius was the first of the scientific anatomists to correct the many errors that had been handed down for a thousand years from Galen's texts.

---

1. Julius Comroe (1911–1984) was Director of the Cardiovascular Research Institute in San Francisco and one of the great pulmonary physiologists of the past century.

The first investigator ever to observe the function of the capillary network was Jan Swammerdam. As a medical student, he first noted the small cylindrical objects floating through the capillaries, namely, the red blood cells.

The entire story of the development of anesthesia is another example of basic observations by a bright medical student. In 1799, Humphry Davy was a nineteen-year-old medical student when he prepared and inhaled large quantities of nitrous oxide and discovered its marked analgesic effect. In connection with a very painful, inflamed wisdom tooth, he said, "One day when the inflammation was most troublesome, I breathed three large doses of nitrous oxide. The pain always diminished after the first four or five inspirations. As nitrous oxide in its extensive effect appears capable of destroying physical pain, it may probably be used with advantage during surgical operations" (2).

Moreover, William T. O. Morton was a medical student when he administered the first ether anesthetic at the Massachusetts General Hospital in Boston in 1846. Also, while a medical student, Poiseuille, the famous biophysicist, was the first to devise the mercury manometer for measuring arterial blood pressure. Later, he developed the equation for determination of blood flow, now termed "Poiseuille's Law." As the thesis for his medical degree, Raynaud in 1862 wrote the classic description of his now famous syndrome.

The cells in the pancreas that secrete insulin were first described by Paul Langerhans, a student under the tutelage of the father of modern pathology, Rudolf Virchow. Langerhans was provided a laboratory and encouragement to pursue his work on the pancreas. These islets now bear his name. Similarly, in Sweden in 1888, a medical student at the University of Uppsala, Ivar Sandstrom, identified for the first time the parathyroid glands and wrote a monograph documenting his observations. The discovery of insulin is the product of two investigators, Banting and Best, the latter being a medical student at the time of their extraordinary work.

America's greatest physiologist, the late Walter B. Cannon, entered the Harvard Medical School in 1896, the year following the discovery of X rays by Röentgen. He went to work at once on the use of this technique in the study of gastrointestinal motility and presented his initial experiments as a first-year medical student before the prestigious American Physiological Society in 1897. His classic paper on the influence of emotion on gastric motility was published when he was a third-year medical student, and with those landmark achievements, his career was well on its successful path.

Jay MacLean, while a second-year medical student in the laboratory of William H. Howell, who expressly directed him to identify a thromboplastic substance, actually found the opposite, namely, an anticoagulant which he later named "heparin" in recognition of its source in the liver. Today, there hangs in the Johns Hopkins Medical School a bronze plaque stating, "To Jay MacLean in recognition of his contribution in the discovery of heparin in 1916 as a second year medical student."

Finally, two surgeons received the Nobel Prize for achievements initiated in their medical school days. While a second-year medical student at the University of Lyons, Alexis Carrel was greatly saddened by the fact that while visiting the city, the president of France was attacked and stabbed in the abdomen with a dagger, after giving a major address at the Palace of Commerce. The dagger was thrust deep into the right upper quadrant, causing massive intraperitoneal hemorrhage. He was operated upon as an emergency, and the surgeon found a large incised wound in the portal vein. At that time, all attempts to directly suture blood vessels had been unsuccessful and were followed either by massive infection and hemorrhage or by thrombosis. The operating surgeon feared ligation of the portal vein because of the high mortality associated with such a procedure and, therefore, chose simply to drain the abdomen. The president continued to hemorrhage and died a short time later.

The young medical student, Carrel, was stimulated by this event to begin his painstaking efforts at successful vascular anastomosis. Using exacting surgical technique, with fine bites of tissue, and using tiny, highly polished needles with small sutures, he was able to successfully reanastomose small vessels with a diameter as small as one millimeter. Because of jealousy and lack of support in his own medical school, he later came to the Rockefeller Institute where he was provided excellent facilities. Using his basic vascular techniques, he transplanted organs and tissues, and for this work he received the Nobel Prize in 1912.

Similarly, Werner Forssmann in 1929, while a first-year resident in surgery in Germany, captured the concept of passing a catheter through an arm vein into the heart. He first sought a volunteer for the procedure but was unsuccessful. Therefore, with great courage, he passed the catheter into his own arm and into the heart. Once the catheter was in the heart, he pondered whether or not he would later be believed unless he had some objective proof of this daring human experiment. Therefore, he arose from the operating table, walked upstairs, had a chest film taken, and then walked back down the stairs to remove the catheter. His painstaking honesty is reflected in the last sentence of his report, in which he apologized to his readers since, a week later when he removed the bandage from his forearm, he had superficial wound infection. He admitted he must have inadvertently broken surgical technique during this historic procedure.

Of course there are many other examples, and only a few have been selected to emphasize that recognition of such achievements underscores the significance of Comroe's admonition to all those who have an opportunity to stimulate medical students.

As a key part of preparing students for original investigation, continuing efforts must be directed toward improvement in medical education. Earlier this month, Dean Daniel Tosteson presented to the Harvard Medical Faculty a new proposal for a seven-year demonstration project to provide a new pathway to the M.D. degree. Twenty-five students are to be accepted each year, beginning in the fall of 1983, in an effort that this pathway would be the "beginning of a general transformation of the style of learning at the Harvard Medical School." Throughout the experience, the students will have a mix of electives and shared courses. The shared part of the curriculum will comprise about half the students' time and will stress problem solving through the case-method approach, self-learning, and self-assessment using computer-assisted audiovisual devices. Acquiring the skills together with analysis of clinical data is to be an important goal.

The other half of the program is to be elective and will allow students to enroll in courses throughout Harvard University and the

Massachusetts Institute of Technology. The program consists of two segments, the first four years devoted to the arts and sciences basic to medicine, and the second three years to clinical arts and sciences. Both basic and clinical materials will be interwoven throughout the curriculum, and a thesis describing an independent study will be required in both the basic and clinical segments of the program.

In approaching the future of medical education, we must face a number of dilemmas. The general features of these problems apply to all of academic medicine, and specific ones are of primary significance to the field of surgery and the surgical specialties.

The number of medical schools in this country rose from 79 in 1950 to 126 in 1981, a rapid increase requiring a number of additional faculty in all specialties, including surgery. During this period, the number of medical students has climbed precipitously from 25,000 in 1950 to more than 65,000 in 1981. This increase has created what many believe to be a "glut" of physicians and is quite apt to be responsible for increasing economic problems in the entire health field of the future.

This problem is further reflected in the total numbers of approved residency positions in all specialties, rising from 17,000 in 1950 to nearly 62,000 in 1981. The total number of applicants for first-year residency positions will soon exceed the number of approved residencies, thus creating a further dilemma. Although the number of graduates of foreign medical schools has been leveling off in the recent past, for the 1982 National Residency Matching Program, the percentage is again increasing, representing yet another serious problem.

For many reasons, including increased numbers of physicians, the annual admissions to hospitals in the United States have risen sharply, from 18 million in 1950 to nearly 39 million in 1980. Similarly, the number of surgical procedures has risen dramatically from 17 million in 1972 to almost 24 million in 1979.

The specific features that primarily affect surgery include the diminishing number of outstanding residency training programs as well as the most significant feature of these programs, that is, the number of patients who can be assigned primarily to the resident staff under the supervision of the faculty. In recent years, this group of patients has diminished sharply in all areas of the United States, and many believe this factor has had a serious effect on the quality of these training programs and on the competence of the surgical resident.

Another feature of considerable significance is the length of time necessary to meet the requirements of the various surgical boards. In surgery and the surgical specialties, this ranges from a minimum of four years to a maximum of seven years. The seven-year program is in cardiothoracic surgery and is the absolute minimum of required training in order to meet the standards of the American Board of Thoracic Surgery. Moreover, in such programs in which young surgeons are being trained for academic posts with additional time devoted to research, the length of the training period is eight or even ten years.

Finally, in recent surveys of current medical students, considerable apprehension and concern are being expressed about the quality and numbers of medical student applicants in the immediate years ahead. Moreover, the ratio of applicants to available first-year openings in medical schools throughout the nation has begun to decline, thus emphasizing another significant factor.

In summary, while a number of challenges facing the future of academic surgery have been successfully met, there are clearly a series of problems that deserve our concerted immediate attention and thoughtful solution.

References

1. Comroe, J. H., Jr. *Retrospectroscope. Insights into Medical Discovery.* Menlo Park, California: Von Gehr Press, 1977.
2. Davy, H. *Researches, Chemical and Philosophical: Chiefly concerning Nitrous Oxide, or Dephlogisticated Nitrous Air, and Its Respiration.* London: J. Johnson, 1800.

Chapter 16 ☞

The Effect of the Three-Year Medical School Curriculum on Undergraduate Surgical Education: A Professor's Point of View

*I*n the recent past a growing number of educators have advocated a three-year medical school curriculum. Only a few years ago, three-year graduates were quite uncommon in the United States, whereas today a significant number of medical schools have adopted three-year programs as the standard curriculum. Moreover, an even larger number has made this shortened program available on an optional basis.

In any discussion of medical curricula, the year 1910 is a very significant one. In that year Flexner made his epochal report and drew the conclusion that a four-year curriculum was essential for proper medical education. Following acceptance of the Flexner report, most medical schools designed the curriculum such that essentially two years were devoted to basic sciences and two years to clinical science. This format remained essentially unchanged, except during the Second World War, until 1952, when Case Western Reserve University School of Medicine initiated an innovative experiment in interdisciplinary teaching throughout its medical curriculum. One clearly recognizes that the amount of information medical students bring from college today is greatly expanded over that of sixty years ago, and moreover, much more is included in the current standard medical curriculum. In other words, an arbitrary figure of four years is not necessarily relevant to present standards.

In considering a reduction in total curriculum time, the absolute minimum of time required is an important feature. This has recently been established as thirty-two months, a figure set jointly by the Liaison Committee on Medical Education, the executive council of the American Association of Medical Colleges, and the Council on Medical Education of the American Medical Association. Thus for the immediate future, it would appear that the concept embraced in current programs of eight months or each academic year of the standard four years has been reaffirmed. If schools wish to eliminate or greatly reduce vacations, it is possible to earn an M.D. degree within three calendar years. A problem in some schools which permit a three-year curriculum is the fact that with classes entering in September, graduation is apt not to occur until July 1, a time of critical importance to those seeking internships and residencies.

During a recent Macy conference at which the three-year medical education curriculum was discussed, a detailed consideration of the experience at the Dartmouth Medical School was reviewed with emphasis upon its new program (1). Under the segment, "Shortened Medical School Curricula," it was brought out that the Dartmouth curriculum was established on the premise that not only the specially qualified or gifted students, but also the average undergraduate medical students could be well educated in three years.

The three-year program at Dartmouth begins in the first year at the end of August and terminates after thirty-three-and-a-half months. The curriculum consists of a first year of approximately forty weeks devoted to basic medical science, eight weeks of which are elective. In the second year some forty-three weeks are devoted to what is termed the scientific basis of medicine and clinical diagnosis, and in this period ten weeks are elective. The final experience consists of fifty-one weeks termed "the principal clinical year" in which there are seven weeks of clinical electives. Thus far, the faculty appears quite pleased with this curriculum.

Boston University and Johns Hopkins have developed special programs designed to save a year, although in these curricula emphasis is placed upon accepting gifted and exceptionally qualified students. For many years the University of Tennessee has had an accelerated program open to all students, with a class admitted each six months, and with graduation thirty-nine months later. This faculty has, therefore, been a pioneer in maximal utilization of its educational facilities as well as in the acceleration of the graduation of classes.

According to current records of the American Association of Medical Colleges, there are at least sixteen medical schools in the country in which the standard program of medical education is accomplished in three years. These schools include Alabama, Baylor, Dartmouth, Einstein, Loyola (Chicago), Nebraska, New York Medical College, New York at Stonybrook, Ohio Medical College at Toledo, Ohio State, Rush, Rutgers, South Florida, Tennessee, Texas at Houston, and Texas at Lubbock. In other words, these schools place primary emphasis upon the three-year medical graduate, and in most of these curricula the standard four-year course is taken in three calendar years, largely by the elimination of vacations. In addition to these, twenty-four schools allow three-year graduation on an elective basis should the student elect it. Thus, one can see that within a short period of time a number of schools have adopted three-year programs with strong advocates among the faculty and administration. It should also be recognized that recent federal legislation has encouraged three-year programs with an incentive offered to each school of $6,000 per student. Such financial inducements are of obvious significance.

As might be expected, other medical educators have posed important questions concerning the three-year programs. Writing persuasively is DeWitt Stetten, director of the National Institute of General Medical Sciences at the NIH (2). In considering the advantages and disadvantages of altering the length of the term in medical school and the likely impact of such changes upon the quality and quantity of physicians produced, Dr. Stetten has emphasized that first and foremost is the question of education achieved in four years as compared with that in three. He emphasizes the role of the accelerated pace and its relationship to increased fatigue with its subsequent effects on the teaching-learning process. Attention is called to the accelerated programs during World War II when increased student tension led to frank increases in the incidence of psychoneurosis. He concludes that it is imperative that the quality of the student and that of the educational process not revert to the condition of the so-called trade schools in medicine before Flexner.

An additional practice that deserves mention is the early internship or residency program. At present, several institutions are selecting candidates for these programs from students in the standard curricula during their third year. In other words, the fourth year of medical school may be taken as the first year of graduate training. Three years ago such a program was adopted at Duke, and there have since been eleven appointees in surgery for this type of training. It is of interest that in the Duke medical curriculum the third year is totally elective for basic science, and students generally choose courses appropriate for future career plans. The fourth year is also totally elective, but in clinical science, and qualified students may apply for a first-year postgraduate training program in lieu of the clinical electives. It must be admitted that the students in these programs both here and elsewhere are carefully selected both from the point of view of their academic scholarship and suitability for a surgical career by individual appraisal. Our faculty has carefully examined the progress of these trainees and has found them thus far indistinguishable from their peers. Moreover, each of the candidates has by multiple assessments expressed enthusiasm for the program.

From present evidence, it is apparent that programs leading to the M.D. degree in three calendar years are useful and even desirable for appropriate students. Equally valid is the fact that for many other students the four-year program is best suited for individual needs. Thus, the introduction of flexibility into the basic medical curriculum can clearly be extended to flexibility in the number of calendar years required to obtain the M.D. degree. With the passage of time, it seems both likely and appropriate that the majority of medical schools will permit graduation as early as three years with four-year programs for others. With this combination, it seems quite certain that a logical and judicious solution to a current problem in medical education will have been achieved.

In conclusion, it seems apparent that all teachers of medicine should bear particular responsibility for transmitting an understanding of the approach and methodology of science to developing physicians. Moreover, with the passage of time more and not less research and laboratory investigation will be required for further advances in medicine.

If one surveys the amazing progress of medicine from the time of William Harvey, one immediately accepts the fact that basic scientific observation and investigation have been responsible for the present status of medicine and bear heavily on the motivation of students to pursue new discoveries. This concept was aptly expressed by Claude Bernard and bears repeating:

> Experimental medicine, as we conceive it, includes the problem of medicine as a whole and comprises both the theory and the practice of medicine. But when I said that every physician should be an experimenter, I did not mean to suggest that each one should cultivate the whole extent of experimental medicine. Of necessity there will always be physicians especially devoting themselves to physiological experiments, others to investigation of normal and pathological anatomy, others to surgical or medical practice, etc. This splitting up is not bad for the progress of science; on the contrary, practical specialties are an excellent thing for science, properly speaking, but on the condition that men devoting themselves to the investigation of a special part of medicine be so educated as to be conversant with experimental medicine as a whole, and to know the place which the special science they cultivate should occupy in that whole. By specializing in this way, they will direct their studies so as to contribute to the progress of scientific or experimental medicine. Practical studies and theoretic studies will thus work toward the same object; that is all that we can ask in a science like medicine, which is forced to be ceaselessly in action before it is fully established.

References

1. Lippard, V. W. and Purcell, E., eds. The changing medial curriculum. Report of a Macy Conference; Josiah Macy, Jr. Foundation. Philadelphia: William F. Fell Company, 1972.
2. Stetten, Jr., D. Projected changes in medical school curriculum. Are three years really better than four? *Science* 174: 1303, 1971.

Chapter 17 ☞

The Surgical Medical Student Curriculum at Duke

*W*ith the adoption of the elective curriculum of Duke Medical School in 1966, the alterations in the surgical curriculum were substantial. All of the required work in surgery is currently given in an eight-week period, thus making it necessary to critically select the topics that are included. The faculty of the Department of Surgery at Duke chose to place primary emphasis upon those principles which characterize the discipline of surgery and its specialties.

The required course in surgery is given in the second year, and emphasis is placed upon those basic principles that form the foundation of surgical diagnosis and treatment. Stress is placed upon those subjects which have their origins in objective laboratory and clinical documentation. These include surgical antisepsis and bacteriology, the management of wounds, inflammation, shock, fluid and electrolyte balance, the metabolic response to trauma, the biology of neoplastic disease including chemotherapy and immunotherapy, gastrointestinal physiology and its derangement, and disorders of blood coagulation, thrombosis, and embolism. These subjects are applicable equally to general and cardiothoracic surgery as well as to neurosurgery, orthopaedics, otolaryngology, plastic surgery, and urology (1). Throughout the surgery clerkship, emphasis is placed upon the most meaningful and lasting form of clinical instruction, that is, individual study of the patient. Each student is assigned patients in rotation, and each patient's case is reviewed in detail with members of the resident and senior staff. Maximal student participation is sought in the establishment of the diagnosis and planning of therapy for all patients.

The primary goals of the required course in surgery are to acquaint the student with the basic principles in surgery and to provide a basis for application in actual practice. Primary emphasis is placed upon the study of each patient, and this experience is supplemented by a series of informal seminars. It is intended that the course provide a basic foundation in surgery and prepare the students for a wide variety of elective courses in surgery and the surgical specialties available in their fourth year. A block schedule showing daily assignments is depicted in Table 1.

The students are divided into equal groups with ten to twelve in each, one group being assigned to the service at the Duke Hospital and the other to the Durham Veterans Administration Hospital. In each hospital, the Chief Resident is responsible for the distribution of patients on a posted roster with planning to assure maximal variety in types of clinical disorders. All students are assigned to a residency team with the intention of providing the student maximal participation in patient care. The history and the physical examination as recorded by the student are carefully reviewed and annotated by the team resident. The student is encouraged to participate actively in diagnosis and treatment. The changing of dressings, removal of sutures, care of drains, insertion on nasogastric tubes, administration of intravenous fluids, thoracenteses, spinal puncture, and similar procedures are performed by students under the supervision of the resident and senior staff.

In the past it has been difficult to have an instructor continuously available for the students on the surgery rotation, since the operating room requires nearly every surgeon's presence sometime during the day and often for prolonged periods. In order to alleviate the problem, a resident is assigned each term with the sole responsibility of teaching. This resident is available throughout the day to assist in any manner desired by the students. Specifically, the teaching resident reviews the history and physical examination of each patient assigned on an appointment basis with each student. This provides a continuing basis for teaching. This resident also conducts teaching sessions with the students concerning the practical aspects of pre- and postoperative care and is available for instruction and assistance in the care of wounds, drains, thoracenteses, intubations, and related subjects. The students have found the Teaching Resident to be a very valuable and in fact an essential part of the teaching team. Moreover, it has been gratifying to note the response of the Teaching Residents, as this rotation is considered a very desirable one, by their own assessment.

Table 1 Department of Surgery: Required Course in Surgery— Second Year

Monday	Tuesday	Wednesday	Thursday	Friday	Saturday
7:00–8:00 Resident Rounds	7:00–8:00 Resident Rounds	7:00–8:00 Resident Rounds	7:00–8:00 Resident Rounds	7:00–8:00 Resident Rounds	Surgical Grand Rounds 7:30–9:30
	Teaching Rounds 8:00–9:30		Teaching Rounds 8:00–9:30		Teaching Rounds 9:30–11:00
		Work with patients, general operating rooms, reference reading.			
Surgical Seminar 1:00–3:00		Surgical Seminar 1:00–3:00		Surgical Seminar 1:00–3:00	
			Dr. Sabiston's Conference 2:00–3:00		
Surg. Specialty Demonstration 3:00–4:00	Surg. Specialty Demonstration 3:00–4:00	Surg. Specialty Demonstration 3:00–4:00	Surg. Specialty Demonstration 3:00–4:00	Surg. Specialty Demonstration 3:00–4:00	
		Surgical Staff Conference 4:00–5:30		Combined Cardiac Conference 4:00–5:30	

Each group of students is assigned two members of the senior surgical faculty who make bedside rounds for an hour and a half on three mornings weekly throughout the course. At these rounds, the Teaching Resident selects patients for presentation, and the student presents from memory the history, physical findings, and laboratory data. It is considered essential that the student learn from the beginning the significance of committing to memory all pertinent data about each patient in order that it be instantaneously available, as for example in an emergency situation, without need to consult the chart. Thus, on ward rounds each student is expected to be sufficiently prepared at all times to present, from memory alone, a patient assigned him or her. The instructor generally asks questions concerning the patients with queries directed to all students in the group and especially to that student assigned to the patient. He then proceeds to present a rather complete discussion of the specific illness.

While the broad principles of surgery are emphasized during information seminars three times each week, at the bedside ward rounds the diagnosis and management of specific surgical problems such as acute appendicitis, intestinal obstruction, carcinoma of the breast, empyema, peripheral arterial insufficiency, cardiac defects, pancreatitis, etc., are discussed in detail. Since ward rounds are conducted three days each week and two patients are presented each morning, it is possible to discuss some fifty specific surgical entities during the course. Provision is made to present different disorders on these rounds in order to prevent repetition.

The students meet each morning with the Teaching Resident to discuss specific patient diagnoses and management problems. In these sessions the students have a daily opportunity to ask specific questions regarding details of diagnostic tests, uses and dosages of drugs, wound management and other details of management.

Three times weekly a two-hour seminar is held in which the topics of broad relevance to surgery are discussed. Presentations of these topics are made by members of the faculty most closely associated with the subject. In most instances, the instructors have pursued the subject both in the experimental laboratory and in the clinical situation and are recognized for their contributions in the field. The format of these seminars is arranged such that the instructor presents the subject in the first hour, often with the use of appropriate visual aids. After a ten-minute coffee break, the session continues, with the remainder being devoted to student participation as a dialogue. The student is prepared in advance for the session by means of a reading list with several suggested references for each seminar. Each student is asked to be prepared sufficiently to make the seminars a stimulating exchange of ideas.

It is apparent that in the eight-week period assigned to the Department of Surgery for its required course, it is not possible to cover thoroughly each of the specialties in surgery. Nevertheless, the surgical faculty agreed that it would be unwise for students to graduate from medical school without having been exposed in some way to such important areas of surgery as neurosurgery, orthopaedics, otolaryngology, plastic surgery, and urology. In the structure of the required course, the chiefs of the respective disciplines provide a demonstration, given as a one-hour session each day for a week for each specialty. In these sessions, the student is provided an opportunity to understand the basis of each specialty together with a concept of its scope with specific patient examples.

Our concepts of the relationship of instruction of students to subsequent residency training in surgery have been previously published (2). The faculty in each of the surgical specialties places considerable care in the preparation of these sessions. Since it is possible that a student might graduate from medical school without electing further experience in one or more of these surgical disciplines, attendance at these sessions is mandatory. The demonstrations are given daily, are one hour in length, and each of the surgical specialties is assigned one week during the course. Because of the broad scope of these sessions, the surgical faculty believes that the students are more apt to obtain a better experience if the material presented in these sessions is not included in the final oral and written examinations in the course. Experience has shown that these sessions are both well attended and well received. Moreover, each of these disciplines attracts significant numbers of students into electives in the fourth year and subsequently into their respective residency programs.

Each week a surgical staff conference is held, during which the two most interesting patients in the hospital at the time are presented with a planned discussion by various members of the staff not only in the Department of Surgery but throughout the Medical Center. After each presentation adequate time is allowed for discussion and the students are encouraged to participate in these sessions.

Each week the deaths and complications that have occurred in the department are reviewed. A member of the staff of the Department of Pathology is present to discuss the postmortem findings, and a thoroughly critical presentation of each case is made. The intent of these sessions first is to establish clearly the cause of death or complication, and then to decide if an alternate approach might have been preferable. Every attempt is made to emphasize possible prevention of complications or death, especially as might relate to future similar cases. A critical analysis of each death and complication on the service is an unusually meaningful teaching experience, and the students find this conference to be both informative and challenging.

On alternate weeks various members of the department and at times guest speakers present research work in progress. These are important sessions to students as they obtain an understanding of current laboratory investigation. The resident staff contributes original work, and student participation has been open and helpful. The students attend grand rounds each Saturday morning, a two-hour session of clinical presentations with brief, concise remarks being made by the faculty on a number of interesting patients. This is a popular conference and is well attended by students and residents.

At the end of the course, an objective, multiple-choice written examination is given. The more important features of this examination are: (1) the examination is prepared solely from material covered with the students in the course, i.e., the seminars, conferences, and ward rounds, and (2) since it is recognized that students may at times wish to be present in the operating room, causing conflicts with rounds or seminars, any five questions on the examination can be omitted.

An oral examination also is given by a member of the faculty at the end of the course. Each student provides the examiner a list of patients assigned during the course with the appropriate diagnoses, and the oral examination is taken solely from the disorders on the list.

Following completion of the core course in the second year, students are eligible to select from among thirty elective courses offered in general surgery and the surgical specialties. In most of these courses emphasis is placed upon the student's being delegated considerable responsibilities in patient management. In view of the fact that medical students are better prepared on entry into medical school today than before and maintain this superiority as the course progresses, fourth-year students are now found to perform at a level formerly achieved by interns. In other words, the senior student functions largely as an intern, which is an actual experience since the internship is no longer offered in the department and appointments are made upon graduation from medical school directly to the first year of surgical residency. Experience has shown that this has been a fully justified move.

In addition to clinical responsibilities, a series of advanced seminars for senior students is designed appropriate for the course. Generally, three seminars are given weekly with advance reference reading assigned for informal discussion with a member of this faculty. Particular stress is placed upon the prerogative of students to arrange with the department chairman or division chief any course they may desire that is not specifically listed in the catalog. A number of students utilize this approach in curricular planning, and the surgical faculty has been quite pleased with this flexible approach.

A considerable increase in faculty time has been found necessary in the elective curriculum, as compared with the traditional one. Formerly, a number of subjects were presented in sessions for the entire class. In addition, a number of new sessions and clinical rounds have been created involving small groups. Moreover, nearly all of the electives contain only a few students, and a single student often takes an elective as the only member of the course. Thus, individualized teaching has become much more common today than previously.

In considering the problems and difficulties that introduction of the elective curriculum has reduced or eliminated, one could cite the fact that former problems associated with impersonal and whole-class exercises have been eliminated. This has clearly been a positive feature, both for the students and faculty. Moreover, it has allowed them to become considerably better acquainted, and exchange of information is now much more frequently on a personal basis. The primary problem which has been introduced by the elective curriculum relates to the increased time demands imposed upon the faculty to teach relatively small groups. This also requires considerable repetition of discussion of the same subjects, but in general this has been quite well tolerated by the faculty. Generally, those instructors who enjoy teaching draw the larger numbers of students into their elective courses.

References

1. Anlyan, W. G. and Sabiston, Jr., D. C. A new approach to medical education. *Surgery,* 62: 134–140, 1967.
2. Sabiston, Jr., D. C. A continuum in surgical education. *Surgery,* 66: 1–14, 1969.

Chapter 18 ⌒

Specialization in Surgery

*T*hrough the stimulus of Dr. Francis D. Moore, Moseley Professor of Surgery at Harvard, it has been my privilege to work with the American Board of Surgery and indeed with all the surgical boards in assembling objective data concerning the needs for surgical specialists in the future. These data are impressive and emphasize the marked increase in surgical specialties in the United States since 1950. For example, in that year the American Board of Neurosurgery certified 27 in this field, whereas in 1971 the number had risen to 82. In thoracic surgery, the number was 25 in 1950 and 148 in 1971. For orthopaedic surgery, the most rapidly growing of our specialties, the figure rose from 180 in 1950 to 420 in 1971! The importance of these statistics is emphasized by the fact that these board-certified graduates in the surgical specialties outnumber certified general surgeons by some two to one.

An additional important aspect of contemporary specialty training concerns special interest fields now included in general surgery, which currently seek special recognition. Pediatric surgery and vascular surgery are at the forefront, and the American Board of Surgery is now considering the awarding of a special certificate of competence in these fields. This is being done with a strong hope that these specialties will remain a part of general surgery.

The American Board of Surgery has been quite active in the recent past and some of its decisions have not always been properly understood. For example, elimination of the requirement of internship was one of its actions, but simultaneously it became essential that there be a minimum of four clinical years of surgical training. In other words, the former year in the laboratory may not be used as one of the required years. In essence, one can say that the principles and standards of the Board really have not changed appreciably.

At the time I was a member of the surgical residency staff at Johns Hopkins, most of us thought it was not only the best in this country but one that had been traditional and with little change since the opening of the hospital in 1889. Of course, while the former was true, the latter was not. William Halsted, during his thirty-three years as Chief of Surgery at Hopkins, a rather long period of tenure by today's standards, made numerous changes, and others were added later by Dean Lewis and Alfred Blalock. I believe firmly in the concept that many different programs are healthy and achieve a real need. Fortunately, there are now many quite sound programs throughout the country available to surgical trainees, each of which is often significantly different from the other.

Several years ago in our own program at the Duke University Hospital we adopted a plan whereby the internship was abandoned and eighteen first-year residents were appointed annually upon graduation from medical school. Some six or eight of the appointees are selected as potential candidates for the residency program in general and in cardiothoracic surgery, and in this group also may be appointed those who are undecided about the specific residency to be pursued in the future. The remaining first-year residencies are available for candidates who have decided firmly upon a career in one of the surgical specialties, including orthopedics, otolaryngology, neurosurgery, plastic surgery, and urology. These appointments are made in conjunction with and upon approval of the chief of the respective division with the tentative understanding that the applicant's desire and performance will merit continued training in this specialty residency. It is therefore possible to provide complete residency training for nearly all those selected for the first-year program in the field of their choice.

For the residents who choose the fields of general and cardiothoracic surgery, each is encouraged to select a special field of interest to pursue in depth in addition to the broader training which encompasses the field. For example, a special interest might be either peripheral vascular surgery, children's surgery, transplantation, endocrine surgery, cardiac surgery, or cancer and tumor immunology. Such training is augmented further by a period of one or usually two years in the experimental laboratory, primarily in the basic science departments. In this way, a firm basis is provided to trainees by the time of their completion of the program. The minimum training period for general surgery in the present program is five years, but if cardiothoracic surgery or other specialties are included, the total time is increased appropriately.

Chapter 19 ∜

The University Teaching Hospital

The remarkable advances in medicine occurring in the past several decades have reemphasized the importance of the teaching hospital and its role in medical education. Strides that have been made in the clinical, biomedical, and social sciences have placed increasing emphasis upon the role of the teaching hospital in patient care, education, and research. In the United States today, the responsibility of the teaching hospital includes not only the education of medical students and residents, but also includes the care of increasingly complex medical problems requiring advanced diagnostic and therapeutic resources.

The importance of this problem was emphasized by the Surgeon General Dr. William H. Stewart, in his recent address to the participants in the White House Conference on Health. He noted that one of every twenty-five gainfully employed persons in the United States today serves the cause of health. This represents a dramatic increase over figures during the past several decades. Dr. Stewart chose this occasion to emphasize the fact that the immediate needs are greater than can be logistically supplied on the basis of current development and training programs. For example, there are currently in the United States some 7,138 hospitals, of which 5,684 are short-term general hospitals for the care of predominantly acute problems. Of this total, only 9 percent have more than 300 beds and only 2 percent have 500 or more. These figures help bring into focus the number of teaching hospitals, since the majority of these are found among the larger hospitals.

The Directory of Internships and Residencies shows a total of 227 hospitals that are defined as "major" teaching hospitals. Thus, there are only a relatively few hospitals that can be classified as "teaching hospitals" in the United States today. However, in these hospitals, the majority of the severely ill patients are seen.

The development of medical schools associated with teaching hospitals as we recognize them today appears to have had origin in Italy and France during the Middle Ages. Such institutions were largely for the care of the indigent sick and were supported by civic means. This type of hospital spread to Germany and England, gradually becoming increasingly important in medical education. Of special significance is the fact that the hospital of that period had very little to offer in the way of specific medical care, since the body of medical knowledge remained quite meager until the midnineteenth century. It was at this time that the scientific and biologic approach to medicine was initiated and was followed shortly by the introduction of major surgery. The latter had become increasingly safe due in large part to the advent of understanding of sterile techniques and as a result of the development of anesthesia.

In the United States, the first medical school was established in 1785 in Philadelphia, and in 1768 the King's College Medical School was founded in New York. The Harvard Medical School began in Cambridge in 1783 and was subsequently to demonstrate the value of a close connection between a teaching hospital, the Massachusetts General Hospital, and a medical school.

Despite these advances, it remained for the opening of the Johns Hopkins Hospital (1889) and its Medical School (1893) to emphasize the common bond that must be maintained between medical education and patient care. Dr. William H. Welch, the first Dean of the Hopkins Medical School, forged a strong bond between the Hospital and the Medical School. Moreover, he appointed two young and exceptionally strong clinical chiefs, one in Medicine and the other in Surgery. It was William Osler, the Professor of Medicine, who placed maximal emphasis on the importance of teaching medicine at the patient's bedside. The importance of direct observation in the clinical situation was emphasized in his admonition, "To study medicine without books is to sail an uncharted sea, while the study of medicine only from books is not to go to sea at all." His advice to evaluate the patient first and then to seek additional information from literature is summarized in his comment, "Do not waste the hours of daylight in listening to that which you can read by night, but when you have seen, read. And when you can, read the original descriptions of the masters who with crude methods of study saw so clearly." The Professor of Surgery, Willliam S. Halsted, enunciated the principles of residency training in surgery that have since been so successful in this country and elsewhere. It was his view that residents learned first by adequate examples and assistance at operations and later by actually performing the procedure themselves at a time when they were fully qualified to do so.

The early part of the twentieth century saw massive strides in close alliances between medical schools and teaching hospitals in several centers in the United States. However, the general quality of medical education throughout the country was notoriously inadequate, a fact which led to the detailed study by Flexner that was published in 1910. At that time, the second-rate medical schools represented the major portion of medical education in the country and were in essence providing only diplomas. The Flexner Report succeeded in closing many of the poor schools and placed increased emphasis upon the necessity for quality. A further factor that strengthened the hand of those schools that emphasized excellence was the establishment of the Rockefeller Foundation, which through its general education board made significant grants to such schools as Johns Hopkins, Washington University, and the University of Rochester School of Medicine. It was the influence of these Institutions, together with those at Harvard, Pennsylvania, and Columbia, that were already fully established, that strengthened the foundations of modern university medicine.

The Educational Responsibility of the Teaching Hospital

Following the lead of the more outstanding medical schools, most medical schools in the United States today maintain a strong relationship with a teaching hospital. Recognition of the fact that students need close contact with patients and require liberal patient responsibilities has had a strongly positive effect on the student's educational experience. In the better medical schools, the student is part of the team that cares for the patient and has become identified with the group rather than being solely a student in the eye and mind of the patient. One of the most important advances in medical education in the recent past has been the complete integration of students in their clinical years into the medical team.

Since World War II, the role of postdoctoral education in specialized residency systems has expanded rapidly. Thus, in recent years the
trend for medical students has been to seek postgraduate education in
university hospitals. As an example, the graduating class of the Duke
University Medical School of 1967 showed a marked tendency in this
direction. Of seventy-four graduates, sixty chose internships in university hospitals; four received assignments to federal hospitals and four
selected nonuniversity hospitals. The discrepancy between the number
of interns needed in hospitals throughout the country as compared
with those available is shown in the statistics for 1961 provided by the
National Internship Matching Plan, in which 14,178 positions were
available' with only 7,753 positions actually filled. These statistics are
quite meaningful in terms of adequate recognition of the problem
which exists in the training of physicians in medical schools today.

Research Responsibilities of Teaching Hospitals

Advances in medicine have traditionally taken place in the teaching hospitals affiliated with universities. It is apparent that the proximi-
ty of the laboratories of the various medical schools' departments, the
availability of medical scientists trained in investigative techniques, and
the presence of sufficient patients under study provide adequate reasons for this fact. During the past fifteen years, the importance of the
National Institutes of Health in providing research grants for worthy
investigations has been of unparalleled importance. It is fully recognized that this source of funds has been materially responsible for
research as well as for teaching. Moreover, many students have been
attracted into investigative medicine as a direct result of these programs. Of special significance are the programs sponsored by the
National Institutes of Health for Clinical Research Units. These units
are now established in eighty-one teaching hospitals and funds are provided for the study of patients with interesting disorders for whom
diagnosis and therapy remain a problem. Operating under a policy
which is both broad and wise, directors of these units in the various
teaching hospitals are permitted to authorize qualified members of the
faculty to engage in clinical research on the basis of protocols approved
by local committees. Much important information has already been

obtained in such units, and the prospects for the future are quite impressive. It has already been noted that in addition to the physicians in charge of these investigations, medical students, interns, residents, postdoctoral fellows, dietetic interns, and student nurses participate actively in these investigations.

Economic Aspects of Teaching Hospitals

Advances in medicine have been accompanied by increasing costs, especially in university teaching hospitals. Moreover, the teaching hospitals characteristically have a higher percentage of indigent patients who can afford to pay little or nothing. Although the increasing responsibility of social welfare groups for at least partial payment of hospital expenses has made a favorable impact, the fact remains that the spiraling cost of medical care has created distinct problems for teaching institutions. Virtually all teaching hospitals report deficits in these patient groups. For example, during the five years of 1959–1964, the Duke University Medical Center sustained a loss of $4,871,000 from the hospitalization of non-private patients. In addition, there was a loss of $859,000 in the treatment of outpatients. Such deficits must be sustained by endowment gifts and funds earned in other parts of the hospital. While the hospital administration is quite sympathetic to the teaching needs, it is quite clear that these requirements pose difficult and serious problems on the financial structure of teaching hospitals. The advent of Medicare has helped in some respects since the actual cost is paid on all patients over the age of sixty-five. However, many teaching hospitals depend upon the charges which are slightly above costs for private patients in order to diminish the deficit on the part-pay patients. Thus, it is no longer possible to realize this slight gain from patients who are supported by Medicare.

It has become increasingly apparent that the traditional classes of patients (private and public[1]) will both be required for teaching in the future. Moreover, as government-sponsored insurance becomes increasingly available for all age groups, it is highly likely that the indi-

---

1. The designations "public" and "private" patients are no longer made at Duke.

gent patient will disappear. Clearly, both medical schools and the government have an obligation to produce adequately trained physicians, and the participation of patients is essential.

References

1. Knowles, J. H. *The Teaching Hospital: Evolution and Contemporary Issues.* Harvard University Press: Cambridge, Massachusetts, 1966.
2. Flexner, A. *Medical Education: A Comparative Study.* New York: McMillon, 1925.
3. Smiley, D. F. Medical education today: Its aims, problems and trends, *The Journal of the American Medical Association and Association of American Medical Colleges*, 1953.
4. Hammond, K. R., and Kern, F. *Teaching Comprehensive Medical Care.* Cambridge, Mass.: Harvard University Press, the Commonwealth Fund, 1959.

V

The Heart

*T*he effect of organized cardiac contraction on flow through the capillary bed of the myocardium remains unsettled despite much work that has been done to elucidate this basic problem. Evidence has accumulated in support of two opposing viewpoints. One concept is that the shortening of the muscle fibers during systole compresses the vascular bed in the myocardium and acts as a "throttling" mechanism. The opposing view is that cardiac contraction "massages" or "kneads" the blood through the vascular bed and increases coronary flow.

Chapter 20 ☞

The Coronary Circulation

*I*n discussing the coronary circulation, I will discuss primarily the work that my colleagues and I have performed in the laboratory and in a series of patients with coronary disorders. I am indebted to many coworkers at Hopkins, Walter Reed, Oxford, and Duke for their stimulation and assistance. To my chief, Alfred Blalock, I owe much for his teaching, his assistance in many ways, and his friendship. Following residency training, it was my privilege to spend two years in the laboratory of Donald F. Gregg, who taught me much concerning proper methods of obtaining and interpreting physiological data, and I am greatly indebted to him. Therefore, it is with much gratitude to these teachers and many others that I make these comments on some of the anatomical, physiological, and clinical features of the coronary circulation.

The right and left coronary arteries are the first branches of the aorta and are relatively small vessels, particularly in view of the volume of blood they conduct. While the entire body normally receives an average of 7 ml of blood per 100 gm of tissue per minute, the comparable figure for the heart is 25 ml, or some 300 percent greater than for the body as a whole. The coronary circulation also has a number of unique features that make it quite different from that of other organs. First, except for the heart, blood flow is generally maximal during systole, since arterial perfusion pressure is greatest during this period of the cardiac cycle. However, during systole the intramyocardial coronaries are compressed and blood flow is greatly reduced. During diastolic relaxation of the myocardium, the pressure surrounding the coronary vessels is minimal and therefore coronary flow increases. This phenomenon was demonstrated in experiments with Dr. Gregg by perfusion of the coronary circulation at a constant pressure through an in-dwelling cannula in the coronary orifice (23). Control flows were determined during a period in the normally beating heart and following a period of asystole, and during the latter, coronary blood flow was continued by perfusion. When asystole is induced and the heart enters a prolonged period of diastole, the coronary arterial inflow rises to 170 ml per minute.

Another interesting feature of myocardial metabolism is its high oxygen utilization. For the body as a whole, approximately 25 percent of the oxygen in the arterial blood normally is removed during passage from the arterial to the venous circulation through the capillary bed. In the heart, however, some 65 to 70 percent of the available oxygen is removed in the myocardial capillaries. This is also reflected in the total oxygen consumption of the heart and bears a significant role both in cardiac physiology and in cardiac surgery. In other words, the necessity to perfuse the coronary arteries during open heart surgery at times when the proximal aorta is occluded or open becomes apparent.

The oxygen consumption of the beating heart with a normal cardiac output is approximately 5 to 10 ml per 100 gm of heart muscle per minute. This is compared with the average oxygen utilization of the body as a whole, which is only 0.3 ml per 100 gm per minute. If myocardial oxygen consumption is determined during open heart surgery at a time when the heart is beating but not pumping blood, it is consuming nevertheless an appreciable amount of oxygen, approximately 3 to 4 ml per 100 gm per minute. Moreover, if the heart is in a state of ventricular fibrillation, again without any cardiac output, the oxygen utilization is approximately the same as when the heart is beating in sinus rhythm and without a cardiac output. Finally, when the heart is in a state of arrest with no contraction of any kind, its basal metabolism is appreciable, the oxygen requirements being approximately 25 percent of that required for a normal cardiac output. In other words, the need for at least nearly continuous perfusion of the coronary circulation during cardiac surgery is obvious unless cellular changes occur, which may lead to cardiac decompensation.

Another highly distinctive feature of the coronary circulation is its ability to vasodilate massively and almost instantaneously in response to hypoxia. Thus, nature has provided the heart with a mechanism such that, if the arterial saturation of oxygen becomes reduced, the arterial vessels immediately respond by vasodilation. Within a very short period coronary blood flow can increase to surprising proportions even though the perfusion pressure remains constant. This physiological response is a very rapid one, as can be demonstrated by examination of the oxygen usage of the heart. Thus, myocardial oxygen demands are suddenly reduced by the induction of asystole.

One of the most fascinating and yet paradoxical aspects of the coronary circulation is the fact that nature has provided it with a minimum of collateral vessels. To draw a sharp contrast, one might consider the fact that, during a subclavian pulmonary anastomosis (Blalock-Taussig procedure) for pulmonary stenosis, one can totally ligate the first portion of the subclavian artery without fear of arterial insufficiency in the upper extremity. There are many other examples in the arterial circulation in which a major vessel can be permanently occluded without fear of ischemia. This is because there is an adequate number of natural collateral vessels present that can immediately become functional upon sudden demand. On the contrary, acute proximal occlusion of any of the four major coronary vessels is generally associated with acute coronary insufficiency and myocardial infarction. Thus, in the normal state the heart has very few collateral channels that can become immediately functional. The marked differences between the collateral beds of different tissues are appropriately illustrated by pressure studies proximal and distal to acute arterial occlusion (26). If the femoral artery is suddenly occluded and the pressure is measured both above and below the occlusion, an appreciable pressure can be demonstrated in the distal artery. For example, if the proximal pressure is 120/80 mm Hg, with a mean pressure of 100, the distal pressure would be approximately 75/65 mm Hg, with a mean pressure of 70 mm Hg. The distal blood flow and pressure are, of course, supplied by the natural collaterals that communicate with the artery above and below the occlusion. It is recognized that considerable differences occur among individuals, and generally collateral circulation is more effective in the young. If the same hemodynamic study is performed in a major coronary artery, the results are quite different. With a proximal pressure of 120/80 mm Hg and mean pressure of 100, the pressure in the anterior descending coronary following acute occlusion is apt to show a distal mean pressure of only 20 to 25 mm Hg. Thus, it is obvious that in the coronary circulation the collaterals are quite inadequate to meet the immediate metabolic needs of a segment of myocardium supplied by this vessel, and infarction generally ensues.

In our own studies, and those of many others, collateral vessels are rarely demonstrable by coronary arteriography in hearts that do not have significant coronary arterial stenosis. At least a 50 percent occlusion is necessary and generally 75 percent or more of a major coronary vessel must be occluded in order to produce coronary collaterals. In fact, coronary collaterals of respectable size and number are uncommonly present unless the stenosis of a major coronary artery approaches 90 percent.

Coronary atherosclerosis clearly has become a problem of major national importance, and currently is responsible for over 600,000 deaths annually in the United States.[1] It is recognized that the earliest changes of atherosclerosis may begin in infancy (14) and in routine autopsies on children by the age of ten, grossly apparent lesions are present in 10 percent. Pathological studies of hearts of otherwise healthy, young soldiers in the Korean and Vietnam conflicts, who were killed in combat, have shown a high incidence of unsuspected coronary atherosclerosis (6). A surprising 77 percent of these young men had gross lesions in the coronary arteries easily apparent to the naked eye, and an amazing 10 percent had 70 percent or more occlusions of one of the coronary vessels.

Angina pectoris is a frequent clinical manifestation of coronary atherosclerosis and was first described by Heberden in 1759 (9). This superb and classic description, which is as pertinent today as when written more than 200 years ago, was first called to my attention by Dr. Benjamin Baker in his effective teaching manner on fourth-year Osler medical ward rounds. Heberden was not aware of the basic pathological changes responsible for this symptom complex, but his original description can hardly be improved upon today for its accuracy and incisiveness. It is interesting to reflect upon Osler's observations concerning the pathogenesis of angina pectoris, which were published in a monograph before the turn of the century (15). His observations at that early period are astonishing and deserving of direct quotation:

---

1. This paper was published in 1974.

"It is easy to suppose that a narrowing of the orifices of the coronary arteries, or of the lumen of a main branch, can bring about conditions most favorable for the production of this intermittent claudication — i.e., a state in which, so long as the heart is acting quietly, sufficient blood reaches its muscle; but if called upon to act more forcibly, by exertion or emotion, the larger supply, then needful to maintain the nutrition, might not he forthcoming, with the result of a relative ischemia and disturbance of function. What is the condition of the heart muscle in this ischemia? Is it likely to be the same in the narrowing of atheroma and in the blocking from thrombosis and embolism?" One must admire Osler's brilliance and ability to clearly correlate clinical and pathological findings as evidenced by this classic statement.

The potential role of surgery in the management of myocardial ischemia was first proposed by Francois-Franck, a professor of physiology in Paris in 1899 (8). He recommended cervical sympathectomy, which was first performed by Jonnesco in 1916 with clinical relief of angina (11). During the ensuing years other workers, including Beck (3) and Vineberg (27), made clinical attempts to improve coronary blood flow. Most now agree that the first major advance was the introduction of coronary endarterectomy by Bailey (2) and Longmire (13). A number of these procedures were done in the late 1950s and early 1960s, including a series at Hopkins.

I especially remember a forty-one-year-old gentleman with severe angina in whom a complete occlusion of the right coronary artery was demonstrated by arteriography. A right coronary endarterectomy was performed and the patient was relieved of angina for a period of a year, but then typical symptoms suddenly recurred. Repeat coronary arteriography demonstrated occlusion of the previously endarterectomized segment, a complication which was soon recognized as one of the limitations of this technique. On April 4, 1962, this patient was reoperated upon and a saphenous vein graft was obtained from the leg and anastomosed from the ascending aorta with the use of a partial occlusion clamp. This was illustrated at the time by Leon Schlossberg, the great medical illustrator, whose impact upon surgical teaching has been immense (See figure 1).

The procedure was performed with the use of a partially occluding clamp on the aorta for the proximal anastomosis, thus allowing the

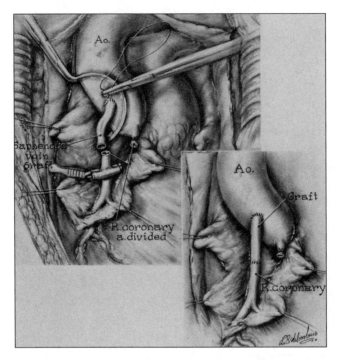

FIGURE 1.
Illustration of use
of saphenous vein
autograft anasto-
mosed from the
ascending aorta to
the right coronary
artery to treat
proximal coronary
arterial occlusion
by Sabiston.

heart to maintain cardiac output (See figure 1). The distal end of the
graft was anastomosed to the right coronary artery, and we were quite
pleased with the immediate results and were hopeful that this technique might open a new approach in the management of patients with
coronary atherosclerosis and myocardial ischemia. We were disappointed, however, that in the postoperative period the patient developed a
cerebrovascular accident and died three days later. At autopsy, thrombus was present at the aortic end of the coronary anastomosis, and we
presumed that an embolus from this site had been swept into the cerebral circulation. Although in retrospect it is obvious that we should
not have been discouraged by this initial experience, nevertheless we
did not repeat it until the notable contributions of Favaloro (7) and
Johnson (10) some six years later. Their successful use of vein grafts in
the coronary circulation has greatly expanded the direct approach to
the management of myocardial ischemia and they are deserving of
much credit for this contribution. This procedure currently constitutes
the greatest single indication for cardiac surgery and of the some

50,000 open-heart cardiac operations performed in 1972. In a survey by the Joint Commission on the Accreditation of Hospitals, 25,000 of these operations were for coronary bypass surgery.

It is now recognized that lesions of the left main coronary artery are especially hazardous, and the incidence of sudden death in this group of patients is quite high. Mortality from this lesion during the first year after discovery has been reported to range from 20 to 50 per-cent, and all groups now recognize the seriousness of this lesion. Ten years ago Dr. Richard S. Ross was referred a thirty-nine-year-old lady with severe angina pectoris. At the time of coronary arteriography, the tip of the catheter could not be made to enter the left coronary orifice and on injection of dye the proximal left coronary was almost totally occluded with only a thread-like lumen remaining (figure 2).

It was elected to relieve this stenosis surgically by excision and enlargement of the lumen by a pericardial graft (figure 3). During the procedure, the anterior descending and circumflex coronary arteries were continuously perfused.

Postoperative coronary arteriography five months later revealed that the left main coronary was quite patent (figure 4). This patient has

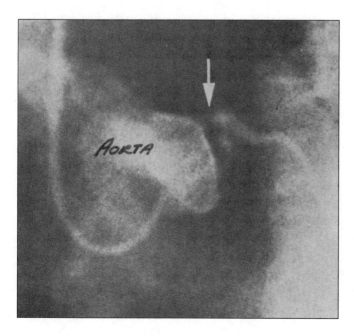

FIGURE 2. Coronary arteri-ogram demon-strating severe stenosis of left main coronary artery. The catheter tip could not be made to enter the coro-nary due to the severity of the stenosis. Contrast medium injected into the arota fills the left coronary artery.

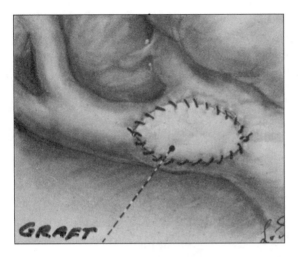

FIGURE 3.   Illustration of operative procedure performed for severe stenosis of left main coronary artery employing extracorporeal circulation. An aortotomy was made for excision of stenotic lesion from within the aorta and with the placement of a coronary-perfusion cannula for constant pefusion while the stenotic lesion was further managed by excision and insertion of a pericardial graft.

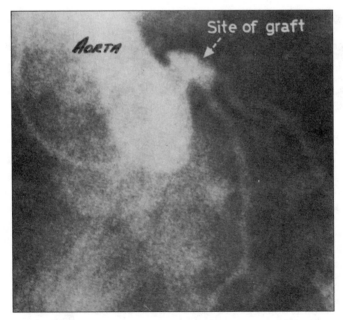

FIGURE 4. Postoperative coronary arteriogram from patient demonstrated in figure 2, showing correction of the stenosis of the left main coronary artery.

remained well during the past ten years and continues to work daily. She represents an example of a long-term follow-up of a direct operation for this serious lesion.

Among more than 500 patients operated on at Duke for coronary arterial occlusion with bypass grafts, approximately two-thirds have been completely relieved of angina, and in an additional 20 percent the symptoms are greatly improved. Similar results have been reported in a number of series from other centers. At present, one of the challenging problems is the appropriate selection of patients for surgery. Generally, the procedure is performed for severe angina, but in selected circumstances the procedure may also be performed for intractable arrhythmias or preinfarction angina. The procedure can be performed as well in association with operations for ventricular aneurysms, mitral insufficiency due to infarction of the papillary muscle, or for revascularization during closure of postinfarction ventricular septal defects.

We have been quite interested in the assessment of a variety of preoperative physiological variables that might aid in developing an accurate prognostic prediction of the operative results (17). In our patients we have found that the ejection fraction of the left ventricle is a very reliable index of prognostic significance. The ejection fraction represents the percentage of blood ejected from the left ventricle into the aorta with each systolic contraction of the heart. In our computerized series, Dr. Robert Rosati[2] at Duke recently informed me that, in a group of patients in whom the ejection fraction was greater than 25 percent, the mortality of the operation was 4 percent, whereas in a group of 20 patients with severe cardiac decompensation in whom the ejection fraction was less than 25 percent, the mortality rate was 40 percent (22). Thus, if the ejection fraction falls below 25 percent, left ventricular function is markedly impaired and revascularization is attended with an appreciably increased risk.

The conventional method for determining left ventricular ejection fraction is the measurement of left ventricular volume by contrast medium during angiography using views in the anteroposterior and lateral positions. This technique, however, requires cardiac catheteriza-

---

2. Dr. Robert Rosati was a member of the Department of Medicine at Duke and played a key role in developing the Duke cardiovascular database.

tion as well as the injection of contrast medium. Dr. Robert Jones[3] in
our department has been interested in determining the ejection fraction by a noninvasive technique which requires only an intravenous
injection of radioactive tracer. The simplicity of this method makes it
suitable for repeated determinations before and after surgery. The
detector of a multicrystal gamma camera is positioned anterior to the
precordium and counts are recorded at 0.1 second intervals for a
minute following intravenous injection of 20 mCi of technetiurn-99
pertechnetate. Computer analysis of the data separates counts arising
from the structures adjacent to the left ventricle from counts observed
within the left ventricular cavity. The change in counts of each contraction of the left ventricle relates directly to the fraction of blood
leaving the left ventricle with each systole and provides a method for
determination of the ejection fraction. Moreover, comparison of the
radionuclide method of ejection fraction with that of the standard
angiographic determination in twenty-four patients shows a close correlation efficient between the two techniques, and the ease of this
study makes it quite useful.

It is well known, as demonstrated by postoperative coronary arteriography following bypass surgery, that previously developed collateral
channels may disappear when the need for them no longer exists.
Moreover, there is recent evidence that this may occur within a very
short period. We have been interested in the rapidity with which
coronary collaterals can develop in the various anatomical areas of the
myocardium.

Drs. Cox, Pass, Wechsler, Oldham,[4] and I performed a series of
experiments in dogs, and observations were made following acute
coronary occlusion in an effort to determine coronary flow and
appearance of functional coronary collaterals to each layer of the
myocardium. Two weeks prior to the experiment, a left thoracotomy
was performed and an inflatable balloon cuff was placed around the

---

3. Dr. Robert Jones, Professor of Surgery at Duke University School of
Medicine.

4. Drs. Andrew Wechsler and Newland Oldham were on the senior staff at
Duke in 1974. Drs. J.L. Cox and H.I. Pass were surgical residents.

anterior descending coronary at its origin and a polyethylene catheter was positioned in the left atrium. The lips of the left atrial catheter and the balloon cuff were buried subcutaneously. Subsequently, each animal was trained daily for two weeks to lie quietly on a padded table for three hours without premedication. On the day prior to the study, the subcutaneous ends of the atrial catheter and balloon cuff were extracted under local anesthesia, and a catheter was also placed in the femoral artery with all incisions being closed. The following day the study was performed in a control state without premedication or local anesthetic since the animals had been trained over a prolonged period to lie quietly.

Myocardial blood flow was measured with injection of radioactive carbonized microspheres with diameters of 8 to 10μ labeled with either scandium 46, strontium 84, or cesium 141. This technique allows injections to be made at varying times with measurement of the specific radioactivity of each of these three substances. Prior to coronary occlusion, cerium 141 was injected into the left atrium and reference sampling was performed. The coronary artery then was occluded by inflation of the peri-arterial cuff, and strontium 85 was injected through the left atrial cannula into the systemic circulation. The coronary artery remained totally occluded through the remainder of each experiment. At either 6, 12, 15, or 24 hours after the coronary occlusion, scandium 46 was injected into the left atrium. The animal then was sacrificed and the heart excised. Both main coronary arteries of the excised heart were perfused with basic fuchsin to demonstrate the ischemic zones of the left ventricle. Perfused areas of the myocardium were stained a brilliant red color and the area distal to the balloon occlusion remained unstained. The unstained ischemic region was removed and designated as the "central" zone of the infarct. A half-centimeter wide portion of the myocardium around the central zone was excised and designated as the "marginal" zone of the infarct. These two tissue specimens were divided into the subepicardial (outer two thirds) and the subendocardial (inner one third) layers and the radioactivity was determined.

The twenty-two surviving animals in this study were hemodynamically stable through the 24-hour period of the study. After coronary occlusion, they showed no evidence of pain, although electrocardio-

graphic changes, consisting of occasional premature ventricular con-
tractions and ST segment depression in lead II, were observed in most
of the animals within several minutes after occlusion.

Immediately after coronary occlusion, the subepicardial flow
decreased but subendocardial flow dropped to a much lower level.
There was no significant increase in the level of collateral flow to the
deepest layer of the subendocardium of the central zone during the
next 24 hours. In contrast, a marked increase in subepicardial flow
occurred, so that by 24 hours after coronary occlusion, central subepicardial flow had returned to almost normal. Although blood flow in
the marginal subendocardium had dropped to 36 percent of control
levels by 12 hours after occlusion, it had returned to 77 percent of
control by 24 hours. The marginal subepicardium was affected least by
coronary occlusion, and blood flow in that area was 97 percent of
control by 24 hours after the coronary had been occluded.

From such studies, it was demonstrated that under normal circumstances subendocardial flow was slightly greater than that in the subepicardium. However, the subendocardium was more vulnerable than the
subepicardium to ischemic injury, and the collateral circulation was not
as effective in returning blood flow to this zone after coronary occlusion. Vessels in the subendocardium must traverse greater intramyocardial distances than those in the subepicardium. Moreover, subendocardial pressure has been demonstrated to be greater than both
subepicardial and intracavitary left ventricular pressure. In all probability, these findings significantly alter the immediate transmural distribution of blood flow following acute coronary occlusion.

Although coronary atherosclerosis is the greatest single cause of
angina pectoris and myocardial ischemia, there are a number of additional lesions that may present a similar clinical situation. Increasing
experience has shown the necessity of being familiar with a variety of
specific causes of myocardial insufficiency.

Origin of the left coronary artery from the pulmonary artery was
first described in 1911 by Abrikossoff in a five-month-old infant who
died of a myocardial infarction and congestive heart failure (1). In
1959 a two-month-old infant was seen at Johns Hopkins by Drs.
Helen Taussig and Catherine Neil with an enlarged heart and signs of
congestive heart failure (24). The electrocardiogram revealed evidence

of a recent anterior myocardial infarction, and on the basis of these findings, origin of the left coronary artery from the pulmonary artery was diagnosed. At operation the heart was shown to have an area of recent infarction. Until that time there was considerable controversy concerning the direction of flow in the coronary artery, and many agreed with the traditional view that it came from the pulmonary artery. However, at operation on this infant samples of blood were simultaneously removed from the anterior descending coronary artery and from the pulmonary artery, with the finding that the oxygen saturation in the pulmonary artery blood was 75 percent as would have been expected, whereas the saturation in the blood from the anterior coronary descending artery was 100 percent. In addition it could be shown that, by occluding the anterior descending coronary artery at its origin, the pressure in it rose from 25 mm Hg to 75 mm Hg. Both these observations indicated that the blood in the left coronary artery must have arisen from the right coronary artery and passed through collateral channels connecting the two circulations. Thus, ligation of the left coronary artery was performed. Following ligation, the blood in the left coronary artery was forced to the capillary bed of the left ventricle rather than allowing it to reflux back into the pulmonary artery. This child is now asymptomatic fifteen years later. Among our group of twenty-four patients with origins of the left coronary artery from the pulonary artery, three have been adults (25). It is interesting that, although symptoms did not develop until adulthood, angina pectoris appeared in each in the twenties. Today, the modern treatment of this condition is the anastomosis of a vein graft from the aorta to the left coronary artery in those patients in whom the size of the coronaries is sufficient to permit it.

Another interesting example of a surgically correctable lesion of the coronary circulation is a coronary arteriovenous fistula. Since the first description by Krause in 1865 (12) more than 200 of these fistulae have been reported in the world literature (5). We have reported a series of twelve patients with this lesion (16). One of our most interesting patients was a one-month-old infant referred to us in congestive heart failure. A continuous murmur was heard low over the precordium, and a coronary arteriogram demonstrated a massively dilated left anterior descending coronary which drained directly into the right ventricle at the apex of the heart. In this infant, it was calculated that more blood was passing through the fistula than was being ejected into the aortic arch. The anterior descending coronary measured 11 mm in diameter with an aneurysm at the site of entry into the right ventricle. It was possible to close this directly at operation, and the child has since remained well.

There is another interesting type of angina that is physiologically related to origin of the left coronary artery from the pulmonary artery (28). We recently saw a sixteen-year-old girl with severe angina pectoris associated with marked aortic insufficiency. At the time of coronary arteriography, it was not possible to enter the left coronary orifice, but injection of the right coronary showed tremendous collaterals that connected with the left coronary circulation. The blood flow was reversed in the left coronary and coursed in retrograde direction to the aorta. The dye accumulated in the left sinus of Valsalva but stopped there in a cul-de-sac and did not enter the aorta. It was concluded that the free margin of the left aortic cusp had become fused to the aortic wall, thus trapping the retrograde coronary flow at that point and at the same time explaining the severe aortic regurgitation. At operation exactly this was found. It was quite easy to dissect the free margin of the cusp away from the aortic wall and to see at this point massive regurgitation of blood from the left coronary orifice. Fortunately, this simple operation has completely relieved this patient of aortic insufficiency, with disappearance of the angina pectoris and syncope attacks that she had previously experienced. This patient adds to the growing spectrum of nonatherosclerotic coronary abnormalities capable of producing myocardial ischemia and that are relievable by direct surgical attack.

At this point attention should be drawn to a patient report in the literature, which is one of the most interesting cases ever to be published. In 1935 Dr. Rienhoff and the late Dr. Louis Hamman described a thirty-six-year-old male admitted to the Johns Hopkins Hospital with the history of having sustained a right inguinal gunshot wound seventeen years previously. He had had an intermittent fever for six months, associated with anorexia and weight loss. Numerous blood cultures obtained at his local hospital had been negative. On examination a mass in the right lower quadrant and a continuous murmur were present, and a diagnosis of an arteriovenous fistula was made. *Streptococcus viridans* was obtained in three blood cultures, and these observations demonstrated conclusively that the patient was ill with *Streptococcus viridans* septicemia. Drs. Rienhoff and Hamman concluded that the most likely source of the bacteremia was the arteriovenous aneurysm, and accordingly it was exposed at operation. Dr. Rienhoff performed proximal and distal ligations of both the common iliac artery and common iliac vein (21). The entire specimen was excised and contained thrombus which was infected, and the same *streptococcus* organism found in the blood was cultured from it. The patient made an uneventful recovery. This represents the first instance of a chronic *Streptococcus viridans* bloodstream infection being cured by any means and, interestingly enough, by surgery. The brilliance of this observation led to the subsequent use of surgery to correct bacterial endocarditis in patients with patent ductus arteriosus in the days prior to the availability of effective antibiotics, and many patients were cured of subacute bacterial endocarditis by surgery alone.

References

1. Abrikossoff, A. Aneurysm des linken Herzventrikels mit abnormer Abgangstelle der linken Koronararterie von der Pulmonalis bei einem funfmonatlichen Kinde. *Virchows Arch.* 203: 413, 1911.
2. Bailey, C. P., May, A., and Lemmon, W.M. Survival after coronary endarterectomy in *Man. J.A.M.A.*, 164, 1957.
3. Beck, C. S. The development of a new blood supply to the heart by operation. *Ann. Surg.* 102: 801–813, 1935.
4. Cox, J. L., Pass, H. I., Wechsler, A. S., Oldham, H. N., Jr. and Sabiston, D. C., Jr. Evolution and transmural distribution of collateral blood flow in acute myocardial infarction. *Surg. Forum*, 24: 154, 1973.
5. Daniel, T. M., Graham, T. P. and Sabiston, D. C., Jr. Coronary artery-right ventricular fistula with congestive heart failure: Surgical correction in neonatal period. *Surgery*, 67: 985, 1970.
6. Enos, W. F., Holmes, R. H. and Beyer, Jr. Coronary disease among United States soldiers killed in action in Korea. Preliminary report. *JAMA*, 152: 1090, 1053.

7. Favaloro, R. G., Effler, D. B., and Groves, L. K. Severe segmental obstruction of the left main coronary artery and its divisions: Surgical treatment by the saphenous vein graft technic. *J. Thorac. Cardiovasc. Surg.*, 60: 469, 1970.

8. Francois-Franck, C. A. Signification physiologique de la resection du sympathique dans la maladie de Basedow, L'epilepsie, l'idiotie et le glaucome. *Bull. Acad. Natl. Med.* (Paris), 41: 565, 1899; cited by White, J. C.: Cardiac pain-anatomic pathways and physiologic mechanisms. Circulation, 16: 644, 1957.

9. Heberden, W. *Commentaries on the History and Cure of Diseases.* Boston: Wells and Lilly, 1818, p. 292.

10. Johnson, W. D., Flemma, R. J., Lepley, D., Jr. and Ellison, E. H. Extended treatment of severe coronary artery disease: A total surgical approach. *Ann. Surg.*, 170:460, 1969.

11. Jonnesco, T. Angine de poitrine guerie par Ia resection du sympathique cervico-thoracique. *Bull. Acad. Med.*, 84: 93, 1920.

12. Krause, W. Uber den Ursprungeiner accessorischen A. coroneria cordis aus der A. pulmonalis. *Z. Rat. Med.* 3rd series, 24: 225, 1965.

13. Longmire, W. P., Jr., Cannon, J. A., Kattus, A.A. Direct-vision coronary endarterectomy for angina pectoris. *N. Engl. J. Med.* 259: 993–999, 1958.

14. Moon, H. D. Coronary arteries in infants and juveniles. *Circulation*, 16: 263, 1957.

15. Osler, W. *Lectures on Angina Pectoris and Allied States.* New York: D. Appleton & Co., 1897.

16. Oldham, H. N., Jr., Ebert, P. A., Young, W. G. and Sabiston, D. C., Jr. Surgical management of congenital coronary artery fistula. *Ann. Thorac. Surg.* 12: 503, 1971.

17. Oldham, H. N., Jr., Kong, Y., Bartel, A. G., Morris, J. J., Jr., Behar, V. S., Peter, R. H., Rosati, R. A., Young, W. G., Jr. and Sabiston, D. C., Jr. Risk factors in coronary artery bypass surgery. *Arch. Surg.*, 105: 918, 1972.

18. Rienhoft, W. F., Jr.: Development and growth of the metanephros or permanent kidney in chick embryos (eight to ten days' incubation). *Johns Hopkins Hosp. Bull.*, 33: 392, 1922.

19. Rienhoff, W. F., Jr.: The histological changes brought about in cases of exophthalmic goitre by the administration of iodine. *Bull. Johns Hopkins Hosp.*, 37: 285, 1925.
20. Rienhoff, W. F., Jr. Pneumonectomy. A preliminary report of the operative technique in two successful cases. *Bull. Johns Hopkins Hosp.*, 53: 390, 1933.
21. Rienhoff, W. F., Jr. and Hamman, L. Subacute streptococcus viridans septicemia. Cured by the excision of an arteriovenous aneurysm of the external iliac artery and vein. *Ann. Surg.*, 102: 905, 1935.
22. Rosati, R. A. (personal communication).
23. Sabiston, D. C., Jr. and Gregg, D. E.: Effect of cardiac contraction on coronary blood flow. *Circulation*, 15:14, 1957.
24. Sabiston, D. C., Jr., Neil, C. A. and Taussig, H.B. The direction of blood flow in anomalous left coronary artery arising from the pulmonary artery. *Circulation*, 22: 591, 1960.
25. Sabiston, D. C., Jr. and Orme, S. K. Congenital origin of the left coronary artery from the pulmonary artery. *J. Cardiovasc. Surg.*, 9: 543, 1968.
26. Smith, G.W., and Sabiston, D.C., Jr. A study of collateral circulation in vascular beds. *Arch. Surg.*, 83: 702, 1961.
27. Vineberg, A. M. Development of an anastomosis between the coronary vessels and a transplanted internal mammary artery. *Can. Med. Assoc. J.*, 55: 117, 1946.
28. Waxman, M. B., Kong, Y., Behar, V. S., Sabiston, D. C., Jr. and Morris, J. J., Jr. Fusion of the left aortic cusp to the aortic wall with occlusion of the left coronary ostium, and aortic stenosis and insufficiency. *Circulation*, 41: 849, 1970.

Chapter 21 ☞

Coronary Endarterectomy

E ndarterectomy has become an accepted and established method of therapy in the management of a variety of clinical conditions that are the result of atherosclerotic arterial occlusion. Removal of lesions by this method from the aortic, iliac, and femoral vessels has been shown to be highly beneficial in the relief of vascular obstruction. Recently the employment of endarterectomy on vessels of smaller caliber, including the internal carotid, vertebral, and superior mesenteric arteries, has also been successful. These encouraging results have stimulated an interest in the use of this procedure in the management of myocardial ischemia produced by coronary atherosclerosis. The present communication concerns a group of clinical observations recently made on several patients with angina pectoris in whom coronary endarterectomy was performed.

A forty-one-year-old-engineer was admitted to The Johns Hopkins Hospital with the complaint of severe chest pain typical of angina pectoris. The family history revealed that the father had angina and died after a cerebral vascular accident. The mother was living and had hypertensive cardiovascular disease. There was nothing significant in the past history. The present illness began seven years before admission with the onset of sudden severe chest pain and prostration. The patient was admitted to a hospital where an electrocardiogram was thought to show evidence of myocardial infarction. He was placed on bed rest for two months and was discharged asymptomatic. Two years later the onset of chest pain was noted on mild exertion. This gradually became more severe and could be induced by walking fifty feet. It was characteristically relieved by sublingual nitroglycerin. The pain ultimately forced him to cease work and remain essentially at rest.

On admission the physical examination was not remarkable. The blood pressure was 120/80, and all peripheral pulses were palpable. Laboratory studies revealed a serum cholesterol of 295 mg. percent. The electrocardiogram at rest was normal, but after exercise the tracing showed ventricular extrasystoles and slight depression of ST1 and marked depression of ST2, ST3, and T4, regarded as evidence of myocardial ischemia. A coronary arteriogram was performed and showed good filling of the left coronary artery and its anterior descending and circumflex branches. The right coronary artery was visualized for distance of approximately 1 cm and a single small branch was patent. There was no filling of the right coronary artery distally, and it was concluded that there was a complete block at this site.

On February 12, 1959, a bilateral anterior thoracotomy with sternal transection was performed using Pentothal and nitrous oxide anesthesia. Both pleural cavities were entered, and the pericardum was opened widely. The left main, anterior descending, and circumflex coronary arteries were each firm but compressible. Palpation of the right coronary artery revealed it to be enlarged and quite hard. It was dissected free of the surrounding fat in the auriculoventricular groove from its aortic origin to the lateral border of the right atrial appendage. It was then occluded with an arterial clamp for five minutes. During this time no change occurred in the systemic arterial pressure, the appearance or action of the heart, or in the electrocardiogram. It was concluded that the right coronary artery was probably totally occluded, and a longitudinal incision was made approximately 2 cm. from the origin. Upon incising the adventitia and entry into the muscular layer, a good cleavage plane was developed. With the coronary arterial dissector the thrombus was freed throughout its circumference, and the dissector was directed toward the aorta. The thrombus was doubly ligated and divided. The proximal ligature was passed through an arterial stripper and the thrombus drawn tightly as the stripper was advanced in the plane of cleavage. As the proximal end of the thrombus was reached, a jet of blood escaped through the arteriotomy. The thrombus was removed and the artery was occluded proximally. With the removal of the distal thrombus an appreciable quantity of back-bleeding occurred. The total length of the specimen was 7 cm. An X ray showed the presence of calcium in the thrombus, and histologic sections demonstrated an area of total occlusion. The arteriotomy was closed with a continuous suture of 6-0 arterial silk with a BV-I needle, and the occluding clamp near the aortic orifice was removed. The chest was closed with catheter drainage of both pleural cavities. The patient recovered without event from the operation. The postoperative electrocardiogram showed minimal ischemic changes. He has since returned to full-time work as an engineer with considerable symptomatic improvement.

Case 2. A forty-nine-year-old man was referred to The Johns Hopkins Hospital with the diagnosis of angina pectoris due to coronary arterial insufficiency. The family and past histories were noncontributory. The present illness began two years before admission with the onset of substernal pain which was characteristically relieved by nitroglycerin. An exercise test performed at the time showed electrocardiographic evidence of myocardial ischemia. The pain became progressively worse and he found it necessary to stop work.

On examination the blood pressure was 140/80. The remainder of the findings were within normal limits except for diminished pulsations in all the arteries of the lower extremities. The serum cholesterol was 365 mg. percent and total lipids 897 mg. percent. The electrocardiographic exercise test was positive. A coronary arteriogram showed satisfactory visualization of the left coronary artery and its branches with no filling of the right coronary artery.

On May 14, 1959, a median sternotomy was performed, and the vessels were palpated. The left coronary and its branches were thickened; the right and hard and uncompressible. The latter was dissected and occluded for five minutes without effect on the systemic pressure or electrocardiogram. The right coronary artery was then opened and a thrombus, 5 cm in length with total occlusion of the lumen, was removed. The technique employed was essentially the same as that in the first patient. It was well tolerated, and the postoperative recovery was unremarkable. The electrocardiogram was normal at rest and after exercise showed ST segment depression. Since discharge the patient has noted a marked reduction in the previous anginal pain and has resumed work.

Case 3. A forty-three-year-old man was referred with a diagnosis of angina pectoris. The family and past histories were noncontributory. Fifteen months before admission the patient had an episode of substernal pain which radiated across the left anterior chest. An electro-cardiogram after exercise was stated to have shown evidence of myocardial insufficiency, and nitroglycerin was found to relieve the pain. The attacks became more frequent, and in April 1958 bilateral ligation of the internal mammary arteries was performed. This did not bring relief, and the use of nitroglycerin was continued in large amounts. Finally he found it necessary to retire completely from work. At the time of admission an attack could be precipitated by walking across the room.

The physical examination was essentially negative. The blood pressure was 125/70, and the laboratory findings included a serum cholesterol of 175 mg. percent and total lipids of 720 mg. percent. The electrocardiogram showed T-wave changes indicative of coronary arterial insufficiency. A coronary arteriogram was performed which demonstrated a block in the left main and circumflex coronary arteries. The right coronary artery filled but was narrowed at its origin.

On September 11, 1959, a left posterolateral thoracotomy was performed. The chest was entered through the bed of the resected fifth rib, and the pericardium was opened widely. The left main coronary artery was quite hard, and the process was found to extend for approximately 2 cm. into the anterior descending and circumflex branches. The main vessel was dissected free of the surrounding tissues, and an occluding clamp was applied for five minutes. No changes occurred in the systemic arterial pressure, heart action, or electrocardiogram. The circumflex artery was opened first, and an attempt was made to dissect the thrombus. It was not possible to withdraw the rather large occluding lesion present in the left main corollary artery through the opening in the circumflex branch, and the wall of the latter was torn in an effort to remove it in this manner. At this point the left main coronary artery was incised, and using the arterial dissector, atheromatous plaques were removed from the origin of the vessel, including its circumflex and anterior descending branches. The involvement in these vessels was extensive, with complete occlusion of the left main coronary artery. It was not possible to remove the obstruction totally, and although the procedure was well tolerated at the time, the patient developed ventricular tachycardia followed by irreversible ventricular fibrillation later on the day of operation. Postmortem examination of the left coronary artery and the anterior descending and circumflex branches showed residual plaques and fresh thrombus. The right corollary artery showed diffuse atherosclerosis with a patent lumen.

The feasibility of direct endarterectomy for the relief of coronary arterial occlusion is dependent upon several factors. These include (1) the anatomical distribution of coronary atheroseleroisis, (2) the status of the arterial vascular bed distal to the occlusion, (3) the technical problem of removal of lesions in the coronary arteries and satisfactory reconstruction, and (4) the predisposition to thrombosis in small arteries after endarterectomy. Although it is possible to answer these points completely, data are presently available concerning each and may be considered in a discussion of the problem.

Distribution of coronary atherosclerosis. Several groups of investigators have studied large numbers of hearts at postmortem examination, and it has shown that in most instances coronary atherosclerosis is a part of generalized arterial disease with involvement of multiple vessels throughout the body. Despite this fact it is well recognized that a considerable degree of atherosclerosis is present throughout the body and yet well tolerated. When serious difficulty occurs, it is usually found to be the result of marked narrowing or complete obstruction of one or more important arteries. Experience has shown that removal of such an occlusion often may provide relief for a prolonged period. Pathologic studies concerning the distribution of atherosclerosis in the coronary arteries indicate that the chief involvement is in the larger, subepicardial vessels while the deeper and smaller intramyocardial vessels are essentially free of disease. In a thorough gross and microscopic study of 400 hearts at postmortem examination, Schlesinger and Zoll (13) concluded that "most zones of occlusion of the coronary arteries are less than 5mm in length." They further observed that "the majority of coronary occlusions are found within 3 cm. of the mouths of these vessels." These and other similar studies (1) confirm the fact that in many instances coronary arterial occlusion is segmental in distribution and occurs near the origin of the vessels.

The arterial bed distal to the site of occlusion. One of the basic principles that determines the success of any endarterectomy is the degree of patency of the vessels distal to the obstruction. The importance of this factor has been observed particularly in the lower extremities where the amount of back-bleeding has been shown to be of great significance in an estimation of the prognosis.

This principle is of added importance in the coronary arteries since these vessels have been termed "end arteries" due to the reduced number of interarterial collateral vessels normally present in the myocardium. Gregg (7) and Gregg and associates (8) have made a significant contribution to this problem in a study of the experimental hemodynamics after chronic occlusion of a major coronary artery. Both back pressure and backflow in the distal portion of the occluded artery were found to be increased greatly after a period of chronic ligation. These studies showed that collateral channels develop and conduct appreciable quantities of blood. Postmortem observations in human hearts have indicated that intercoronary anastomoses greater than 40μm in diameter are not found in normal hearts, whereas collateral vessels measuring 40 to 200μm in diameter regularly develop in the presence of coronary arterial obstruction (3). These collateral vessels supply blood to the coronary circulation distal to the point of occlusion. Further evidence of the patency of the distal coronary bed has been supplied by recent perfusion studies in our laboratory in hearts obtained at autopsy from patients with myocardial infarction. After endarterectomy a marked increase was found in the volume of fluid which could be perfused through the coronary arteries (10). Each of these observations tends to support the view that coronary arteries distal to an obstruction are often patent.

The technical problem of coronary endarterectomy. From the operative viewpoint there is little doubt that endarterectomy is most easily accomplished in vessels of moderate or large size. The initial clinical procedures were performed in vessels of this caliber, but with the passage of time smaller arteries have been attacked and successful results reported. Included in this group are endarterectomies of the internal carotid (6), vertebral (5), and superior mesenteric arteries (14). Widespread interest in the surgical management of occlusive coronary artery disease has led to a consideration of its use for this disease, and Bailey and associates (2) were the first to report a successful coronary endarterectomy. Cannon and coworkers (4) and Longmire and associates (9) have recently presented their results of operation in nine patients. The operative technique employed in the present patients is essentially the one which they developed.

Predisposition of small arteries to thrombosis after endarterectomy. One of the problems that has been encountered in the direct removal of occluding lesions of small arteries has been the predisposition to post-operative thrombosis. The problem is an important one, and further clinical studies are necessary before the final answer to this question is available. In a group of experiments in our laboratory, indirect evidence was obtained on this point. A long segment of the left carotid artery, with the proximal end intact at the brachiocephalic artery, was drawn into a tunnel in the left ventricular myocardium. The branches were allowed to remain open, and the vessel was fixed in place at the cardiac apex by a suture. Under these circumstances the carotid implants remained patent in most of the hearts. However, similar implants of the carotid and femoral arteries into the sternomastoid muscle, liver, and spleen uniformly resulted in thrombosis (11). It is possible that the rhythmic contraction of the heat retards the development of thrombosis. In another experimental study, endarterectomy with removal of the intima and a portion of the muscular layer was performed on the femoral arteries of the dog (12). These vessels were 3.0 to 4.0 mm. in diameter and comparable in size to coronary arteries found in the human. Long term patency of the lumen was demonstrated in 90 percent of the animals by arteriogram and histologic examination. It is recognized that these studies were done on normal vessels, whereas similar procedures on humans are performed in association with atherosclerosis. Current studies are in progress to determine the effect of experimental canine atherosclerosis on the results of experimental endarterectomy in small vessels.

A summary of the several factors considered to be important in the rationale of coronary endarterectomy indicate that the anatomical localization of lesions, status of the distal arterial vascular bed, and feasibility of technical removal are each favorable in selected patients with coronary atherosclerosis. At present it appears that the patient with severe angina pectoris without a proved history of myocardial infarction is the most suitable candidate for the procedure. In our experience coronary arteriograms obtained preoperatively have been of considerable aid in the establishment of an accurate anatomical diagnosis and localization of the lesion. A group of over thirty such studies has been done with no significant morbidity and no mortality.

While experimental and clinical evidence is available that supports the rationale of coronary endarterectomy, the fact remains that in many instances coronary atherosclerosis is an extensive disease and is probably beyond the scope of an excisional therapy. At the present this method should be considered to be in a stage of evaluation, and conclusions regarding its role in the management of coronary atherosclerosis are dependent upon further observation and study.

References

1. Absolon, K. B., Aust, J. B., Varco, R. L., and Lillehei, C. W. Surgical treatment of occlusive coronary artery disease by endartectomy or anastomotic replacement. *Surg. Gynec. & Obst.*, 103: 180, 1956.

2. Bailey, C. P., May, A., and Lemmon, W. M. Survival after coronary endarterectomy in man. *J.A.M.A.*, 164, 1957.

3. Blumgart, H. L., Schlesinger, M. J., and Davis, D. Studies on the relation of clinical manifestations of angia pectoris, coronary thrombosis and myocardial infarction to the pathologic findings with particular reference to significance of collateral circulation. *Am. Heart J.* 19: 1, 1940.

4. Cannon, J. A., Longmire, W. P., Jr., and Kattus, A.A. Consideration of the rationale and technique of coronary endarterectomy for angina pectoris. *Surgery*, 46: 197, 1959.

5. Cate, W. R., Jr., and Scott, H.W., Jr. Cerebral ischemia of central origin: Relief by subclavian-vertebral artery thromboendarterectomy. Surgery, 45: 19, 1959.

6. Debakey, M. E., Crawford, E. S., Cooley, D. A. and Morris, G. C., Jr. Surgical considerations of occlusive disease of the abdominal aorta and iliac and femoral arteries: Analysis of 803 cases. *Ann. Surg.*, 148: 306, 1958.

7. Gregg, D. E. *Coronary Circulation in Health and Disease*. Philadelphia: Lea & Febiger, 1950.

8. Gregg, D. E., Thornton, J. J., and Mautz, F. R. The magnitude adequacy and source of the collateral blood flow and pressure in

chronically occluded coronary arteries. *Am. J. Physiol.*, 127: 161, 1939.

9. Longmire, W. P., Jr., Cannon, J. A., and Kattus, A. A. Direct-vision coronary edartectomy for angina pectoris. *New England J. Med.*, 259: 993, 1958.

10. Sabiston, D. C., Jr., and Blalock, A.: Physiologic and anatomic determinants of coronary blood flow and their relationship to myocardial revascularization. *Surgery*, 44: 406, 1958.

11. Sabiston, D. C., Jr., Fauteux, J. P., and Blalock, A Experimental study of the fate of arterial implants in the left ventricular myocardium with a comparison of similar implants in other organs. *Ann. Surg.*, 145: 927, 1957.

12. Sabiston, D. C., Jr., Smith, G. W., and Talbert, J. L. Evaluation of experimental endarterectomy in vessels of different caliber. *Surg. Gynecol. & Obst.*, 110: 563, 1960.

13. Schlesinger, M. J., and Zoll, P. M. Incidence and localization of coronary artery occlusion. *Arch. Path.*, 32: 178, 1941.

14. Shaw, R. S., and Maynard, E. P. Acute and chronic thrombosis of the mesenteric arteries associated with malabsorption. *New England J. Med.*, 258: 874, 1958.

Chapter 22 ☙

Observations on the Coronary Circulation, With Tributes to My Teachers

*I*n his commentaries published in 1768, the famous English physician William Heberden (1) provided the first clinical description of angina pectoris. Heberden described, in an exceedingly poignant manner, the clinical symptoms of anginia as well as its prognosis. This description is such a classic that it bears frequent repetition. Heberden said:

> There is a disorder of the breast marked with strong and peculiar symptoms, considerable for the kind of danger belonging to it, and not extremely rare, which deserves to be mentioned more at length. The seat of it, and sense of strangling, and anxiety with which it is attended may make it not improperly be called angina pectoris. They who are afflicted with it, are seized while they are walking (more especially if it be uphill, and soon after eating) with a painful and most disagreeable sensation in the breast, which seems as if it would extinguish life, if it were to increase or continue; but the moment they stand still, all this uneasiness vanishes. In all other respects, the patients are, at the beginning of this disorder, perfectly well, and in particular have no shortness of breath from which it is totally different. The pain is sometimes situated in the upper part, sometimes in the middle, sometimes at the bottom of the sternum, and often more inclined to the left than to the right. It likewise very frequently extends from the chest to the middle of the left arm. The pulse is, at least sometimes, not disturbed by this pain, as I have had opportunities of observing by feeling the pulse during the paroxysm. Males are most liable to that disease, especially such as have passed their fiftieth year. After it has continued a year or more, it will not cease so instantaneously upon standing still, and it will come on not only when the persons are walking, but when they are lying down, especially if they lie on their left side, and oblige them to rise up out of their beds. In some inveterate cases it has been brought on by the motion of a horse, or a carriage, and even by swallowing, going to stool, or speaking, or any disturbance of the mind.... The

termination of the angina pectoris is remarkable. For if no accidents inter-
vene, but the disease go on to its height, the patients all suddenly fall down,
and perish almost immediately. Of which indeed their frequent faintness, and
sensations as if all the powers of life were failing, afford no obscure intima-
tion.

Most regard Sir William Osler as being among the greatest physicians of the late nineteenth and early twentieth centuries. In 1897, he
delivered a series of lectures on "Angina Pectoris and Allied States,"
and these were published as a monograph (2). His ability to clearly
associate clinical signs and symptoms with pathological lesions is skillfully illustrated in these presentations. Osler likened the pain of
myocardial ischemia to intermittent claudication of the lower extremities, stating quite simply that claudication is due to obstruction of the
iliofemoral system and appears following excessive muscular contraction. Similarly, he said, angina pectoris occurs in patients with coronary arterial obstructive lesions, and when the heart is forced to over-
work, as during exercise or in the presence of emotional stress, there is
insufficient blood supply to deliver the oxygen needed and anginal
pain results. Osler therefore provided a sound pathophysiological basis
for this very important clinical disorder.

It is rather paradoxical that it was not until 1912 that an ante-
mortem diagnosis of acute myocardial infarction was made. Herrick
(3) described a fifty-five-year-old patient with intractable substernal
pain, pallor, a rapid and weak pulse, and with a low urinary output.
Herrick made a diagnosis of acute coronary occlusion and fifty-two
hours later the patient died. Hektoen, the famous pathologist, performed the posmorten examination and found a severe stenosis of the
left main coronary artery superimposed upon which was a fresh
thrombus. The first suggestion that a surgical approach might have a
role in the treatment of angina pectoris was made by a professor of
physiology at the University of Paris, Francois-Franck (4), in 1899. He
predicted that excision of the cervical sympathetic chain would inter-
rupt the pain fibers to the heart and therefore provide relief for
patients with anginal pain. The procedure was actually performed in
1916 by Jonness (5) of Bucharest with a successful result. Despite the
relief of anginal pain that occurred in some patients undergoing this

procedure, this approach did not provide additional blood supply and was ultimately abandoned.

A number of early pioneers responded to the challenge of augmenting coronary blood flow, including O'Shauhnessy (6) of London, Fauteux (7) of Montreal, Beck (8) of Cleveland, Harken (9) of Boston, and many others who devised procedures designed to revascularize the myocardium in an attempt to increase the number of collaterals and add new vessels to the coronary circulation. Pedicles of tissue such as muscle or omentum were sutured to the surface of the heart, and epicardial abrasion was tried, but none of these techniques ever became widely adopted. Later, Beck and associates (10) attempted to add new arterial blood with a more extensive procedure by creating an aorta-coronary sinus anastomosis with a vein graft designed to perfuse the coronary circulation retrogradely. This approach was also unsuccessful.

In 1946, Vineberg (11) implanted the internal mammary artery into the left ventricular myocardium and showed, to the astonishment of many, that this vessel developed arterial communications with the coronary arteries. Despite the fact that these vessels remained patent for prolonged periods, direct measurement of blood flow in these internal mammary implants performed in patients whose chests were later reopened for other reasons indicated that the blood flow in them was minimal (12). Therefore, this technique became infrequently utilized.

At the time I was a medical student and resident in surgery, Dr. Blalock had surrounded himself with a number of extremely bright young men who were also my teachers, including Drs. Mark Ravitch, William Longmire, William Scott, Rollins Hanlon, William Muller, Denton Cooley, Harry Bahnson, and Andrew Morrow. With each of them I had the privilege of working clinically, both helping them and they assisting me in the operating room. In addition, there were many memorable experiences in the experimental laboratory and in the preparation of clinical and research manuscripts (14–18). Dr. Blalock had taught us all to work together, and this was another of his basic principles that was to remain with us. There were many others in the training program, too numerous to mention individually, but several who have been especially close through the years and are known for their original contributions. They include Dwight McGoon, Jim Maloney, Frank Spencer, and Rainey Williams, and for their positive influence I pay to each grateful tribute.

Shortly thereafter I was called to active duty in the U.S. Army Medical Corps and sent to the Walter Reed Army Medical Center in Washington, D.C. It was fortunate that I was assigned to the Army Medical Service Graduate School there, where I had the privilege of spending two full-time years working with the world-recognized leader in coronary physiology, Donald E. Gregg. He had written the most respected and most frequently cited monograph on the subject, and this book was considered the most authoritative reference in the field (19).

At the outset, he thought my first task should be a review of those basic physiological and metabolic features of the coronary circulation that had become accepted as established facts. He had just been invited by a leading journal to contribute an in-depth review of the coronary circulation and asked me to join him in preparing it (20). Then came a study of those specific aspects of the coronary circulation that were quite unlike the anatomic, physiological, and metabolic features of other body organs. These included the fact that the large arteries are primarily on the surface of the heart and that quite paradoxically the most important organ in the body is endowed by nature with exceedingly few collateral vessels of much functional significance. Moreover, the oxygen extraction of the heart is quite remarkable, since even at rest, some three quarters of all oxygen delivered to the capillary bed is extracted. Finally, the coronary arteries are known to have an extraordinary capacity to undergo massive vasodilation even at a constant arterial perfusion pressure, and this major compensatory feature has often been underemphasized. Much has been written concerning arterial collaterals, and it is generally accepted that arterial stenosis throughout the body favors the development of collateral channels. However, in the human heart this is usually minimal. In studies conducted with my colleagues, Newland Oldham,[1] Joseph C. Greenfield,[2]

---

1. Newland Oldham, Professor of Surgery at Duke University School of Medicine.

2. Joseph C. Greenfield, Professor of Medicine and Fifth Chair of Medicine at Duke University School of Medicine.

and others, the pressures in the coronary arteries were directly measured distal to severe stenoses at the time of operation in a group of patients undergoing operative procedures for myocardial revascularization (21). It was interesting that the distal pressures were generally low, even in the vessels that were completely occluded proximally with a patent lumen beyond as well as those with a 70 percent or greater occlusion. Thus, even in the vessels with total proximal occlusion the mean distal pressure averaged only 30 mm Hg. In other arterial systems with this magnitude of occlusion, the distal pressure would usually be considerably greater. Of primary importance is an appreciation of the oxygen requirements of the myocardium. During normal cardiac output the heart requires a tremendous amount of oxygen, 5 to 10 ml/100 gm/mm. Moreover, in the beating, nonworking heart such as during extracorporeal circulation with no cardiac output, the oxygen requirement is still quite high, and is even higher during ventricular fibrillation. Finally, when the heart is absolutely motionless, the basal metabolic rate of this organ at normothermia is about one fourth of that required for the normal cardiac output. Donald Gregg was deeply committed to objective and reproducible studies of the moment-to-moment oxygen requirements of the myocardium. For this reason, he suggested development of a device designed to place an indwelling catheter in the coronary sinus, allowing blood in it to be continuously withdrawn through an appropriate recorder such that the oxygen levels in the blood could be continuously recorded. He set me, Edward Khouri, and others to work on the development of the project, and ultimately it was possible to utilize a cuvette densitometer that provided accurate calibration curves for determination of myocardial oxygen consumption (27). Using this instrument, we were able to perform instantaneous measurements of oxygen saturation at varying degrees of cardiac performance. A number of additional studies with him then followed (23–26).

On return to Baltimore to assume the assignment that Dr. Blalock had originally given me,[3] I was soon asked by the cardiologists to see a number of patients with severe angina pectoris. During a short period, a series of epicardial operations and Vineberg procedures were per-

---

3. The task was to lead a program in cardiac revascularization.

formed, but the results were disappointing. However, in 1958, Bailey and, independently, Longmire (28) described direct coronary thromboendarterectomy. When Longmire published his early results, I felt that we should attempt this procedure, and we used this technique in a series of patients in Baltimore (29).

In 1962, Connolly and associates (30) reported successful transaortic endarterectomy of the right coronary ostium using cardiopulmonary bypass, and Effler and colleagues (31) did a similar procedure the same year. Our enthusiasm with endarterectomy, as well as that of others, was to greatly diminish, however, within a year or so because of the recurrence of anginal pain in a number of the patients, and when repeat arteriograms were performed there was evidence of occlusion of the previously endarterectomized site in most instances.

After our disappointment with endarterectomy, we turned our attention to the basic problem of the pathogenesis of atherosclerosis and the effects of endarterectomy in healing of such lesions after surgical intervention. In order to achieve this, canine, and, later primate colonies were established for experimental production of severe experimental coronary atherosclerosis (32). Lesions quite similar to those in man developed in these animals. It was also interesting that with the creation of experimental supravalvular aortic stenosis, such that the pressures in the proximal aorta rose as high as 300 mm, the coronary lesions were much more severe.

While the experimental studies were being conducted on the pathogenesis of atherosclerosis, I was fortunate in being able to obtain a Fulbright Research Scholarship to study in England at the University of Oxford. The work there was in association with the Department of Surgery with Professor Philip Allison, the Nuffield Professor of Surgery, and with Sir Howard Florey, the Sir William Dunn Professor of Pathology at Oxford. Florey had expressed an interest in our studies on experimental atherosclerosis, and the work with his group was another unique and unparalleled privilege. At the time I was in Oxford, Florey had directed his research interest to the field of atherosclerosis and its effect upon the healing process. I worked with him and his associates, primarily John C. F. Poole, on endothelium and its growth in atherosclerosis and in the lining of prosthetic grafts (33). In these studies, it was found that endothelium usually spread by replicating itself cell by cell over the endarterectomized or grafted site. The endothelium grew from the native vessels proximally and distally, ultimately meeting in the center of the graft or the endarterectomy site. In addition, islands of endothelial growth in these specimens were observed, which enlarged concentricially and could be demonstrated to originate from vasa vasora spreading through the wall of the endarterectomized site. The ingrowth of endothelium from vasa vasora was demonstrated by phase microscopy. While I was working with Florey, he received the highest honor that can be accorded a British academician, namely, election to the presidency of the Royal Society. I had already learned from him, as I had from Drs. Blalock and Gregg, that great people are basically very kind and thoughtful, and he consistently showed this characteristic to me.

Upon my return from Oxford a great contribution, selective coronary arteriography, had recently been introduced in the United States. It is interesting that the first coronary arteriogram was reported experimentally in 1932 by Rousthoi (34), and he predicted at the time that the technique would ultimately have clinical use. However, to Mason Sones (35) is due tremendous credit for the pioneering technique of selective coronary arteriography, and for this work he was subsequently chosen to receive the Lasker Award. The advent of coronary arteriography refocused attention on a direct surgical approach to the coronary circulation, and we and others turned attention to direct vascular anastomoses of the coronary vessels. In a series of experiments, the left subclavian artery of the dog was ligated distally and the proximal end was rotated inferiorly for direct anastomosis with the severed end of the left main coronary artery. Similarly, the left subclavian was anastomosed to the circumflex coronary artery (36). After many studies on animals, and with the results usually showing patent anastomoses, we felt prepared to apply these principles clinically.

On April 5, 1962, we operated upon a patient with severe angina pectoris and total occlusion of the right coronary artery (see figure 1, Chapter 20). A saphenous vein graft was obtained from the leg and anastomosed from the ascending aorta with the use of a partial occlusion clamp. We were quite pleased with the immediate results and were hopeful that this technique might open an entirely new approach in the management of such patients. However, our optimism was dampened when the patient developed a cerebrovascular accident postoperatively and died, and we unwisely did not pursue this procedure until several years later.

The first successful bypass for a left main lesion was performed by Garrett, Dennis, and DeBakey (38) in 1964. Great credit is due Favaloro (39) and Johnson (40) for bringing this procedure to full fruition, since both championed the coronary bypass procedure simultaneously in the late 1960s.

In 1964, we saw a patient with severe, unremitting angina and a 95 percent stenosis of the left main coronay artery, who was in obvious need of an urgent procedure that would provide additional blood flow to the myocardium immediately. It was elected to correct the stenosis by placing the patient on cardiopulmonary bypass and, through a direct aortotomy, excising the lesion of the left main ostium from within the aorta (37). Our earlier experimental work had emphasized the necessity for continuous coronary perfusion to protect the myocardium, and it will be noted that the right and left coronary arteries were continuously perfused while the procedure was being performed. The stenosis in the left main coronary artery was an extensive one, and after excision a large defect on the anterior surface of the left main coronary artery was apparent. Therefore, a pericardial graft was used to close this defect to prevent narrowing of the arterial lumen. Postoperatively, the patient did very well and a late postoperative arteriogram showed excellent patency of the left main coronary artery (see Chapter 20). This patient has been followed at the Vanderbilt University Medical Center. The most recent report, received in 1984, indicated that there were no cardiovascular complaints, there were only nonspecific changes in the electrocardiogram, and there were no ventricular wall abnormalities seen on the radionuclide angiocardiogram. A personal telephone call quite recently, twenty-one years after the operation, revealed the patient to be asymptomatic and working daily in managing a business. This may be the longest survival of a direct coronary procedure, and one wonders if this technique might not be reconsidered for some patients with this lesion in view of the late results of occlusion of bypass grafts.

At that time we were unaware of the unfavorable prognosis of severe left main coronary lesions, but in 1972, J. Willis Hurst and I were asked to be the medical and surgical consultants to the Veterans

Administration's randomized study conducted by Dr. Timothy Takaro and associates. The results were exceedingly impressive, and since then coronary bypass grafts have generally been recommended for significant left main lesions (41).

In recent years, the improvements in myocardial protection, the conduct of the anesthesia, the technique used for anastomosis, the choice of graft, the use of inotropic agents, and more complete revascularization have each contributed to a striking lowering of surgical mortality. A major advance was made in 1955 by Melrose and associates (42) with the introduction of potassium arrest. In retrospect, perhaps the high dosage employed and lack of sufficient topical hypothermia might have accounted for the discontinuance of the procedure at that time.

However, later the work of Bretschneider and colleagues (43) in Germany, Hearse, Stewart, and Braimbridge (44) in England, and Gay and Ebert (45) in this country each provided sound metabolic evidence of the advantages of placing each cardiac cell in diastolic arrest. Under these circumstances and in the presence of topical hypothermia, oxygen metabolism is reduced to a very low level. My colleagues and I (46) obtained data indicating that potassium alone achieves a great reduction in metabolism, but nevertheless it remains sufficiently high that it is clear that the metabolic activity of the heart must be further diminished by lowering the temperature of the heart.

To Bigelow goes much credit for his original concepts of hypothermia so well expressed in his recent monograph entitled, "Cold Hearts — The Story of Hypothermia and the Pacemaker in Heart Surgery." In this superb work, he (47) states: "What would be the effects of general hypothermia on the metabolism of the body? I could hardly wait to return to Toronto in 1947 to investigate this simple and enchanting theory. The thinking may not sound particularly courageous today. However, one must realize that in those days a fall in body temperature was considered dangerous—something to be carefully avoided in surgery and in the treatment of injury." His contributions will remain of epic proportion.

Many improvements have been made in the technical aspects, including more generalized acceptance of the fundamental contribution of Green (48) in 1970, emphasizing the superiority of the internal

mammary artery as a graft, particularly in relation to long-term patency. This has been fully documented in several clinics, including a
recent publication from the Cleveland Clinic (49). In our institution,
Rankin[4] and associates (50) have performed some interesting recent
studies using internal mammary grafts and have also demonstrated that
early patency is quite high in addition to the fact that improvement in
ventricular function can be demonstrated within several weeks following the operative procedure.

Among the recent advances in cardiac surgery, the fine work that
has been established in the surgical approach to intractable arrythmias
has been dramatic. Guiraudon,[5] Harken,[6] Cox,[7] Lowe,[8] and other have
been pioneers in this field, and the results of therapy for ischemic ventricular tachycardia have been impressive.

Radionuclide angiocardiography has brought much objective,
practical, and useful data in the daily practice of cardiac surgery. Moreover, its potential for the future is apt to be great, especially in view of
some of the new technical advances that are currently available.

Studies on performance of the left ventricle in normal and diseased hearts have been of paramount interest to cardiac surgeons, particularly in selection of patients for myocardial revascularization and in
objectively assessing the postoperative results.

My interest in this field began twenty-five years ago while working in Oxford with Philip Allison, another teacher who taught me
much and who became a close counselor and friend. During the
course of studies on experimental pulmonary embolism it was apparent that a simple, safe, noninvasive, and relatively inexpensive assess-

---

4. Scott Rankin was Professor of Surgery at Duke University School of
Medicine, and now is Clinical Professor at Vanderbilt University.

5. Gerard M. Guiraudon, former Chairman, Department of Thoracic and
Cardiovascular Surgery, Millard Fillmore Health System, and Professor of
Surgery, Assoc. Chief, Division of Cardiothoracic Surgery, State University of
New York at Buffalo, Buffalo, N.Y.

6. Alden H. Harken trained at Duke University and now is Professor of
Surgery, University of Colorado Health Science Center.

7. James L. Cox trained at Duke University and is now in private practice in
Naples, Florida.

8. James Lowe is Professor of Surgery at Duke University School of Medicine.

ment of the pulmonary circulation was much needed. On return from Oxford to Baltimore, I had the good fortune to work with Henry Wagner, a pioneer in nuclear techniques, in development of the pulmonary scan using radioactive microaggregates of human serum albumin (51, 52). After many studies in the experimental laboratory assessing its reliability and safety, the procedure was then employed clinically and has since remained the primary screening technique for the identification of pulmonary embolism in most instances.

In the past several years, my colleagues and I have had an increasing interest in chronic, recurring pulmonary embolism with progressive development of cor pulmonale and right ventricular failure. The radionuclide scan has been of considerable use in the preoperative diagnosis and postoperative follow-up of these patients (53). Our experience with the surgical management of chronic pulmonary embolism has recently been reviewed with my colleagues, W. Randolph Chitwood[9] and H. Kim Lyerly[10] (54).

One of our brightest and most effective members of the faculty, Robert H. Jones,[11] was a medical student in Baltimore and worked with Henry Wagner and me in the laboratory at the time the pulmonary scan was being developed. Fortunately, Robert Jones chose Duke for his residency training, and he has become a world leader in the development of radionucide angiocardiography. This technique provides accurate measurement of cardiac function and images of cardiac chambers at rest and especially during exercise. Dr. Jones has had an immense impact on the use of the radioactive angiocardiogram in assessment of a variety of cardiac disorders. One of his most interesting studies has been a multivariable analysis, which has documented the prognosis of 386 patients with coronary disease treated medically up to $4^{1}/_{2}$ years. It was interesting that the ejection fraction during exercise was the single most important variable that could predict the survival of the patient as well as freedom from a future myocardial infarction.

---

9. W. Randolph Chitwood, former trainee at Duke and Chief of Surgery at East Carolina University School of Medicine.

10. H. Kim Lyerly, Professor of Surgery at Duke University School of Medicine and Director of the Duke Comprehensive Cancer Center.

11. Robert H. Jones, Professor of Surgery at Duke University School of Medicine.

Moreover, recent data show this test to be more important than data about the coronary anatomy as seen on arterlograms in documenting the natural history of patients with coronary disease. In 386 patients with a left ventricular ejection fraction greater than 50 percent during exercise, a very good event-free survival is seen (55). As the ejection fraction decreases below this level, there is a progressive worsening in prognosis such that patients with an ejection fraction of 20 percent during exercise had a 40 percent chance of death within two years. Moreover, these patients had a greater than 50 percent chance of myocardial infarction or death during this period. Such data are quite important in identifying patients likely to have a stable course in the future contrasted with those who are very apt to have potential instability, complications, and death.

In selecting optimal therapy for patients with coronary artery disease, the Duke computerized data base has been repeatedly utilized. A group of 857 patients were identified who had stable coronary artery disease by coronary angiography. These patients were further subdivided into the 208 who showed no ischemia during exercise and compared with the 649 who did demonstrate ischemia during exercise. The survival curves show no difference in the outcome of medical or surgical therapy in patients with anatomic coronary disease who had no physiological ischemia by radionuclide angiography. Even patients with three-vessel and left main coronary disease did not benefit by bypass grafting if their preoperative radionuclide studies were normal. Moreover, relief of pain was not improved by coronary bypass in this subgroup of patients who had no documented physiological ischemia by scan. Therefore, one can draw the conclusion that exercise testing reveals potential problems based upon physiological alterations, whereas anatomic evidence alone is insufficient to predict outcome correctly.

Exercise angiocardiography can also be used to evaluate the influence of coronary artery bypass grafting on left ventricular function postoperatively, as shown by the work of two of our residents, Richard Floyd and Erle Austin. In a study of patients following coronary artery bypass grafting, there is a very slight influence on resting function but a dramatic influence during exercise (56).

Another resident, Richard Peterson, studied a group of patients with Fontan procedures and showed that the cardiac index during exercise is not reduced in these individuals who do not have a functioning right ventricle. John Kirklin[12] wrote this resident a highly complimentary letter which stimulated him to work ever harder to further extend these basic observations. John Kirklin's thoughtfulness in praising work he regards as deserving is another of his many sterling characteristics. His contributions in introducing quantitative and objective data in final assessment rank second to none and have set a high standard for everyone.

The use of radionuclide angiography in determining normal cardiac function during peak exercise has been quite revealing. One of our residents, Stephen Rerych, has attracted a group of world-class athletes to the laboratory for study of their cardiac function at rest and during peak exercise. As an example, he persuaded a silver medalist at the Montreal Olympics to have rest and exercise studies performed (57). The heart rate rose from 51 at rest to 210 beats/mm, the blood pressure increased as would be expected during exercise, and the ejection fraction, which was already a high 74 percent at rest, increased to an almost perfect 97 percent at peak exercise. Moreover, the end-systolic volume was extraordinary in the left ventricle since it was 52 ml at rest with only 5 ml in the left ventricle at the end of systole during exercise. Finally, the cardiac output rose from 7.64 L/min at rest to an extraordinary level of 56.6 L/min at maximal exercise, the highest ever recorded in the literature. In turning toward the future, through much hard work and dedicated commitment, and with the cooperation of the Baird Corporation, Robert Jones has recently been able to devise a new, highly refined multicrystal gamma camera, of which I am confident much will soon be heard.

This instrument can be used in the operating room to obtain measurements of cardiac function immediately after discontinuation of cardiopulmonary bypass and at varying times thereafter. These data permit construction of pressure-volume loops for each individual heartbeat, from both the right and left ventricles. This type of measurement, which can be done early after coronary bypass grafting or other cardiac proce-

---

12. John Kirklin, Chief of Surgery at University of Alabama-Birmingham School of Medicine.

dures, provides a new dimension of objective data available to the cardio-vascular surgeon in the immediate situation in the operating room. This approach should be quite useful in providing objective end points for clinical studies, including the effectiveness of myocardial preservation and the technical aspects of the operative procedure. It also may provide information concerning the clinical benefit that can be predicted following operation. Further studies are being conducted in the operating room and in the intensive care unit at this time on the important changes that occur immediately after surgical procedures.

References

1. Heberden, W. *Commentaries on the History of Cure of Diseases*. London: T. Payne, 1802.
2. Osler, W. *Lectures on Angina Pectoris and Allied States*. New York: D. Appleton & Co., 1897.
3. Herrick, J. B. Clinical features of sudden obstruction of coronary arteries. *JAMA*, 59: 2015–2020, 1912.
4. Francois-Franck, C. A. Signification physiologique de la resection du sympathique dans la maladie de Basedow, l'epilepsie, l'idiotie et le glaucome. *Bull Acad Natl Med*. 41: 565, 1899.
5. Jonnesco, T. Angine de poitrine guerie par la resection due sympathique cervico-thoracique. *Bull. Acad. Med*. 84: 93, 1920.
6. O'Shaughnessy, L. An experimental method of providing a collateral circulation to the heart. Br J Surg. 23: 665–670, 1936.
7. Fauteux, M. Experimental study of the surgical treatment of coronary disease. *Surg. Synecol Obstet*. 71: 151–155, 1940
8. Beck, C. S. The development of a new blood supply to the heart by operation. *Ann. Surg*. 102: 801–813, 1935.
9. Harken, D. E., Black, H., Dickson, J. F., III, Wilson, H. E., III. De-epicardialization. A simple, effective surgical treatment for angina pectoris. *Circulation*, 12: 955–9662, 1955.
10. Beck, C. S., Stanton, E., Batiuchok, W., Leiter, E. Revascularization of the heart by grafting a systemic artery or a new branch from the aorta into the coronary sinus. *JAMA*, 137: 436–442, 1948.

11. Vineberg, A. M. Development of an anatomosis between the coronary vessels and a transplanted internal mammary artery. *Can. Med. Assoc. J.* 55: 117–119, 1946.

12. Sethi, G. K., Scott, S. M., Takaro, T. Myocardial revascularization by internal Thoracic arterial implants. Long-term follow-up. *Chest*, 64: 235–240, 1973.

13. Sabiston, D. C., Jr. Alfred Blalock. Presidential Address. *Ann Surg.*, 188: 255–270, 1978.

14. Ravitch, M. M., Sabiston, D. C., Jr. Anal ileostomy with preservation of sphincter. A proposed operation in patients requiring total colectomy for benign lesions. *Surg. Gynecol. Obstet.* 84: 1095–1099, 1947.

15. Hanlon, C. R., Sabiston, D. C., Jr., Burke, D. R. Experimental pulmonary venous occlusion. *J. Thorac. Surg.* 24: 190–200, 1952.

16. Sabiston, D. C., Jr., Scott, H. W., Jr. Primary neoplasms and cysts of the mediastinum. *Ann. Surg.*, 136: 777–797, 1952

17. Scott, H. W. Jr., Sabiston, D. C., Jr. Surgical treatment for congenital aorticopulmonary fistula. Experimental and clinical aspects. *J. Thorac Surg.*, 25: 26–39, 1953.

18. Sabiston, D. C., Jr., William, G. R. The experimental production of infundibular pulmonic stenosis. *Ann. Surg.*, 139: 325–329, 1954.

19. Gregg, D. E.: *Coronary Circulation in Health and Disease.* Philadelphia: Lea & Febiger, 1950.

20. Gregg, D. E., Sabiston, D. C., Jr. Current research and problems of the coronary circulation. *Circulation*, 13: 916–927, 1956.

21. Oldham, H. N., Jr., Rembert, J. C., Greenfield, J. C., Jr., Wechsler A. S., Sabiston, D. C., Jr. Intraoperative relationships between aorto-coronary bypass graft blood flow, peripheral coronary artery pressure and reactive hyperemia. *Primary and Secondary Angina Pectoris.* A. Maseri, G.A. Klassen, M. Lesch, Eds. New York: Grune & Stratton, Inc., 1978.

22. Sabiston, D. C., Jr., Khouri, E. M., Gregg, D. E. Use and application of the cuvette densitometer as an oximeter. *Circ. Res.*, 5: 125–128, 1957.

23. Sabiston, D. C. Jr., Gregg, D. E. Coronary arterial inflow, coronary sinus drainage, and myocardial oxygen consumption in asystole and ventricular fibrillation. *Fed. Proc.*, 14: 127, 1955.

24. Sabiston, D. C., Jr., Theilen, E. O., Gregg, D. E. The relationship of coronary blood flow and cardiac output and other parameters in hypothermia. *Surgery*, 38: 498–505, 1955.

25. Sabiston, D. C., Jr., Theilen, E. O., Gregg, D. E. Physiologic studies in experimental high output cardiac failure produced by aortic-caval fistula. *Surg. Forum*, 6: 233–237, 1956.

26. Shadle, O. W., Ferguson, T. B., Sabiston, D. C., Jr., Gregg, D. E. The hemodynamic response to lantoside C of Dogs with experimental aortic-caval firstulas. *J. Clin. Invest.*, 36: 336–339, 1957.

27. Bailey, C. P., May, A., Lemmon, W. M: Survival after coronary endarterectomy in man. *JAMA*, 164: 641–646, 1957.

28. Longmire, W. P., Jr., Cannon, J.A., Kattus, A. A. Direct-vision coronary endarterectomy for angina pectoris. *N. Engl. J. Med.*, 259: 993–999, 1958.

29. Sabiston, D. C., Jr.: Coronary endarterectomy. *Am. Surg.*, 26: 217–226, 1960.

30. Connolly, J. E., Eldridge, F. L., Calvin, J. W., Stemmer, E. A. Proximal coronary-artery obstruction. Its etiology and treatment by transaortic endarterectomy. *N. Engl. J. Med.*, 271: 213–219, 1964.

31. Effler, D. B., Groves, L. K., Sones, F. M., Jr., Shirey, E. K. Endarterectomy in the treatment of coronary artery disease. *J. Thorac Cardiovasc Surg.*, 47: 98–108, 1964.

32. Sabiston, D. C., Jr., Smith, G. W., Talbert, J. L., Gutelius, J., Vasko J.S. Experimental production of canine coronary atero-sclerosis. *Ann. Surg.*, 153: 13–22, 1961.

33. Poole, J. C. F., Sabiston, D. C., Jr., Florey, H. W., Allison P. R. Growth of endothelium in arterial prosthetic grafts and following endarterectomy. *Surg. Forum*, 13: 225–227, 1962.

34. Rousthoi: Über Angiokardiographie. Vorlaufige Mittei-lung. *Acta Radiol.*, 14: 419–423, 1933.

35. Sones, F. M., Jr., Shirey, E. K. Cine coronary arteriography. *Mod. Conc. Cardiovasc.*, Dis. 31: 735–738, 1962.

36. Sabiston, D. C., Jr., Blalock, A. Physiologic and anatomic determinants of coronary blood flow and their relationship to myocardial revascularization. *Surgery*, 44: 406–423, 1958.
37. Sabiston, D. C., Jr. The coronary circulation. The William F. Rienhoff, Jr., Lecture. *Johns Hopkins Med. J.*, 134: 314–329, 1974.
38. Garrett, H. E., Dennis, E. W., DeBakey, M. E. Aortocoronary bypass with saphenous vein graft. Seven-year follow-up. *JAMA*, 223: 792–794, 1973.
39. Favaloro, R. G. Saphenous vein autograft replacement of severe segmental coronary artery occlusion. Operative repair. *Ann. Thorac. Surg.*, 5: 334–339, 1968.
40. Johnson, W. D., Flemma, R. J., Lepley, D., Jr. Direct coronary surgery utilizing multiple-vein bypass grafts. *Ann. Thorac. Surg.*, 9: 436–444, 1970.
41. Takaro, T., Hultgren, H. N., Lipton, M. J., Detre, K. M. Participants in the Study Group: The VA cooperative randomized study of surgery for coronary arterial occlusive disease. II. Subgroup with significant left main lesions. *Circulation*, 54: Suppl 3: 107–117, 1976.
42. Melrose, D. G., Dreyer, B., Bentall, H. H., Baker, J. B. E. Elective cardiac arrest. *Lancent*, 2: 21–22, 1955.
43. Bretschneider, H. J., Hubner, G., Knoll, D., Lohr, B., Nordbeck H., Spieckermann, P. G. Myocardial resistance and tolerance to ischemia. Physiological and biochemical basis. *J. Cardiovasc. Surg.*, 16: 241–260, 1975.
44. Hearse, D. J., Stewart, D. A., Brimbridge, M. V. Cellular protection during myocardial ischemia. The development and characterization of a procedure for the induction of reversible ischemic arrest. *Circulation*, 54: 193–202, 1976.
45. Gay, W. A., Jr., Ebert, P. A. Functional, metabolic, and morphologic effects of potassium-induced cardioplegia. *Surgery*, 74: 284–290, 1973.
46. Chitwood, W. R., Jr., Sink, J. D., Hill, R. C., Weschsler, A. S. Oxygen consumption and transmural coronary blood flow in the potassium-arrested heart. *Ann. Surg.*, 190: 106–116, 1979.

47. Bigelow, W. G. Cold Hearts — *The Story of Hypothermia and the Pacemaker in Heart Surgery.* Toronto, Ontario: McClelland and Stewart, Ltd., 1984.

48. Green G. E., Stertzer, S. H., Gordon R. B., Tice D. D. Anastomosis of the internal mammary artery to the distal left anterior descending coronary artery. *Circulation,* 42: Suppl. 2: 79, 1970.

49. Lytle, B. W., Loop, F. D., Cosgrove, D. M., Ratliff, N. B., Easley, K., Taylor, P. C. Long-term (5 to 12 years) serial studies of internal mammary artery and saphenous vein coronary bypass grafts. *J. Thorac. Cardiovasc. Surg.,* 89: 248–258, 1985.

50. Rankin, J. S., Newman, G. E., Muhlbaier, L. H., Behar, V. S., Phillips, H. R., Sabiston, D. C., Jr. The effects of coronary revascularization on left ventricular function in ischemic heart disease. *J. Thorac. Cardiovasc. Surg.,* 90: 818–832, 1985.

51. Wagner, H. N., Jr., Sabiston, D. C., Jr., McAfee, J. G., Tow, D., Stern, H. S. Diagnosis of massive pulmonary embolism in man by radioisotope scanning. *N. Engl. J. Med.,* 271: 377–384, 1964.

52. Sabiston, D. C., Jr. , Wagner, H. N., Jr. The diagnosis of pulmonary embolism by radioisotope scanning. *Ann. Surg.,* 160: 575–588, 1964.

53. Sabiston, D. C., Jr., Wolfe, W. G., Oldham, H. N., Jr., Wechsler, A. S., Crawford, F. A., Jr., Jones, K. W., Jones, R. H. Surgical management of chronic pulmonary embolism, *Ann. Surg.,* 185: 699–712, 1977.

54. Chitwood, W. R. Jr., Lyerly, H. K., Sabiston, D. C., Jr. Surgical management of chronic pulmonary embolism. *Ann. Surg.,* 201: 11–26, 1985.

55. Pryor, D. B., Harrell, F. E., Jr., Lee, K. L., Rosati, R. A., Coleman, R. E., Cobb, F. R., Califf, R. M., Jones, R. H. Prognostic indicators from radionuclide angiography in medically treated patients with coronary artery disease. *Am. J. Cardiol.,* 53: 18–22, 1984.

56. Floyd, R. D., Wagner, G. S., Austin, E. H., Sabiston, D. C., Jr., Jones, R. H. Relation between QRS changes and left ventricular function after coronary artery bypass grafting. *Am. J. Cardiol.,* 52: 943–949, 1983.

57. Rerych, S. K., Scholz, P. M., Newman, G. E., Sabiston, D. C., Jr., Jones, R. H.: Cardiac function at rest and during exercise in normals and in patients with coronary heart disease. Evaluation by radionuclide angiocardiography. *Ann Surg.*, 187: 449–464, 1978.

Chapter 23 ☙

Effect of Cardiac Contraction on Coronary Blood Flow[1]

*T*he effect of organized cardiac contraction on flow through the capillary bed of the myocardium remains unsettled despite much work that has been done to elucidate this basic problem. Evidence has accumulated in support of two opposing viewpoints. One concept is that the shortening of the muscle fibers during systole compresses the vascular bed in the myocardium and acts as a "throttling" mechanism. The opposing view is that cardiac contraction "massages" or "kneads" the blood through the vascular bed and increases coronary flow. The primary objective in this study has been an evaluation of the effect of organized myocardial contraction on coronary flow in the intact animal. This problem has been attacked by the elimination of this factor by the induction of ventricular asystole or ventricular fibrillation.

In the experimental animal the basic and controversial problem was studied of the influence of cardiac contraction on coronary blood flow. Normally beating hearts were perfused at a constant pressure, and coronary inflow and outflow were determined. In order to assess the role of systole, prolonged periods of ventricular asystole and fibrillation were induced and observations were made of the changes in coronary flow. With the cessation of cardiac contraction, blood flow in the coronary arteries and coronary sinus rose appreciably.

The results of these studies support the concept that contraction of the heart muscle, by compression of the myocardial vascular bed,

---

1. Coauthored with Donald E. Gregg, M.D., Ph.D. in 1957.

behaves as a throttling mechanism and impedes coronary flow. The method employed permitted a separation and quantitation of the effects on coronary flow resulting from cardiac contraction and the vasomotor state of the coronary vessels.

For nearly three centuries physiologists have debated the question of the direction and magnitude of the effect of ventricular systole on coronary blood flow. In 1689 Scaramucci expressed the view that the coronary vessels filled during ventricular relaxation and emptied during ventricular contraction (3). The names of Thebesius, Vieussens, and Morgagni are associated with those who maintained that the coronary arteries are prevented from filling during systole due to closure of their orifices by the aortic valves (3). While now all agree that the latter mechanism is untenable, there is much less certainty regarding the effect of organized contraction of cardiac muscle fibers on coronary blood flow. With skeletal muscle the analogous situation is more clearly understood and the experimental results have been in closer agreement. Many observers have reported increased venous outflow during the contraction of this type of muscle. Blalock first made simultaneous observations of arterial inflow and venous drainage in the gastrocnemius before, during, and after contraction. These studies clearly demonstrated a reduction in flow in the artery during and after contraction (4). By use of the technic of direct transillumination, Knisely and associates have observed flow in the capillary bed of the frog and its relationship to muscular contraction (5). It was observed that the striated muscle fibers became wider and compressed the capillaries enough to stop flow at the beginning of a powerful contraction. As individual fibers began to relax, flow began again. Studies on the myocardial vascular bed with this technic have shown compression of the capillaries by ventricular contraction to the point of erythrocyte standstill.

The importance of ventricular systole in the control of coronary flow is illustrated in a number of studies. In the left coronary artery perfused during systole at a pressure approximately equal to the prevailing mean aortic pressure, arterial inflow approaches (7). Other studies have shown that for an equivalent time period, left coronary artery systolic inflow is less than diastolic inflow (7–9). These observations lend support to the concept that organized ventricular contraction results in diminished coronary flow. However, in other studies the systolic flow in the coronary sinus has been observed to be much greater than the diastolic flow, which might suggest that ventricular systole augments coronary flow (10) and coronary sinus drainage has been noted to decrease during ventricular fibrillation. From the available data there is evident a lack of agreement as to the net effect of systolic contraction on flow in the coronary bed.

It is a difficult task to assess the factor of the extravascular myocardial support, and several groups of investigators have made attempts to evaluate its role in the regulation of flow in the heart-lung preparation. Various methods have been employed in an effort to clarify this problem. Hilton and Eichholtz (12), Hammouda and Kinosita (13), and Anrep and Hausler (14) have employed ventricular fibrillation to remove, at least in part, the effect of cardiac contraction and have determined the changes that occur in coronary flow. These investigators found that in this preparation coronary arterial inflow increased during fibrillation. In contradistinction to this, Osher (15), in studying the pressure-coronary sinus flow relationships of perfused hearts both beating and fibrillating, found a decreased flow during ventricular fibrillation. Garcia Ramos (11) also noted less flow during ventricular fibrilliation in the isolated mammalian heart perfused by the circulating blood of another animal. Recently Wiggers (10) has presented an evaluation of the effect of ventricular contraction on coronary flow by integrating phasic flow curves recorded from the coronary sinus. Measurements were made of instantaneous flow in the coronary sinus in late diastole when the effects of myocardial compression and volume elasticity were minimal. From these data it was concluded that systole results in an augmentation in coronary flow. The validity of an analysis based upon phasic flow data rests upon the assumption that flow in the epicardial arteries and veins represents actual flow in the myocardial capillary bed. This point remains to be proved.

A method has been devised in the present studies that is thought to measure separately the magnitude and direction of the effect of mechanical ventricular activity on flow through the coronary bed and that also permits simultaneous quantitation of the vasomotor state of the coronary vessels. This method consists essentially of the simultaneous recording of blood flow in the left coronary artery and coronary sinus together with the mean coronary perfusion pressure and mean aortic pressure. The coronary system was perfused at a constant pressure approximating the prevailing mean aortic pressure, and measurements were made in the normally beating heart and then during ventricular asystole induced by vagal stimulation. The possible effect of vagal stimulation *per se* on the coronary vessels is a factor deserving comment. Anrep (3) has shown that section of the vagi leads to an increase in coronary flow even when the heart rate is kept constant. Stimulation of the peripheral end of the vagus with rhythmically interrupted faradic current resulted in a slower heart rate with little change in coronary flow during the first 30 seconds. Flow then began to diminish, reaching a minimum in 1 to $1\frac{1}{2}$ minutes. The important point relative to the studies reported here is that vagal stimulation would not be expected to have a direct intrinsic effect on the vessel wall that would result in an increase in coronary flow. A flow change, if any, would presumably be opposite in direction from that following the reduction or removal of the extravascular support. For comparison, similar determinations were made before and after ventricular fibrillation, and it was demonstrated that coronary flow was increased under the latter circumstances.

The induction of ventricular asystole invariably has been associated with a marked rise in coronary arterial inflow and coronary sinus drainage. The level of coronary flow reached during ventricular asystole is thought to represent that due to the vasomotor state of the coronary bed alone at the prevailing aortic pressure and the increase in flow that occurs during asystole to indicate the magnitude and direction of the effect of myocardial contraction on blood flow through the myocardial wall. Trends of the same direction but of smaller magnitude occurred when the ventricle was in a state of fibrillation.

In summary, coronary arterial inflow and coronary sinus drainage have been determined in the perfused heart in both the beating state and after withdrawal of the extravascular support by the induction of asystole or ventricular fibrillation. The removal of the extravascular support by this means invariably resulted in an increase in flow in the coronary arterial bed and in the venous drainage from the coronary sinus. Evidence is presented to advance the concept that the net effect of ventricular contraction is to impede coronary flow. Contrariwise, the removal of this factor results in an increase in flow through the myocardial vascular bed. It is believed that this approach supplies a method for the separation and quantitation of the effects on the left coronary flow of myocardial contraction and of the smooth muscle in the walls of the coronary vessels.

References

1. Shipley, R. E., and Wilson, C. An improved recording rotameter. *Proc. Soc. Exper. Biol. & Med.*, 78: 724, 1951.

2. Anrep, G. V. The circulation in striated and plain muscles in relation to their activity. *The Harvey Lectures*, XXX. Baltimore: The Williams & Wilkins Company, 1936, p. 146.

3. Anrep, G. V. *Lane Medical Lectures: Studies in Cardiovascular Regulation*. California: Stanford University Press, 1936.

4. Blalock, A. Observations upon the blood flow through skeletal muscles by the use of the hot wire anemometer. *Am. J. Physiol.*, 95: 554, 1930.

5. Knisely, M. K. Mechanical effects of ventricular systole on coronary flow. In *Shock and Circulatory Homeostasis*. Transactions of the Forth Conference, Dec., 6–8, 1954. New York, Josiah Macy, Jr., Foundation, 1955, p. 255.

6. Gregg, D. E., and Green, H. D. Effects of viscosity, ischemia, cardiac output and aortic pressure on coronary blood flow measured under a constant perfusion pressure. *Am. J. Physiol.*, 130: 114, 1940.

7. Gregg, D. E., and Green, H. D. Phasic changes in flow through different coronary branches. In *Blood, Heart and Circulation*. Publication of the American Association for the Advancement of Science, No. 13. Lancaster, Pa.: The Science Press, 1940, p. 81.

8. Gregg, D. E., and Green, H. D., and Green, H. D. Registration and interpretation of normal phasic inflow into a left coronary artery by an improved differential manometric method. *Am. J. Physiol.*, 130: 114, 1940.

9. Gregg, D. E., and Green, H. D. *The Coronary Circulation in Health and Disease*. Philadelphia: Lea & Febiger, 1950.

10. Wiggers, C. J. The interplay of coronary vascular resistance and myocardial compression in regulating coronary flow. Circulation Research 2: 271, 1954.

11. Garcia Ramos, J., Alanis, J., and Rosenbluth, A. Estudios sobrela circulacion coronaria. *Arch. Inst. Cardiol. Mexico*, 4: 474, 1950.

12. Hilton, R., and Eichholtz, F. Influences of chemical factors on coronary circulation. *J. Physiol.*, 59: 413, 1924.

13. Hammouda, M., and Kinosita, R. The coronary circulation in the isolated heart. *J. Physiol.*, 61: 615, 1926.

14. Anrep, G. V., and Hausler, H. The coronary circulation. II. The effect of changes of temperature and of heart rate. *J. Physiol.*, 67: 299, 1929.

15. Osher, W. J. Pressure-flow relationship of the coronary system. *Am. J. Physiol.*, 172: 403, 1953.

Chapter 24

The Direction of Blood Flow in Anomalous Left Coronary Artery Arising from the Pulmonary Artery[1]

M yocardial infarction in infancy secondary to the anomalous origin of the left coronary artery from the pulmonary artery is now a condition that is being recognized with increasing frequency during life.

One of the more interesting aspects of this congenital abnormality is the problem of the direction of the blood flow in the left coronary artery. In 1886 St. John Brooks (1) first postulated that the flow in an anomalous corollary artery was retrograde. Following an anatomic dissection in two cases in which the right coronary artery arose from the pulmonary artery, he concluded that arterial blood flowed from the normal left coronary artery, which arose from the aorta, through anastomotic collateral vessels into the right coronary artery, with ultimate drainage into the pulmonary artery. If the flow is retrograde, it is apparent that one of the coronary arteries is not only failing to supply the myocardium but is actually draining fully oxygenated blood from the heart into the pulmonary artery. Recently Edwards (2) and others have presented further evidence in support of this view. The present communication concerns a patient with anomalous origin of the left coronary artery from the pulmonary artery in whom the direction of blood flow in this vessel was studied and demonstrated conclusively.

---

1. Coauthored with Catherine A. Neill M.D. and Helen B. Taussig M.D. in 1960.

Case Report

A two-and-a-half-month-old male infant was referred to the Harriet Lane Home Cardiac Clinic of the Johns Hopkins Hospital on June 3, 1959. He was originally examined at the Memorial Hospital of the University of North Carolina, where a diagnosis of an anomalous origin of the left coronary artery from the pulmonary artery had been made by Drs. Herbert Harned and George Summer. The family history was not contributory. The child had a four-year-old sibling, who was healthy and normal. The mother had noted considerable vomiting toward the end of the pregnancy and her weight gain had been twenty-eight pounds. Delivery was performed by Cesarean section twelve days prior to term and an excessive amount of amniotic fluid was noted. The birth weight was seven pounds eleven ounces. He was a slow feeder from the beginning, and had slightly grunting respirations. An examination at the end of one month was normal. When the infant was approximately six weeks of age, he suddenly became quite red in the face and vomited during a feeding and was dyspneic for a short time. Approximately two weeks prior to admission he became irritable and had a deep reddish-blue color of the skin. He was very dyspneic and vomited several times. Shortly thereafter the attending pediatrician noted a heart murmur. Chest films were interpreted as showing cardiomegaly, and the child was referred to the Memorial Hospital of the University of North Carolina. Marked cardiac enlargement was noted, and a grade-I systolic murmur was present along the left sternal border and at the apex. An electrocardiogram showed sinus tachycardia and the pattern of a recent anterior myocardial infarction. A cineangiocardiogram showed the left ventricle to he markedly enlarged, with a very thin wall. There was no evidence of an intracardiac shunt. A diagnosis of anomalous origin of the left coronary artery from the pulmonary artery was made.

On admission to the Johns Hopkins Hospital the infant's weight was eleven pounds, eleven ounces. He appeared well developed and well nourished. He was active, alert, and without cyanosis. The respirations were forty-four per minute and had a grunting quality, but there was no marked respiratory distress. The heart was enlarged to the left anterior axillary line and the sounds were somewhat distant.

The second aortic and pulmonary sounds were equal. A grade-IT, slightly harsh, systolic murmur was heard along the left sternal border and radiated over the precordium. The blood pressure in the right arm by the flush technic was 90. The femoral pulses were easily palpable. The lungs were clear to percussion and auscultation. The liver was palpable 1.5 cm. below the right costal margin and the spleen was felt 2 cm. below the left costal margin. The remainder of the examination was not remarkable.

Laboratory data: The hematocrit value was 32, the hemoglobin 10.1 gm. per 100 ml., and the leukocyte count was 13,550 per mm. An electrocardiogram showed sinus tachycardia at 140 per minute, left axis deviation, deep Q in leads I, aVl, V3, and V5 elevation of the S-T segments and inverted T waves in V5 and V6. The diagnosis was made of recent anterior infarction.

A review of the chest films showed marked cardiomegaly with normal pulmonary vascular markings. The cineangiocardiogram revealed a small right heart with a massively dilated left ventricle. The left ventricular wall was quite thin and pulsations were barely discernible. No evidence of filling of the left coronary artery from the pulmonary artery was seen. The diagnosis of anomalous origin of the left coronary artery from the pulmonary artery was confirmed and it was decided that an operation should be performed. On June 6 the infant was lightly anesthetized with cyclopropane and a left anterior thoracotomy was performed with entrance into the chest through the fourth intercostal space. A considerable amount of fluid escaped from the pericardium. The left ventricle was greatly dilated.

A definite myocardial infarct was present on the anterolateral surface of the left ventricle measuring approximately 3 by 4 cm. With each beat of the heart the area of the infarct bulged paradoxically. A chest retractor was poorly tolerated, producing arrhythmias, bradycardia, and hypotension.

It was removed and most of the operative procedure was done without it. The left coronary artery was dissected and was found to arise from the pulmonary artery. It was a vessel of normal size and its anterior descending and circumflex branches were also visualized. The pressure in the left coronary artery was recorded at 30/15 mm Hg. An arterial clamp was then applied to the proximal portion of the artery at its origin and the distal pressure was found to be 75 mm Hg systolic. A simultaneous local pressure from the pulmonary artery was 25 mm. Hg. A sample of blood from the anomalous left coronary artery was found to have 100 percent oxygen saturation. At the same time saturation of a sample from the pulmonary artery was 76 percent. These observations were considered to demonstrate conclusively that the flow in the anomalous coronary artery was retrograde into the pulmonary artery. The anomalous artery was then ligated with three suture ligatures proximal to its division into anterior descending and circumflex branches. At this the time systolic systemic arterial pressure rose from 90 to 120 mms. Hg, and it was thought that movement of the left ventricular infarct was less paradoxical. Concentrated phenol was then applied to the entire surface of the heart for de-epicardialization. The pericardium was left open and the chest was closed with catheter drainage of the pleural cavity. The patient tolerated the procedure well. An electrocardiogram was recorded continuously during the procedure and no significant or persistent changes occurred. Following operation the child made an uneventful recovery. The mother noted a marked difference in his appetite and in ability to eat without respiratory distress. Six months after operation his physician reported that he was gaining weight and doing well. A recent electrocardiogram definitely showed less evidence of left ventricular myocardial ischemia, and a chest film showed a slight decrease in the size of the heart.

In 1911, Abrikossoff first reported anomalous origin of the left coronary artery from the pulmonary artery. Little interest was shown in this condition except for occasional reports, until 1933, when Bland, White, and Garland (4) first recorded an electrocardiogram in an infant with this condition and described the clinical and pathologic features. More than sixty cases are now recorded in the literature. Early diagnosis of anomalous origin of the left coronary artery from the pulmonary artery is essential if successful therapy is to be employed. In many infants with this anomaly myocardial damage may become so extensive that the changes become largely irreversible within a relatively short period. For this reason early recognition and diagnosis is imperative if the most successful results are to be obtained by surgical therapy. The condition should be suspected in an infant having cardiomegaly associated with electrocardiographic evidence of left ventricular infarction. Further confirmation may be obtained by angiocardiography with demonstration of a normal right ventricle and a massively enlarged, thin-walled, left ventricle. It has been noted previously that the anomalous left coronary does not usually fill from the pulmonary artery when contrast media are injected into the right side of the heart, but the normal right coronary artery arising from the aorta may be demonstrated by the performance of a retrograde aortogram. The seriousness of this anomaly is emphasized by the fact that in untreated cases death secondary to myocardial infarction and cardiac failure usually occurs within the first five months. An excellent review of the clinical manifestations and course of infants with this anomaly has been published recently by Keith (5).

In the past, various forms of surgical therapy have been advocated. Gasul and Loeffler (6) first suggested the creation of an aortic-pulmonary fistula in an effort to increase the arterial pressure and oxygen content of the blood in the pulmonary artery. This was attempted by Potts (7) on two occasions but was unsuccessful. In 1955 Kittle and associates (8) planned a constriction of the pulmonary artery just distal to the origin of the anomalous left coronary artery in an effort to increase the pressure within it, but the infant died while the incision was being made. Others have recognized that the ideal surgical approach to this condition is transplantation of the anomalous coronary artery into a systemic artery by direct anastomosis. Such a procedure is necessarily tedious and difficult, and infants with this condition have an extremely limited myocardial reserve. This procedure was attempted by Mustard (9) in 1953 but the child did not survive. Apley and associates (10) advocated resection of the infarct as a means of reducing the paradoxical motions of the left ventricle as well as ligation of the left coronary artery. Paul and Robbins have employed talc poudrage and recommend its use. In our own experience two infants have been treated by chemical de-epicardialization (phenol) in an effort to revascularize the left ventricle. This procedure has appeared to provide real benefit, since both children are surprisingly well two and four years following operation, although cardiomegaly persists.

Within the past several years there has been increased interest in the direction of blood flow in an anomalous coronary artery arising from the pulmonary artery. In 1886 St. John Brooks (1) reported

observations on two hearts with this condition, which he found inci-
dentally in the anatomic dissecting laboratory. In both instances the
right coronary artery arose from the pulmonary artery and his dissec-
tions led him to make the following observation:

> A consideration of this case will show that a very interesting question is con-
> nected with it. There are two arteries belonging to the different circula-
> tions—the pulmonary and the systemic anastomosing with each other. In
> these circulations, as is well known, the arterial pressure is very much greater
> in the systemic than in the pulmonary; how then did the blood flow in the
> anomalous coronary artery?

There cannot be doubt that it acted very much after the manner
of a vein and that blood flowed through it towards the pulmonary
artery and thence into the lungs (11). Later, Maude Abbott (12) also
endorsed this theory of retrograde flow of blood under these circumstances. Recently Edwards (2) has renewed interest in a recon-
sideration of this problem and has called attention to the fact that
infants with congenital cyanotic cardiac disease often have all arterial oxygen saturation that is below that of the venous blood in
patients without right-to-left shunts. Yet these patients do not show
clinical or pathologic evidence of myocardial ischemia. For this reason he concludes that the reduced perfusion pressure in the anomalous left coronary artery is the most important feature and has
advocated ligation of this vessel as the therapeutic method of choice.
This has been performed by Morrow (13), Jahnke (14), and others.
Edwards (15) offered the following points in support of the theory
of retrograde flow: (1) In both normal and anomalous coronary
arteries anastomoses exist between the branches; (2) in anomalous
origin of the left coronary artery from the pulmonary artery both
the right and left coronary arteries have been observed to have been
extremely dilated and tortuous in a manner similar to that occurring
in other situations in which arterial venous communications are
known to be present; (3) clinical evidence of myocardial ischemia is
usually not apparent until several months after birth, at a time when
the difference between the pressures in the systemic and pulmonary
circuits become established; (4) perfusion studies on postmortem

specimens with these anomalous vessels show evidence of large communications between the anomalous and normal coronary arteries; and (5) an observation by Apley and associates that "when the coronary artery which arose from the pulmonary trunk was divided at operation bright red blood flowed freely from its distal end."

We have also been able to demonstrate free communication between the left and right coronary arteries in two autopsy specimens of the heart from infants with anomalous origin of the left coronary artery from the pulmonary artery. Radiopaque contrast media injected into the right coronary artery completely filled the left coronary artery immediately and actually prior to the filling of the coronary veins. Similarly, methylene blue injected into the right coronary artery quickly filled the left coronary artery and was noted to flow into the pulmonary artery in significant amounts. In the present case it was possible to isolate the anomalous coronary artery that arose from the pulmonary artery and to measure the pressure within it. This was first done with the vessel open and later with it occluded at its origin. With proximal occlusion of the vessel the pressure rose sharply in the artery, thus suggesting strongly that the source of blood was from the collateral branches. In addition, a sample of blood drawn from the anomalous artery showed full oxygen saturation (100 percent), whereas a simultaneous sample from the pulmonary artery showed a saturation of 76 percent. These observations appear to demonstrate conclusively that the blood in an anomalous left coronary artery arising from the pulmonary artery does in fact flow in a retrograde manner. It lends further support to the concept that ligation of the vessel at its origin is a rational method of treatment.

References

1. Brooks, H. St. J. Two cases of an abnormal coronary artery of the heart arising from the pulmonary artery; with some remarks upon the effect of the anomaly in producing cirsoid dilatation of the vessels. *J. Anat. & Physiol.*, 20: 26, 1886.

2. Edwards, J. E. Symposium on cardiovascular diseases: Functional pathology of congenital cardiac disease. *Pediat. Clin., North America*, 1: 13, 1954.

3. Abrikossoff, A. Aneurysm des linken Herzventrikels mit abnormer Abgangstelle der linken Koronararterie von der Pulmonalis bei einem funfmonatlichen Kinde. *Virchows Arch.*, 203: 413, 1911.

4. Bland, E. F., White, P. D., and Garland, J. Congenital anomalies of coronary arteries: Report of an unusual case associated with cardiac hypertrophy. *Am. Heart J.*, 8: 787, 1933.

5. Keith, J. D. The anomalous origin of the left coronary artery from the pulmonary artery. *Brit. Heart J.*, 21: 149, 1959.

6. Gasul, B. M., and Loeffler, E. Anomalous origin of the left coronary artery from the pulmonary artery (Bland-White-Garland syndrome). *Pediatrics*, 4: 498, 1949.

7. Potts, W. J. Cited by Gasul and Loeffler.

8. Kittle, C. F., Diehl, A. M., and Heilbrunn, A. Anomalous left coronary artery arising from the pulmonary artery: Report of a case and a surgical consideration. *J. Pediat.*, 47: 198, 1955.

9. Mustard, W. T., cited by Keith.

10. Apley, J., Horton, R. E., and Wilson, M. G. The possible role of surgery in the treatment of anomalous left coronary artery. Thorax 12: 28, 1957.

11. Paul, R. N. M., and Robbins, S. G. A surgical treatment for either endocordial fibroelastosis or anomalous origin of the left coronary artery. *Pediatrics*, 16: 147, 195.

12. Abbott, M. E. Congenital cardiac disease. In Osler, W. *Modern Medicine*, 3rd ed. Philadelphia: Lea & Febiger, 1927, p. 794.

13. Case, R. B., Morrow, A. G., Stainsby, W., and Nestor, J. O. Anomalous origin of the left coronary artery: The physiologic defect and suggested surgical treatment. *Circulation*, 17: 1062, 1958.

14. Jahnke, E. J., Cited by Case, et al.

15. Edwards, J. E.: Anomalous coronary arteries with special reference to arteriovenous-like communications. *Circulation*, 17: 1001, 1958.

Chapter 25 &

Coronary Arteriography in the Selection of Patients for Surgery[1]

*T*he management of patients with coronary artery disease has proved to be one of the most difficult problems in clinical medicine. In the recent past, increasing interest has been shown in the surgical treatment of this condition, and the direct removal of obstructing lesions from the coronary arteries by thromboendarterectomy has been successfully performed (1, 5, 13). The selection of patients for this procedure is facilitated by the accurate preoperative localization of the site of obstruction. Coronary arteriography provides the surgeon with this much-needed information.

Rousthoi was probably the first investigator to demonstrate the coronary arteries in the intact experimental animal (12). Since then, many methods have been devised for their visualization. Intravenous angiocardiography reveals the coronary arteries only rarely. Furthermore, the detail with this technic is usually unsatisfactory, as a result of the residual filling of the underlying ventricular system with opaque material. The first successful method of coronary visualization was described in 1952 by Diguglielmo and coworkers, who injected opaque material through a catheter placed in the ascending aorta. In their series, however, approximately one-third of the patients failed to show satisfactory visualization of the coronary arteries due to the uncertainties in the filling of the coronary cusps by means of the flushing technic (3). Many modifications of Diguglielmo's method have been proposed in order to eliminate this difficulty. Lehman, for example, has utilized direct needle puncture of the ascending aorta, but this

---

1. Coauthored with Erich K. Lang.

has not substantially improved the percentage of satisfactory studies (9). Williams and his coworkers developed a ring-like catheter with multiple openings, which, if properly placed above the coronary cusps, will effect homogeneous filling of these structures (15, 2). Sones at the Cleveland Clinic advocates introduction of the catheter tip into the coronary ostium. While this technic certainly guarantees consistently successful studies, considerable dexterity is required to manipulate the catheter tip into the orifice of the coronary artery. A special tapered catheter is necessary to allow constant perfusion of the coronary arteries with blood during the procedure. Particular care has to be exercised to avoid complete occlusion of the coronary orifice by the catheter tip. The procedure is particularly useful for cinefluorographic demonstration of the coronary arteries with multiple small manual injections of contrast medium. In our hands, this method, while giving excellent results, has proved to be technically difficult in some cases.

Acetylcholine-induced arrest with subsequent injection of a contrast substance has also been advocated by some as the most successful means of demonstrating the coronary arteries (9). This method, however, has the disadvantage that the cardiac arrest often results in failure of the contrast column to be propagated to the more peripheral branches of the coronary arteries. A balloon-catheter technic has been described by Dotter to increase the concentration of the medium in the ascending aorta and to retain it in this segment for a prolonged time (4). While, theoretically, this should offer many advantages, the placement of the balloon is quite critical and its maintenance in the ascending aorta during the injection phase is often difficult. Another modification of the flushing technic uses an Odman catheter, which is introduced into the arterial system via percutaneous puncture of the femoral artery, with the aid of a Seldinger guide wire (8). This procedure has the advantage of a simple percutaneous introduction of the catheter, but also has the disadvantage of an abnormally long catheter stretching throughout the entire aorta, increasing the surface friction considerably and tending to slow down the rate of injection of the contrast medium.

A series of sixty-three examinations has been evaluated for this discussion. The majority of these were of the type described as a

TABLE I   Sixty-three Examinations and Their Results

Flush Technic	
Satisfactory	32
Unsatisfactory	8
Seldinger Technic	
Satisfactory	1
Unsatisfactory	9
Fush with Acetylcholine-induced arrest	
Satisfactory	1
Unsatisfactory	4
Selective Coronary Artery Injection	
Satisfactory	8
Unsatisfactory	0

flushing technic (Table I). In a few of the more recent cases, and particularly in the cinefluorographic examinations, direct injection into the coronary cusps or ostium of the coronary artery was carried out.

The procedure employed in the present series adapts routine catheter aortography to examination of the coronary vessels. An end-hole catheter of the Coumand type is advanced into the ascending aorta via an incision in the right ulnar artery. The tip of the catheter is placed approximately 1 inch above the aortic cusps. The relative position of the catheter tip in the middle of the ascending aorta is of critical importance, since only an adequately distant position assures proper mixing of the injected medium with the residual blood and effects homogeneous filling of all aortic cusps. Approximately 45 cc of 90 per cent ditrizoate methylglucamine (Hypaque) is injected with a pressure syringe under a pressure of approximately 140 to 160 pounds per square inch. The speed of the injection is a function of the lumen of the catheter, the viscosity of the medium, and the pressure under which it is introduced. For optimal visualization, the entire amount of the contrast agent should be delivered in a time not exceeding three seconds. For the average adult patient, a 9-gauge catheter or larger should be for this reason, no attempt has been made used. To effect optimal filling of the to reduce the injection time to less than two main as well as peripheral branches of the seconds. Films are exposed at a rate of coronary arteries, prolonged filling of the 3 or 4 per second for a total period of four coronary cusps has been found desirable to five seconds. The exposure time of each film is critical and determines the detail of the study. Due to the rapid motion of the heart, exposures exceeding one-fifteenth of a second result in undesirable blurring of the coronary artery images. High-speed films and screens are essential for this examination. The films are taken in both the anteroposterior and lateral positions on a double plane Sehbnander film changer. Thirty-two of forty cases thus examined have shown adequate visualization of the coronary arteries, allowing proper interpretation. Eight examinations were found to be inadequate due either to only unilateral filling or to bluffing of the coronary arteries from motion (Table I).

In five cases, a temporary arrest of the heart action was achieved by preloading the catheter with acetyleholine. In only one patient examined with this technic, however, was an adequate study obtained. In the four other cases, there was filling only of the main coronary arteries without propagation of the contrast column into the distal branches. It became apparent that the systolic and diastolic action of the heart muscle is desirable to help transport the medium to the more peripheral branches and allow demonstration of these areas on the later films of the serial examination. For this reason, this method was discontinued in spite of its apparent merits in the demonstration of the main branches of the coronary arteries, particularly under the adverse circumstances of necessarily long exposure times (9, 1). In ten patients, coronary arteriography by a percutaneous retrograde arterial route was performed (8, 10). An Odman catheter was advanced over a Seldinger guide wire which had been introduced into the right femoral artery via a percutaneous puncture. Under fluoroscopic control, this radiopaque polyethylene catheter is advanced into the midportion of the ascending aorta and an injection is carried out, again with utilization of the flushing technic. The ease of the percutaneous introduction of the catheter by this method is most desirable. However, this benefit was unfortunately offset, in our experience, by rather poor results. In only one of the patients examined was a diagnostic study obtained. The great length of the catheter and the attendant surface friction to the flow of the opaque medium resulted in an abnormally slow injection. In five cases, the coronary arteries were selectively injected after the catheter tip had been engaged in the ostium of the artery. This type of examination lends itself particularly well to cinefluorographic studies. Once the tip of the catheter is engaged, it may remain in position for only a very short time, since the normal coronary circulation and blood flow are embarrassed and ischemia of the supplied heart muscle may result. Even the introduction of side-holes in the catheter does not guarantee adequate perfusion of the partially occluded coronary artery via the communicating catheter segment. Recently, a very fine tapered end-hole catheter has been made available which does not appear to produce occlusion of the coronary artery after its tip has been inserted into the orifice. The method is therefore most adaptable to short movie exposures in which the artery is occluded only momentarily by the catheter tip during hand injection of a small amount of contrast medium. Compared to the flush technic, this method offers the advantage of an unimpaired view of the entire course of one coronary artery. With the flush technic, the temporary obscuration of portions of the coronary arteries by the contrast-filled aorta may be compensated by information derived from the latter films of the run. Tracings of the entire course of the arteries from various films may afford excellent information on the presence or absence of some of the peripheral branches. The selective injection of a coronary cusp is technically much easier and offers the advantage that the placement of the catheter tip does not embarrass the blood supply to the heart muscle. The tip may be maintained in the cusp for an almost indefinite period and it is therefore possible to examine the patient on a Schonander film changer. The detail of the films thus obtained is considerably better than that on 16-mm. movies; in at least two cases a proper diagnosis of small plaques could be made only with the help of the large films. In the recent past, combined examinations by cinefluorographic technics and the Schonander film changer have been performed. In these cases, the coronary ostium was first selectively engaged and injected, and the catheter tip was then placed in the coronary cusp and the patient moved to the Schonander film changer for a second contrast injection and examination. Comparison of the examinations done by these two methods strongly supports the opinion that both cinefluorography and large detail film are necessary for a correct diagnosis. Electrocardiographic monitoring during the entire procedure is regarded as imperative. Both arterial and venous pressure tracings were obtained on the first patients of this series. These data were particularly useful in the interpretation of patient reaction to the injected medium.

Clinical Experience

In this series, coronary arteriography was primarily employed in the selection of patients for coronary end arterectomy (13). The examination supplied important information concerning the site and extent of arterial occlusion and indicated the feasibility of a surgical procedure. In fact, the decision for the performance of coronary endarterectomy is determined almost exclusively by the findings of coronary arteriography (1, 5, 13). In general, localized segments of occlusion are the most suitable for end-arterectomy; patients who are shown to have multiple areas of occlusion or occlusion of the more peripheral branches of the coronary arteries are not subjected to coronary endarterectomy. Forty-one patients have been examined by coronary arteriography in this series with the following findings:

Localized lesions (amenable to endarterectomy)	9
Multiple lesions and peripheral lesions (generally unsuitable for endarterectomy)	26
Normal coronary artery	6

In nine cases localized lesions were demonstrated that were felt to be suitable for endarterectomy. Six patients have been operated upon and an endarterectomy has been performed, with removal of the obstruction. Five of these patients showed good postoperative results. One died in the immediate postoperative period. Three of the patients found suitable for coronary endarterectomy have not yet been operated upon. In at least six patients, the coronary arteriogram failed to show any anatomical lesion or narrowing; the electrocardiographic

findings were also equivocal and the Master's exercise test was negative. The rather severe "anginal" attacks that these patients experienced were therefore felt to be on a functional basis. Two of this
group could be rehabilitated by psychotherapy and were asymptomatic
when last seen. In one patient, a large sliding hiatus hernia was subsequently demonstrated and successfully managed by operation.

The most important contribution of coronary arteriography is
probably the possibility of selection of those patients with localized
narrowing of one of the main coronary arteries by arteriosclerotic
plaques that may be successfully subjected to endarterectomy. This
procedure has produced encouraging results in the initial series, and
continuance in selected patients appears indicated.

References

1. Bailey, C. P., Musser, B. G., and Lemmon, W. M. Appraisal of
   Current Surgical Procedures for Coronary Heart Disease. *Progr.
   Cardiovas. Dis.*, 1: 219–236, October 1958.
2. Bellman, S., Frank, H. A., Lambert, P. B., Littmann, D., and
   Williams, J. A. Coronary arteriography. I. Differential opacification of the aortic stream by catheters of special design. Experimental development. *New England J. Med.*, 262: 325–328, Feb. 18,
   1960.
3. Di Guglielmo, L., and Guttadauro, M. A roentgenologic study of
   the coronary arteries in the living. *Acta Radiol.*, Suppl. 97, 1952.
4. Dotter, C. T., and Frische, L. H. Visualization of the coronary circulation by occlusion aortography: A practical method. *Radiology*,
   71: 502–523, October 1958.
5. Gottesman, L. Direct surgical relief of coronary artery occlusion.
   Am.J. Cardiol., 2: 315–320, September 1958.
6. Hase, O., Holaday, D. A., and Deterling, R. A., Jr. Studies in
   coronary arteriography: Systolic vs. diastolic appearance of the
   coronary arteries. *Radiology*, 73: 785–786, November 1959.
7. Johnson, A. M. and Logan, W: Coronary artery catheterization
   during thoracic aortography. *Brit. Heart J.*, 20: 411–415, July
   1958.

8. Jonsson, G., and Hellstrom, L. Roentgenographic demonstration of the coronary arteries. *Acta Radiol.*, 53: 273–278, April 1960.

9. Lemmon, W. M., Lehman, J. S., and Boyer, R. A. Suprasternal Transaortic Coronary Arteriography. Circulation 19: 47–54, January 1959.

10. Mouquin, M., Brun, P., Chartrain, E., Bacquet, G. and Pierron, J. Coronary Arteriography by a Percutaneous Retrograde Arterial Route. *Arch. Mal Coeur*, 52: 874–881, August 1959.

11. Nordenstrom, B., Ovenfors, C. O., and Westberg, G. Experimental Stereoangiography of the Coronary and Bronchial Arteries. *Acta chir. scandinav.*, Suppl., 245, 1959, pp. 357–358.

12. Rousthoi, W.: Über Angiokardiographie. Vorlaufige Mitteilung. *Acta Radiol.*, 14: 419–423, 1933.

13. Sabiston, D.C., Jr.: Coronary endarterectomy. *Am. Surgeon*, 26: 217–226, April 1960.

14. West, J. W., and Guzman, S. V. Coronary dilatation and constriction visualized by selective arteriography. *Circulation Res.*, 7: 527–536, July 1959.

15. Williams, J. A., et al. Coronary Arteriography. II. Clinical experiences with the loop-end catheter. *New England J. Med.*, 262: 328–332, Feb. 18, 1960.

Chapter 26

The Diminishing Mortality of Coronary Artery Bypass Grafting for Myocardial Ischemia[1]

N early two decades have passed since the first attempts to direct- ly revascularize the myocardium of patients with ischemic coronary artery disease (1–4). Since then, coronary artery bypass graft- ing (CABG) has emerged both as an effective modality for relieving the symptoms of ischemic heart disease (5, 6) and as a method of improving survival in certain groups with coronary disease (7–9). The number of patients to undergo such procedures has increased each year, and more than 100,000 persons in the United States alone are expected to receive coronary grafts this year.

A significant factor in the improved results of CABG has been a clearer understanding of perioperative ischemic myocardial injury. In the earlier experience with CABG, the obvious technical advantage of operating on a motionless heart in a bloodless operative field was rec- ognized. It is now well understood, however, that normothermic ischemic arrest has a very unfavorable effect on cardiac metabolism. Recognition of this fact led clinical and experimental investigators throughout the world to seek improved techniques for maintaining the metabolic integrity of the heart during intraoperative cardiac arrest (10). The recent, nearly universal acceptance of cold potassium arrest to protect the ischemic myocardium attests to the influence of these investigators.

1. Coauthored with Robert H. Jones, M.D., Steven E. Curtis, Andrew S. Wechsler, M.D., W. Glenn Young, Jr., M.D., H. Newland Oldham, Jr., M.D., Walter G. Wolfe, M.D., Robert Whalen, M.D., James J. Morris, M.D., and Wal- ter L. Floyd, M.D.

Cold potassium cardioplegia was introduced at Duke University Medical Center as an adjunct to CABG in 1976. Since then we have noted a gratifying decline in the operative mortality for myocardial revascularization procedures. While improved myocardial protection has contributed to this decline, other significant factors have been involved as well. A greater understanding of the various physiologic principles which govern the energy needs of the heart, particularly in the presence of diseased vessels, has led to a broader approach that includes improvements in anesthetic management and in the techniques of cardiopulmonary bypass. The purpose of this study was to compare the results of current techniques used in CABG in one institution with the results of approaches used before the introduction of cold potassium cardioplegia and the other techniques in current use.

Clinical Data

The data were obtained from the records of patients who underwent CABG for chronically disabling or unstable angina at Duke University Medical Center. Group I is comprised of 200 consecutive patients operated upon between July 1974 and October 1976, immediately before the introduction of potassium cardioplegia. The patients in Group II consist of 200 consecutive patients undergoing CABG between December 1978 and December 1979. In both groups, patients who underwent concomitant valvular replacement or ventricular aneurysmectomy were excluded.

Surgical Management

Patients in Group I underwent CABG employing one of three techniques. In most, autogenous saphenous veins were anastomosed to the ascending aorta either before cardiopulmonary bypass or during the initial phases of bypass with a partial occlusion clamp. Distal anastomoses were then made using either (1) intermittent ischemia, (2) continuous ischemia, or (3) constant perfusion and induced ventricular fibrillation (29). In each patient the body temperature was maintained between 280 and 320 C by extracorporeal circulation. The vast majority of the patients in Group II received cold potassium cardioplegia and topical hypothermia during coronary artery anastomoses. The proximal coronary anastomoses were made as previously described. For the distal anastomoses the ascending aorta was occluded, and 500 to 700 ml of potassium cardioplegic solution was infused at 40 C into the aortic root producing almost immediate cardiac arrest and a reduction in the myocardial temperature to approximately 100. During ischemic arrest, most of the patients received additional solution every 15 to 20 minutes in order to maintain the myocardial temperature at low levels and to assure complete pharmacologic cardiac arrest. The reason for repetitive infusions of cold potassium solution is to offset the effect of the non-coronary collateral blood flow which tends to rewarm the ischemic myocardium and wash out intracoronary cardioplegic solution. During the final distal anastomosis, the systemic temperature is gradually increased to 370 C and the heart is allowed to rewarm.

Some of the patients in Group II underwent CABG with topical hypothermia alone and others with cardioplegic solution alone. Topical hypothermia is produced by immersing the heart in cold (40) physiologic saline placed in the pericardial sac. A small number of operations in Group II were performed without cardiopulmonary bypass or in one of the manners described in Group I.

In both the groups cardiopulmonary bypass utilizing a disposable bubble oxygenator was used with a right atrial cannula for venous drainage and an ascending aortic cannula for arterial perfusion. Approximately 75 percent of Group I patients had left ventricular venting of some form while the majority of Group II patients were not vented.

Intraaortic Balloon Pumping (IABP) and Pulsatile Bypass Pump (PBP)

IABP may be used to assist in weaning the patient from cardiopulmonary bypass. It has also been used prior to operation in those with poor left ventricular function. The rationale for using the IABP is its ability to reduce systemic afterload and augment diastolic coronary arterial driving pressure. In Group II the pulsatile bypass pump was frequently employed. During extracorporeal circulation the PBP pro-

TABLE I Functional Status of Patients★

Class	Group I (No. Patients)	Group II (No. Patients)
I	11 (5.5%)	4 (2%)
II	13 (6.5%)	26 (13%)
III	46 (23%)	60 (30%)
IV	130 (65%)	110 (55%)

★ *New York Heart Association Classification for angina pectoris*

vides pulsatile flow, which many believe is preferable to the usual mean flow pattern of the bypass pump. The PBP can also be used before and after CPB to augment diastolic pressure.

Postoperative Electrocardiogram

In the two groups, the postoperative development of new, significant Q waves (greater than .04 sec.) was considered suggestive evidence for myocardial infarction. Postoperative EKGs were examined for atrial arrhythmias, intraventricular conduction defects, and ischemic changes by a cardiologist unaware of the conduct of the operation or the recovery period. The data are expressed as mean ± standard deviation or as percentage of the total number of patients within each group.

Preoperative Assessment

Sex and age.   In both groups there were 165 males and 35 females. The mean age for Group I was 50.5 years (range, 26–66), and for Group II it was 53.5 years (range, 20–70).

Operative status.   In Group I, 186 patients (93%) underwent operation on an elective basis and 14 patients (7%) received emergency CABGS. In Group II, 158 patients (79%) were operated upon electively and 42 patients (21%) on an emergency basis. The emergency group was comprised of patients with unstable angina or lesions such as left main disease, for whom it was advisable to proceed promptly with operation.

TABLE II   Data Obtained from Cardiac Catheterization

	Group I (No. Patients)	Group II (No. Patients)
Number Diseased Vessels		
0	1 (.5%)	2 (1%)
1	40 (20%)	31 (16%)
2	56 (28%)	78 (39%)
3	103 (51.5%)	89 (44%)
Left Main Disease		
Subtotal (75–95%)	23 (11.5%)	23 (11.5%)
Total (100%)	2 (.196%)	0
Ejection Fraction		
<25%	4 (2%)	0
25–40%	40 (22%)	40 (23%)
46–60%	85 (48%)	89 (50%)
>60%	49 (28%)	48 (27%)
Left Ventricular **End Diastolic** **Pressure > 18mm Hg**	15 (7.5%)	39 (19.5%)

Angina pectoris.   In Table I, the patients in both groups are categorized according to the New York Heart Association Classification for angina. Six patients (3%) in Group I and two (5%) in Group II had previous histories of congestive heart failure.

Cardiac Catherization and Angiography.   The results of cardiac catheterization are shown in Table II. The average number of diseased vessels in Group I was 2.3 ± .8 and in Group II it was 2.3 ± .8. The values for preoperative ejection fractions and left ventricular end diastolic pressure (LVEDP) are listed for the 178 patients in Group I and the 177 in Group II in whom such data were obtained. As is apparent, both groups were similar in terms of the preoperative injection fractions and number of diseased vessels. Also, the degree of left main disease was similar in both groups. The significantly larger number of individuals with an LVEDP greater than 18 in Group II, however, suggests that there were more patients with poorly functioning ventricles in this group.

TABLE III   Techniques of Coronary Artery Bypass Surgery

Mode of Myocardial Protection	n	Total Ischemia (Mins.)	Ischemic Time Per Graft (Mins.)	Reperfusion Time (Mins.)	Length of CPB (Mins.)
Group I					
Intermittent reperfusion	56 pts (28%)	27.2±13.6	12.53±5.25	31.7±20	102.9±39.5
Moderate hypothermia and single ischemic interval	54 pts (27%)	21.87±18.91	11.01±7.91	30.54±23.28	94.33±43
Ventricular fibrillation	90 pts (45%)				63.9±34.5
Group II					
Cardioplegia and topical hypothermia	171 pts (85.5%)	46.78±25.63	17.36±7.9	29.9±20.2	99.4±43
Cardioplegia alone	10 pts (5%)	38.5±20.8	21.75±12.8	16.3±7.21	75.5±42.3
Topical hypothermia alone	3 pts (1.5%)	16.6±3	6.4±1.7	38.6±8	116±11.6
Moderate hypothermia and single ischemic interval	6 pts (3%)	7.7±3	4.9±2.2	37.2±25	69.3±40
Intermittent reperfusion and topical hypothermia	4 pts (2%)	29.5±4	9.8±1.2	49.2±10	127.5±21.8
Without cardiopulmonary bypass	5 pts (2.5%)				
Ventricular fibrillation	1 pt (.5%)				

Preoperative EKG Evidence of Myocardial Infarction.   Sixty-nine patients (34.5%) in Group I and 72 patients (36%) in Group II had electrocardiographic evidence of a previous myocardial infarction. One patient in Group I and six in Group II had preoperative intraventricular conduction defects.

Myocardial Protection.   The techniques by which coronary artery bypass surgery was performed are shown in Table III.

Completeness of Revascularization.   The mean number of grafts in Group I was 2.0 ± .8, and that for Group II was 2.6 ± .9. The number of patients who received fewer grafts than diseased vessels (completeness of revascularization) was 65 (32.5%) in Group l and 17 (8.5%) in Group II.

Intraaortic Balloon Pumping and Pulsatile Bypass Pump.   The use of the has diminished since 1974. In Group I, 31 patients (15.5%) were placed on intraaortic balloon pump while in Group II only 15 patients (7.5%) had IABP. By contrast, there were no patients in Group I who were placed on the PBP, while 42% (84 patients) of Group II received the pulsatile bypass pump.

Operative Mortality.   In Group 1, 12 of the patients died intraoperatively and 6 died within 30 days. Sixteen of these patients died of cardiac problems. There was only one death in Group II—an operative mortality of 0.5%. This patient died of a cardiac arrhythmia on the third postoperative day.

TABLE IV   Postoperative Complications

	Group I (No. Patients)	Group II (No. Patients)
Superficial Wound	2 (1%)	0
Low Cardiac Output	1 (.5%)	1 (.5%)
Hemorrhage	8 (4%)	4 (2%)
Mediastinitis	1 (.5%)	2 (1%)
Post Card. Synd.	26 (13%)	9 (4.5%)
Rectus Hematoma	2 (1%)	0

Surgical Complications. The postoperative complications in both groups are depicted in Table IV. The incidence of postcardiotomy syndrome (chest pain, pericardial rub, and fever) has diminished in the recent past.

Postoperative Electrocardiogram. Seventeen patients (8.5%) in Group I and 18 patients (9%) in Group II developed significant Q waves postoperatively. Of note is that more patients developed intraventricular conduction defects of some type in Group II, 96% of whom received potassium cardioplegia. Most of these EKG changes were transient, resolving within three days, and were generally of little clinical significance.

The operative mortality for coronary artery bypass graft has progressively diminished and many centers now report rates of less than 3% (11–13). Many ascribe this low surgical mortality to the recent use of improved myocardial protection, more complete revascularization, better anesthetic techniques, and more effective postoperative management. The experience reported in the present study tends to support this. The 0.5% mortality in the 200 patients in Group II is most likely the result of a number of interrelated factors.

One important feature concerns the possibility that improvement in patient selection has reduced operative mortality. While it is possible that fewer patients in Group II succumbed acutely because preoperative ventricular function was better and coronary arterial disease was less extensive, analysis of our data does not support this suggestion. Operative mortality has generally correlated directly with a preoperative LVEDP greater than 18 mm Hg, abnormalities in left ventricular wall-motion, and ejection fractions less than 25 to 30% (14–19). In Groups I and II the distribution of patients with 2 and 3 vessel disease, preoperative ejection fractions (less than 40%), and the number of patients in NYHA Class III and LV were similar and do not indicate that patients currently undergoing CABG are significantly different than previously. In fact, with a greater number of patients with an LVEDP greater than 18 in Group II, it appears that the latter group includes sicker patients. It appears that hypothermic solutions containing moderate concentrations of potassium (20–30 mEq/liter) extend the ischemic tolerance time of the myocardium (20–24). During ischemia the demand for energy by the myocardium is primarily determined by its continued electromechanical activity, basal metabolic functions, and temperature. By producing immediate electromechanical cardiac arrest, cold potassium arrest leads to a decrease in utilization of high energy phosphate during ischemia (25–27). Although the primary reason for adenosine triphosphate (ATP) depletion during ischemia is continued electromechanical activity (28), hypothermia is also critical in reducing utilization of ATP by slowing all intracellular metabolic processes and thereby forestalling significant ischemic injury (29). The ischemic interval notwithstanding, the reperfusion phase is important in determining the ultimate state of the previous ischemic myocardium (30–32). In contrast to normothermic ischemia, blood flow in hearts arrested with potassium and kept cold during ischemia is redistributed toward the subendocardium (28). Ventricular compliance and overall ventricular performance, moreover, are also not affected when hearts are made ischemic with cold pharmacologic arrest (33).

In contrast, earlier use of intermittent coronary reperfusion during ischemia to repay metabolic debt has been associated with deterioration in ventricular compliance as well as maldistribution of flow with underperfusion of the subendocardium (34–36). Of the 56 patients in Group I whose hearts were rendered intermittently ischemic, four died. That induced ventricular fibrillation exerts an adverse effect upon the heart is suggested by the eight deaths among those patients so treated. That fibrillation may create similar flow imbalances and be associated with subendocardial necrosis, especially in hypertrophied hearts (37–40), has led to striking restriction of its use. In addition, there were 54 patients in Group I who underwent coronary arterography 130 during a single ischemic interval under conditions of moderate hypothermia (20° to 32° C). It is now recognized that metabolic deterioration during ischemia is not only related to time but to temperature as well and that deeper hypothermia provides additional protection from severe irreversible injury (41, 42).

The different approaches for protecting the heart during CABG which were formerly used and considered effective have been replaced by sounder methods of myocardial preservation, while changes in perioperative anesthetic management have been significant in reducing operative mortality, as instanced by the current practice of preventing fluctuations in blood pressure of more than 20% of normal. The use of the Swan-Ganz catheter to monitor left as well as right heart pressures throughout the operation has also been effective in providing hemodynamic data upon which more appropriate therapeutic decisions can be made.

Advancements in anesthetic management parallel the improvements in operative skill brought about by a greater experience. A committed effort to bypass all significant lesions is illustrated in the present series by the fewer patients receiving incomplete grafting (9% in Group II vs. 32% in Group I). The completeness of revascularizing significantly obstructed vessels, including branches of the major coronary arteries, is important and has been clearly related to the decline in operative mortality (17, 44).

The relationship of pulsatile perfusion during cardiopulmonary bypass to operative mortality and morbidity is actively debated. The ability of the PBP to improve hemodynamics in a patient with a compromised ventricle is supported by early work with the intraaortic balloon pump. Following cardiopulmonary bypass, IABP can reduce afterload and increase diastolic coronary flow. The effects of reducing metabolic demand while increasing coronary flow are beneficial particularly to those regions of the heart supplied by stenotic or obstructed vessels. The effect of a putsatile arterial pressure on renal and other vital organ functions awaits further study of its role in improving surgical results (45, 46).

In our series postoperative morbidity was minimal in both groups. Of much interest is the strikingly greater number of patients in Group II who developed intraventricular conduction defects. Recent evidence suggests that the use of potassium to protect the ischemic heart is related to the appearance of these changes (47). Fortunately, most of these alterations in conduction were transient and did not appear to retard postoperative recovery. The rise of cold cardioplegia, moreover, has not been associated with deterioration in myocardial function in patients restudied 6 to 18 months after surgery (47).

The use of hypothermia and pharmacologic cardiac arrest to protect the ischemic heart has been important in making coronary artery bypass grafting as safe as many other less complicated major surgical procedures. These techniques should be considered within the context of the expanding role of coronary artery bypass grafting in the management of coronary artery disease. The ultimate aim of myocardial revascularization includes longer life for the patient with ischemic heart disease as well as relief of symptoms. With the marked reduction in immediate mortality and morbidity in such patients, improved survival in certain high-risk patients has been observed.

References

1. Sabiston, D. C. Jr. The coronary circulation. *Johns Hopkins Med J.* 134: 329, 1974.
2. Effler, D. B., Groves, L. K., Sones F. M., Jr., Shirey, E. K.: Endaterectomy in the treatment of coronary artery disease. *J. Thorac. Cardiovascular Surg.*, 47: 98–108, 1964.
3. Connolly, J. E., Eldreidge, F. L. Calvin, J. W., Stemmer, E. A. Proximal coronary artery obstruction: Its etiology and treatment by transaortic endarterectomy. *N. Engl. J. Med.*, 271:213–219, 1964.
4. Garrett, H. E., Dennis, E. W., DeBarkey, M. E. Aortocoronary bypass with saphenous vein graft. *J.A.M.A.*, 223: 792–794, 1973.
5. Mathur, V. S., Guinn, G. A. Prospective randomized study of coronary bypass surgery in stable angina: The first 100 patients. *Circulation*, 51–52(1): 133, 1975.
6. Peduzzi, P. Hultgren H. Effect of medical vs surgical treatment on symptoms in stable angina pectoris: The Veterans Administration cooperative study of surgery for coronary arterial occlusive disease. *Circulation*, 60: 888–900, 1979.
7. Stiles, Q. Lindesmith, G. C., Tucker, B. L. et al. Long term follow up of patients with coronary artery bypass grafts. *Circulation*, 54(111): 32–34, 1976.
8. Takaro, T., Hultgren, H. N. Lipton, M. J., Detre, K. The VA cooperative randomized study of surgery for coronary occlusive disease: Subgroup with significant left main disease. *Circulation*, 54(111): 107–117, 1976.
9. VA cooperative study group for surgery for coronary arterial occlusive disease: use of noninvasive clinical parameters with angi-

na pectoris, treated medically and surgically, *Am. J. Cardiol.*, 45: 456, 1980.

10. Miller, D. W., Hessel, E. A. Winterchied, L. R., et al. Current practice of coronary artery bypass surgery: results of a national survey. *J. Thorac. Cardiovasc. Surg.*, 73: 75, 1977.

11. Cameron, A., Kemp, K. G., Shimomura, S. et al. Coronary artery bypass surgery: A seven year follow-up. *Circulation*, 57–58: 11:19, 1978.

12. Kouchoukos, N. T., Oberman, A. Kirklin J. W., et al. Coronary bypass surgery, analysis of factors affecting hospital mortality. Circulation, 59–60: 11–58, 1979.

13. Greene, D. G., Bunnell, I. L, Arani, D. T. et al. Survival of selected subsets after coronary bypass surgery. *Circulation*, 59–60: 11–58, 1979.

14. Manley, J. C., Johnson, W. D. Effects of surgery on angina (pre- and postinfarction) and myocardial function (failure). *Circulation*, 46: 1208–1221, 1972.

15. Collins, J. J., Cohn, L. H. Sonnenblick, E. H. et al. Determinants of survival after coronary artery bypass surgery. *Circulation*, 48(III): 132–136, 1973.

16. Kay, J. H., Redington, J. V., Mendez, A. M. et al. Coronary artery surgery for the patient with impaired left ventricular function. *Circulation*, 46: 11–49, 1972.

17. Oldham, H. N., Jr., Kong, Y., Bartel, A. G. et al. Risk factors in coronary artery bypass surgery. *Arch. Surg.*, 105: 918–923, 1972.

18. Hammond, G. L. Poirer, R. A. Early and late results of direct coronary reconstructive surgery for angina. *J. Thorac. Cardiovasc. Surg.*, 65: 127–133, 1972.

19. Ruel, G. J., Morris, G. C., Howell, J. F. et al. Experience with coronary artery bypass grafts in the treatment of coronary artery disease. *Surgery*, 71–586–593, 1972.

20. Gay, W. A., Ebert, P. A. Functional, metabolic and morphologic effects of potassium induced cardioplegia. *Surgery*, 74: 284–290, 1973.

21. Carver, J. M., Sams A. B., Hatcher, C. R. Potassium-induced cardioplegia: Additive protection against ischemic myocardial injury

during coronary revascularization. *J. Thorac. Cardiovascular. Surg.*, 76–27, 1978.

22. Gay, W. A. Potassium-induced cardioplegia. *Ann. Thorac. Surg.*, 20: 95–100, 1975.

23. Reitz, B. A., Brody, W. R., Hickey, P. R., Michaelis, L. L. Protection of the heart for 254 hours with intracellular (high K+) solution and hypothermia. *Surg. Form.*, 25: 149–151, 1974.

24. Sink, J. D., Pellom, G. L., Currie, W. D. et al. Protection of mitochondrial function during ischemia by potassium cardioplegia: Correlation with ischemic contracture. *Circulation*, 60: I–158–163, 1977.

25. Roe, R. B., Hutchinson, J. C., Fishman, N. H. et al. Myocardial protection with cold, ischemic potassium induced cardioplegia. *J. Thorac. Cardiovasc. Surg.*, 73: 366–374, 1977.

26. Hearse, D. J., Stewart, D. A., Braimbridge, M.V. Hypothermic arrest and potassium arrest: Metabolica and myocardial protection during elective cardiac arrest. *Circ. Res.*, 36: 481–489, 1975.

27. Bretschneider, H. J. Überlebenszeit und Wiederbelebungszeit des Herzens bei Normo- und Hypothermie. *Vehr. Dtsch. Ges. Kreislaufforsch*, 30: 11–34, 1964.

28. Goldstein, S. M., Nelson, R. L., McConnel, D. H., Buckbery G. D. Effects of conventional hypothermic ischemic arrest and pharmacological arrest on myocardial supply demand balance during aortic cross-clamping. *Ann. Thorac. Surg.*, 23: 520–528, 1977.

29. Jones, R. N., Hill, M. L., Reimer, K. A. et al. Effects of hypothermia on the rate of myocardial ATP and adenine nucleotide degradation in total ischemia. *Fed. Pro.*, 39: III, 1980.

30. Vary, T.C., Angelakos, E. T., Schaffer, S. Relationship between adenine nucleotide metabolism and irreversible ischemic tissue damage in isolated perfused rat heart. *Circ. Res.*, 45: 218–225, 1979.

31. Reimer, K. A., Hill, M. L., Jennings, R. B. ATP and adenine nucleotide resynthesis following episodes of reversible myocardial ischemic injury. *Fed. Pro.*, 39: III, 1980.

32. Bittar, N., Koke J. R., Berkoff, H. A., Kahn D. R. Histochemical and structural changes in human myocardial cells after cardiopulmonary bypass. *Circulation*, 51-52: I: 16-25, 1975.

33. Olsen, C. O., Hill, R. C., Jones, R. N. et al. Dimensional analysis of left ventricular systolic and diastolic properties in man during reperfusion following hypothermic potassium cardioplegia. Unpublished observations.

34. Chitwood, W. R., Jr., Hill, R. C. Kleinman, L. H. Wechsler A.S. The effects of intermittent ischemic arrest on the perfusion of myocardium supplied by collateral coronary arteries. *Ann. Thorac. Surg.*, 26: 535–547, 1978.

35. Chitwood, W.R., Hill R.C., Sink, J.D. et al: Assessment of ventricular diastolic properties and systolic function in man with sonomicrometry. Surg Forum 30:266–268, 1979.

36. Hill, R. C., Chitwood, W. R., Jr., Klienman, L. H. Wechsler, A. S. compressive forces of fibrillation in normal hearts during miasmal coronary dilation by adenosine. *Surg. Form.*, 28: 257. 1977.

37. Kleinman, L. H., Wechsler, A. S. Pressure flow characteristics of coronary collateral circulation during cardiopulmonary bypass: Effects of ventricular fibrillation. *Circulation*, 58: 233, 1978.

38. Hottenrott, C. E., Towers, B. Kurkji, H. J. The hazard of ventricular fibrillation in hypertrophied ventricles during cardiopulmonary bypass. *J. Thorac. Cardiovasc. Surg.*, 66: 742, 1973.

39. Burkberg, G. D., Fixler, D. E. Archie J.P. Experimental subendocardial ischemia in dogs with normal coronary arteries. *Circ. Res.*, 30: 67, 1972.

40. Tyers, G. F. O. Evidence for a safe myocardial hypothermic temperature range between 10°C and 20°C. Presented at Symposium on Myocardial Preservation. New York, N.Y., June 1979.

41. Angell, W. W., Rikkers, L., Dong, E., Shumway, N. Organ viability with hypothermia. *J. Thorac. Cardiovascular. Surg.*, 58: 619–624, 1969.

42. Hutchinson, J. E., Green G. E., Medhjian, H. A, Kemp, H. G. Coronary bypass grafting in 376 consecutive patients with three operative deaths. *J. Thorac. Cardiovasc. Surg.*, 67: 7–16, 1974.

43. Loop, F. D., Cosgrove, D. M., Lytle, B. W. et al. An 11-year evolution of coronary arterial surgery. *Ann. Surg.*, 190: 444–445, 1979.

44. Many, M., Soroff, H. S., Birtwell, W. C. The physiologic role of pulsatile and nonpulsatile blood flow. *Arch. Surg.*, 97: 917–923, 1968.
45. Sink, J. D., Chitwood, W. R., Hill, R. C. Wechsller, A. S. Comparison of nonpulsatile and pulsatile extracorporeal circulation on renal cortical blood flow. *Ann. Thorac. Surg.*, 29: 57–62, 1980.
46. Ellis, R. Marvroudis C., Ullyot D. et al. Relationship between artio-ventricular arrhythmias and the concentration of K+ ion in cardioplegia solution. Presented at the annual meeting of the American Association for Thoracic Surgery, 1980.
47. Ellis, R.J., Gertz, E.W., Wisneski, J., Ebert, P; Analysis of myocardial function following potassium cardioplegia. Presented at the Symposium on Myocardial Preservation, New York, N.Y., June 1979.

Chapter 27 ☞

Radionuclide Angiocardiography in the Diagnosis of Congenital Heart Disorders[1]

C ardiac catheterization and angiography provide anatomic and physiologic information important in the surgical management of patients with congenital heart disorders. However, this procedure is associated with some risk, as well as discomfort and inconvenience, and is not ideal for repetitive serial examinations. Radionuclide angiocardiography is accomplished by intravenous injection of a tracer which passes through the heart and lungs to image blood flow and to obtain hemodynamic measurements (1). This noninvasive procedure appears well suited for confirming a clinical diagnosis and providing serial measurements of cardiac function. Moreover, it is rapid, and relatively inexpensive in comparison with cardiac catheterization and angiocardiography. The purpose of this investigation was to review a three-year experience with the use of radionuclide angiocardiography in patients with congenital heart disorders to define clinical situations which justify the use of this method of diagnosis.

Clinical Data

Since January 1977, radionuclide angiocardiograms have been obtained in 343 patients with a clinical diagnosis of congenital heart disease at the Duke University Medical Center (Table I). Sixty-eight per cent of these patients were 16 years of age or younger, and 19% were under the age of one year. The primary indications for the

1. Coauthored with Robert H. Jones, M.D., Erle H. Austin, M.D., Claude A. Peter, M.D. in 1981.

radionuclide study included documentation of anomalous blood flow, assessment of intracardiac shunting, and measurement of left ventricular function.

Technique of Radionuclide Angiocardiography

A computerized multicrystal gamma camera (System Seventy-Seven, Baird Corporation, Bedford, MA) was used to acquire and process all studies. The detector of the instrument was placed directly anterior to the pericordium, and counts were recorded at 25 msec intervals for a 30 second period during intravenous injection of the tracer bolus. Technetium199m pertechnetate, in a dose of 0.3 mCi/kg with a minimal dose of 2 mCi and a maximal dose of 30 mCi, was used.

Studies were obtained in the supine position at rest in 214 patients, and rest and exercise studies were performed in 129 patients. All rest and exercise studies were performed with patients sitting erect on an isokinetic bicycle ergometer (Fitron, Lumex, Inc., Bay Shore, New York). After acquisition of the resting study, exercise was begun at a workload of 100 kpm/min and increased by 100 kpm every minute. A single bipolar CM-S electrocardiographic lead was continuously monitored, and blood pressure was recorded by a sphygmomanometer at one minute intervals during exercise and recovery. Attainment of 85% predicted maximal heart rate for age or the onset of exercise-limiting fatigue were the endpoints used to time the injection for the exercise study.

Data Processing

After correction of counts for detector uniformity and dead-time, static and dynamic images were generated which detected the passage of tracer through the central circulation. In patients with congenital heart disorders associated with left-to-right shunting, a curve of counts over the lung was used to quantitate the shunt magnitude by previously described techniques (2). Therefore, this approach used extrapolation of the initial decline in counts to separate and quantitate the relative magnitude of the initial circulation and the recirculation of tracer which passed through the lungs. Right-to-left intracardiac shunting was calcu-

TABLE I   Congenital Heart Disease (Diagnosis by Radionuclide Angiocardiography in 343 Patients)

Diagnosis	Number of Patients
Atrial septal defect	76
Vent. septal defect	70
Patent ductus	20
Tetralogy	16
Transposition	6
Ebsteins	4
Tricuspid utresia	2
Congenital arrhythmia	22
Ventricular dysfunction	36
Aortic insufficiency	10
Aortic stenosis	9
Mitral insufficiency	3
LCA from pulmonary artery	4
Functional murmur	65
Total	343

lated in patients with cyanotic congenital heart disorders from curves reflecting radionuclide transit through the carotid arteries (3). The radionuclide curve recorded over a systemic artery has a configuration similar to that of a dye indicator dilution curve obtained by arterial sampling in these patients (4). The forward triangle approach used to calculate right-to-left shunts from dye dilution curves was applied to radionuclide curves recorded over the carotid artery. Counts recorded over the left ventricle were used to assess left ventricular function (5). Data from several individual cardiac beats when tracer was passing through the left ventricle were added together into a single average beat by retaining the phasic relationship of the data to the cardiac cycle. The resulting images of the contracting left ventricle were displayed to permit assessment of regional wall motion. The left ventricular ejection fraction was calculated from curves reflecting count changes and volume throughout the cardiac cycle (6).

The end-diastolic volume was calculated by applying geometric techniques to the end-diastolic image (7). The end-diastolic volume

TABLE 2   Indications for Radionuclide Angiocardiogram in 343 Patients with a Diagnosis of Congenital Heart Disease

Indication	Patients	Percent
Diagnosis of shunt	152	45
Quantitation of shunt	97	28
Anatomical imaging of blood flow	8	2
Ventricular function	86	25
Total	343	100

was multiplied by left ventricular ejection fraction to provide stroke volume. Left ventricular stroke volume was multiplied by heart rate to calculate cardiac output.

The clinical diagnosis and indication for study were known in each patient prior to the radionuclide angiocardiogram. However, the radionuclide study was reported without knowledge of other procedures such as cardiac catheterization. The results of the radionuclide angiocardiogram were subsequently tabulated and compared with the results of cardiac catheterization, with the operative findings, and also with the clinical course to assess the accuracy and clinical importance of each study. Studies were categorized as follows: (1) confirming a previous diagnosis, (2) providing a neces sary measurement, (3) contributing new major diagnostic information, or (4) providing no clinical benefit.

Radionuclide calculation of intracardiac shunt was available in 146 patients who subsequently underwent cardiac catheterization, and this subgroup of patients was used to calculate the sensitivity and specificity of radionuclide detection of intracardiac shunting. In 62 patients with left-to-right shunting, radionuclide and cardiac catheterization were obtained on the same day and a linear regression equation compared shunt measurements by the two techniques.

Radionuclide angiocardiograms are relatively simple to perform and there were no complications in the very young children. The test provided new diagnostic information in 93 patients (27%), confirmed a medical diagnosis in 57 patients (17%), provided a useful measurement in 183 patients (53%), and provided no useful information in 11

(3%) of 343 patients. Therefore, the procedure appeared of benefit in 97% of patients studied. The anatomic configuration of cardiac chambers and the great vessels was readily demonstrated by radionuclide angiocardiography. The study was often useful for documenting abnormal patterns of blood flow, important both for diagnosis and in the conduct of the surgical procedure, such as a persistent left superior vena cava. The presence or absence of an intracardiac shunt was directly identified in 143 of the 146 patients who also underwent cardiac catheterization for shunt assessment. In three patients, a 14%, a 15%, and a 16% shunt were identified by the radionuclide angiocardiogram which was not confirmed by catheterization. Therefore, the sensitivity of the test for both right-to-left and left-to-right intracardiac shunting is 100%. The specificity for excluding the presence of right-to-left shunting was 100% and for excluding left-to-right shunting was 86%. Of the 109 patients studied by radionuclide angiocardiography because of a possible shunt who did not subsequently undergo cardiac catheterization, 18 were found to have intracardiac shunts greater than 35%. Four of these patients underwent closure of a patent ductus arteriosus without cardiac catheterization. The remaining 14 patients with large shunts did not undergo cardiac catheterization because of other complicating illnesses or because they declined further evaluation and treatment. Thirty-four patients had left-to-right cardiac shunts less than 36% of the pulmonary blood flow. Seven of these patients had patent ductus arteriosus ligation without cardiac catheterization. The 27 other patients with small shunts received medical treatment. A normal heart was documented in 57 of the 109 patients studied by radionuclide angiocardiography to exclude intracardiac shunting. Because of a normal radionuclide study, cardiac catheterization was not performed in these patients and none has subsequently been found to have evidence of a shunt.

Eleven patients had previously undergone operation for correction of left-to-right intracardiac shunting, and the study was used to confirm the innocence of postoperative murmurs without the need for cardiac catheterization.

Cardiac catheterization with measurement of left-to-right shunting by the Fick technique was performed in 62 patients with atrial or ventricular septal defects on the same day of the radionuclide angiocardiogram. The radionuclide and Pick measurements correlated well and permitted recognition of shunts as small as 10% of the pulmonary blood flow.

Measurements of left ventricular function at rest and exercise were obtained in 129 patients with congenital heart disorders. Ten of these studies were performed in 1,100 children in whom cardiac disease was suspected but not confirmed. The pattern of responses in these studies in children without cardiac disease was identical to hemodynamic changes observed in a larger number of patients studied as normal volunteers, who were between the ages of 18 and 25 (5). Nine children were studied with the diagnosis of idiopathic left ventricular dysfunction, and this diagnosis was confirmed in four while the remaining had normal left ventricular function. Left ventricular function was assessed at rest and exercise. In 15 patients with congenital aortic or mitral regurgitation, left ventricular function remained normal in 12 of these patients, and the study will be used for serial examination to aid in the appropriate timing of value replacement. Deterioration of left ventricular function during exercise was observed in three patients who underwent successful valve replacement.

Congenital cardiac dysrhythmias occur infrequently in children but represent difficult management problems. Rest and exercise radionuclide angiocardiograms were performed in 22 patients with dysrhythmia. One of these patients, a 16-year-old girl, demonstrated a depressed ejection fraction during rest and exercise, and during a spontaneous episode of supraventricular tachycardia. At the time of operation, epicardial mapping identified a focus of arrhythmia within the right ventricular outflow tract, and exclusion of this region eliminated a recurrent tachycardia. The patient was evaluated again on the tenth day after operation and radionuclide angiocardiography demonstrated a near normal resting ejection fraction and a normal exercise response. This study illustrates, in an objective manner, the use of rest and exercise measurements of left ventricular function to evaluate patients with cardiac dysrhythmias.

Left ventricular function was measured in three children with origin of the left coronary artery from the pulmonary artery. One patient was a seven-year-old boy at the time of study who had undergone ligation of an anomalous left main coronary artery in infancy. A rest and exercise radionuclide angiocardiogram demonstrated a near normal response presumably because of large collaterals communicating with the right coronary arterial system. An 11-year-old boy with an anomalous coronary artery had a resting ejection fraction of 0.55 which increased to only 0.56 during exercise, indicative of functional myocardial ischemia.

Following proximal ligation and division of the left coronary artery, a saphenous vein bypass graft was inserted between the aorta and the left coronary artery; the resting ejection fraction was 0.72 and increased to 0.79 during exercise. This study documented a clear postoperative improvement in this patient.

Congenital heart disease is an important cause of death and disability in children. Hoffman and Christiansen reviewed the records of 19,044 live-born children followed by consistent examinations for a period of five years. In this group, congenital heart disease was definitively diagnosed in 8.8 per thousand and appeared to be a likely diagnosis in 10.4 per thousand. Stillborn fetuses that had autopsy examinations showed a similar incidence of cardiac disease. About one-fourth of the live-born children with congenital heart disease died in infancy and childhood, and one-half of the deaths were judged to have been caused by the heart disease. The diagnosis of congenital heart disease is recognized by the age of one week in 46% of patients, by age one year in 88%, and by four years in 99%. Moreover, the patient groups studied were derived from a health plan which provided frequent examinations of children, which undoubtedly contributed to the early recognition in this group.

The spectrum of severity of congenital heart disease ranges from lesions which can be anticipated to be self-correcting, such as small ventricular septal defects, all the way to complex lesions incompatible with life and not amenable to operative correction. Therefore, the need for anatomic and physiologic characterization of congenital heart defects is related to the type and severity of these manifestations. In patients who will require operative treatment, catheterization is usually required to provide anatomic characterization of the cardiac disorder. In many other children in whom operation is to be delayed, a noninvasive technique for confirming the clinical diagnosis would often obviate the need for a more invasive procedure. In addition, the capability to

obtain repeated hemodynamic measurements can objectively document
the course of the disorder. Studies which use radioactive substances to
measure and image blood flow through the heart appear well suited for
serial evaluation of patients with congenital heart disorders.

The first studies using radioactive tracers to evaluate congenital
heart disease were reported in 1949 (9). A single unshielded Geiger-
Mueller tube monitored radioactivity over the point of maximum cardiac impulse following intravenous injection of Na-24 in an attempt
to measure left-to-light intracardiac shunts.

In the 1950s, a large number of studies were reported using single
detectors to monitor the flow of a radioactive bolus through the heart
of patients with congenital heart disorders. Development of the
gamma camera permitted imaging of blood flow through the heart
using radionuclides (10). Approximately ten years ago, it became feasible to interface a computer to a gamma camera to permit numeric
analysis of data from any selected region of the cardiac image (11).

A major application of radionuclide angiocardiography has been
the diagnosis and quantitation of intracardiac shunting. In 1974 a
method was described using this technique to accurately quantitate
left-to-right intracardiac shunting (2). Functional cardiac murmurs are
common in children and often raise the consideration of congenital
heart disease. Even when the diagnosis of cardiac pathology appears
highly unlikely, the objective documentation of normal blood flow
provides worthwhile information to reassure the patient and family of
the absence of disease. In the present study, 52% of the 109 patients
studied with a functional murmur were documented to have a normal
heart.

However, 52 patients thought to have a low probability of shunting before the study were found to have a shunt, and in 18 of these
patients the shunt was greater than 35% of pulmonary blood flow. In
the group of 103 patients who underwent cardiac catheterization with
the diagnosis of left-to-right intracardiac shunting, 21 were found not
to have a shunt at the time of catheterization. Eighteen of the 21 were
correctly demonstrated by radionuclide angiocardiography not to have
a shunt.

Moreover, none of the patients subsequently undergoing cardiac
catheterization after no shunt was demonstrated by radionuclide

angiocardiography were found to have a shunt by catheterization. Therefore, radionuclide angiocardiography appears to have an important clinical application in the diagnosis and quantitation of left-to-right shunting prior to cardiac catheterization. In children with an absent or small shunt, in whom an operation would not be indicated, cardiac catheterization would be unnecessary. In children with a shunt of moderate size in whom operation might be delayed until a later age, cardiac catheterization could be reserved until immediately prior to the procedure. A study performed in the postoperative period would be useful in documenting the total correction of the disorder causing the shunt. Cyanosis and a cardiac murmur commonly suggest the diagnosis of heart disease in older children. However, cyanosis in the newborn, which occurs frequently with primary lung disorders, may prove difficult to differentiate from cyanotic heart disease. Moreover, development of a technique which serially quantitates the magnitude of right-to-left shunting offers much benefit in the selection of the most appropriate time for surgical correction. Right-to-left intracardiac shunting may frequently be recognized from radionuclide images of blood flow which show transit of tracer from the right atrium or ventricle to the adjacent cardiac chamber. More recently, mathematic techniques have been applied to radionuclide data in 20 children and shown to measure accurately the magnitude of right-to-left intracardiac shunting. In the present study, the presence or absence of right-to-left shunting was correctly recognized in all 43 patients studied with this diagnosis.

Radionuclide measurements of left ventricular volumes have been demonstrated to be quite accurate and reproducible in adults (12, 13). Radionuclide measurements of left ventricular volumes might be less accurate in children because of their small heart size, rapid heart rate, and the relatively low radiopharmaceutical dose which can be used. The accuracy of radionuclide measurements of left ventricular function was examined in 32 children who underwent cardiac catheterization for congenital heart disorders (14). The ages of these children ranged from age four months to 15 years (mean: 5.5 years). The mean ejection fraction by catheterization was $72 \pm 10\%$ and by radionuclide angiocardiogram was $78 \pm 11\%$ for the group. Moreover, the ejection fraction by catheterization and radionuclide angiocardiogram was within 15% in 84% of the patients. The end–diastolic volume and stroke volume correlated quite well with cardiac catheterization over a wide range of values (r 0.96, r 0.86). These data confirm that radionu-clidc measurements of left ventricular function are sufficiently accurate to be of clinical importance in the management of children with con-genital heart disease.

Surgical treatment of congenital heart disorders has progressed so that a majority of patients with these diseases who previously would have died now survive. Therefore, therapy is no longer evaluated by patient survival alone, and attention has recently been focused upon forms of treatment that minimize myocardial tissue loss and optimally preserve cardiac function. Studies in adults with cardiac disease have documented that many patients with normal resting ventricular func-tion showed depressed ejection fractions during exercise. Much of this change appears to be related to exercise-induced myocardial ischemia, but these changes have also been observed in patients with longstanding ventricular volume overload resulting from valvular regurgitation. Therefore, the definition of cardiovascular function should, ideally, describe heart performance both at rest and during the maximum level of activity typical in the daily routine of individual patients. Use of radionuclide techniques for measurement of ventricular function during exercise should provide a valuable index of myocardial reserve in chil-dren with congenital heart disorders.

References

1. Jones, R. H., Scholz, P. M., Anderson, P. A. W. Radionuclide studies in patients with congenital heart disease. In Willerson, J. T. (ed.), *Cardiovascular Clinics*. Philadelphia: F. A. Davis, 1979, p. 225.
2. Anderson, P. W. A., Jones, R. H., Sabiston, D. C. Jr. Quantitation of left-to-right cardiac shunts with radionuclide angiocardiogra-phy. *Circulation*, 49: 512, 1974.
3. Peter, C. A., Jones, R. H. Radionuclide measurement of right-to-left intracardiac shunting. *Surg. Form.*, 30: 219, 1979.
4. Peter, C. A., Armstrong, B. E., Jones R. H. Radionuclide quanti-tation of right-to-left intracardiac shunts in children. *Circulation*, 64: 572–577, 1981.

5. Scholz, P. M., Rerych, S. K, Moran J. F. et al. Quantitative radionuclide angiocardiography. *Cath. Cardiovasc. Diag.*, 6: 265, 1980.

6. Jones, R. H., Douglas, J. M., Jr., Rerych, S. K. et al. Noninvasive radionuclide assessment of cardiac function in patients with peripheral vascular disease. *Surgery*, 85: 59, 1979.

7. Dodge, H. T., Hey, R. E., Sandler, H. An angiocardiographic method for directly determining left ventricular stroke volume in man. *Circ. Res.*, 11: 739, 1962.

8. Hoffman, J. I. E. Congenital heart disease in a cohort of 19,502 births with long-term follow-up. *Am.J. Cardiol.*, 42: 641, 1978.

9. Prinzmetal, M., Corday, E., Spritzler, R. J. et al. Radiocardiography and its clinical applications, *J.A.M.A.*, 139: 617, 1949.

10. Mason, D. T., Ashburn, W. L., Harbert, J. C. et al. Radiocardiography and its clinical applications. *J.A.M.A.*, 139: 617, 1949.

11. Jones, R. R., Lidofsky, L. Bundinger T. Weber, P. Instrumentation. In Pierson, R. N., Jr., Kriss, J. P., Jones R. H., MacIntyre, W. J. (eds.). *Quantitative Nuclear Cardiology*. New York: John Wiley and Sons, Inc., 1975, p. 231.

12. Anderson, P. A. W., Rerych, S. K. Moore, T. E., Jones, R. H. Accuracy of left ventricular end-diastolic dimension determinations obtained by radionuclide angiocardiography. *J. Nuclear Med.*, 22: 500–505, 1981.

13. Upton, M. T., Rerych, S. K., Newman, G. E. et al. The reproducibility of radionuclide angiocardiographic measurements of left ventricular function in normal subjects at rest and during exercise. *Circulation*, 62: 126, 1980.

14. Newman, G. E., Benson D. W., Jr., Anderson P. A. W., Jones R. H. Documentation of the accuracy of radionuclide measurement of left ventricular function in children. *Circulation*, 60: 11-213, 1979.

VI

The Lungs

O ne of the most perplexing aspects of the problem is the difficulty in establishing a definite diagnosis. Since the clinical
manifestations of pulmonary embolism may closely resemble those of
other cardiorespiratory diseases, a simple and reliable method of objective diagnosis constitutes a distinct need. This is of particular importance at the present in view of the recent use of pulmonary embolectomy with extracorporeal circulation in the management of massive
embolism. Furthermore, treatment aimed at prevention of recurrence
is dependent upon accurate recognition of the disease. Consequently, a
group of experimental and clinical studies were undertaken to develop
a useful diagnostic method of employing the principle of pulmonary
scanning with labeled macroaggregated human serum albumin.

Chapter 28 ☞

The Diagnosis of Pulmonary Embolism by Radioisotope Scanning[1]

P ulmonary embolism continues to represent a serious complication of a variety of medical and surgical disorders. Statistics from
large centers in the United States and abroad indicate that the incidence of this condition has remained essentially unchanged during the
past 50 years, a fact which clearly establishes the importance of this
frequent and often fatal complication.

One of the most perplexing aspects of the problem is the difficulty
in establishing a definite diagnosis. Since the clinical manifestations of
pulmonary embolism may closely resemble those of other cardiorespiratory diseases, a simple and reliable method of objective diagnosis
constitutes a distinct need. This is of particular importance at the present in view of the recent use of pulmonary embolectomy with extracorporeal circulation in the management of massive embolism. Furthermore, treatment aimed at prevention of recurrence is dependent
upon accurate recognition of the disease. Consequently, a group of
experimental and clinical studies were undertaken to develop a useful
diagnostic method of employing the principle of pulmonary scanning
with labeled macroaggregated human serum albumin.

A technique for the production of experimental massive pulmonary embolism was devised which could be performed without
entry into the chest using a balloon catheter.

Macroaggregated Human Serum Albumin (MAA). It is well known
that heating causes the aggregation of albumin molecules forming particles of varying size, depending upon the intensity and duration of the
heat as well as the pH of the medium. radioiodinated human serum

1. Coauthored with Henry N. Wagner, Jr., M.D. in 1969.

albumin of high specific activity (approximately 2 millicuries per milligram) was made into a solution with a concentration of 0.1 in 0.9 percent sodium chloride employing a modification of the technic described by Taplin and associates. The pH was adjusted to 5.5 with dilute hydrochloric acid. Since pH profoundly influenced the size of the macroaggregates, it was controlled within 0.1 units. This produced visible macroaggregates, and less than 6 percent of the radioactivity remained in the supernatant following centrifugation for five minutes at 3,000 rpm.

The entire procedure was performed employing sterile conditions. In some of the studies chromic chloride of high specific activity was used to label the human serum albumin. Again, a pH of 5.5 was obtained and aggregation was produced by heating at 100° C for four minutes. Approximately 50 percent of the radioactive chromium was bound to the MAA and the free chromium was removed by centrifugation after several washings in glucose solution at pH 5.5. A small amount of I-131-labeled MAA (0.1 mg. of albumin with an activity of 300 microcuries) was injected intravenously. The labeled material immediately passed through the right heart and into the lung.

Most of the albumin particles become blocked in the arterioles and capillaries permitting an immediate scintiscan to be performed. More than 75 percent of the injected dose could be demonstrated in the lungs and the second highest concentration of radioactivity was in the organs of the reticulo-endothelium system, primarily the liver and the spleen. In the preparation of MAA, some particles of small size are invariably present and pass through the lungs and accumulate in the liver and spleen. It is possible that some particles pass through shunts within the lung, thus entering the left heart and ultimately reaching the systemic circulation. Chromium-labeled MAA was found to have a smaller proportion of small particles than did the iodine-labeled MAA. In man, the rate of disappearance of radioactivity from the lungs following the intravenous injection of MAA was approximately exponential with half times ranging between three and ten hours. Hepatic radioactivity was determined simultaneously and indicated that the particles in the lungs were being broken down to smaller particles which returned to the circulating blood and were phagocytized by the cells of the reticulo-endothelial system. The iodinated MAA was found to be excreted in the urine at a rapid rate, while the Cr51-tagged albumin was more slowly excreted. The chromium-labelled material did not return as promptly to the circulation but remained in the liver and spleen for considerably longer periods of time. When MAA was injected, no radioactivity was found in the lungs 24 hours later, thus permitting frequent repeat scans.

Creation of experimental emboli by the balloon technic was found to be a very satisfactory method of producing selective obstruction of the pulmonary arteries. In the majority of animals, the balloon lodged in the right pulmonary artery or one of its branches, but the left pulmonary and its branches were also the site of localization in some animals. The embolic occlusion may vary from a small middle lobe to complete obstruction of the right or left pulmonary artery. Ciné-radiography with injection of radio-opaque medium into the right heart showed that the pulmonary artery distal to the balloon embolus did not fill with contrast material. In these experiments the site of obstruction could be seen on the plain chest film since the embolus was opaque; further confirmation was obtained by pulmonary arteriography and ultimate proof was established at postmortem examination.

One advantage of this technique is that large emboli may be introduced into the pulmonary circulation and removed at any time without entry into the chest. With the passage of time (24 hours or longer) in situ, thrombosis often occurs in the artery distal to the embolus and to a lesser extent proximal to the embolus. Thus, if the embolus is allowed to remain for a period of 48 hours or longer, the artery may remain occluded after withdrawal of the balloon embolus. Such a preparation is ideally suited for the controlled evaluation of systemically administered fibrinolytic agents. This problem is currently being studied.

Clinical Evaluation of Macroaggregated Human Serum Albumin in Pulmonary Scanning. Pulmonary scans have been performed in more than 100 patients with various forms of pulmonary disease. Of these, 13 patients have subsequently been proven to have pulmonary emboli by either autopsy or pulmonary arteriography. The technic is simple, quick, and has been found to be safe from the viewpoints of toxicity, radiation hazard, and antigenicity. Although the method has proven of considerable diagnostic aid in the evaluation of several pulmonary disorders, the discussion in this communication is limited to the findings in pulmonary embolism. All scans were performed in the anterior-posterior position with the patient lying supine. For quantitation of blood flow, the output of the detection crystal was led to a ratemeter and chart recorder to obtain a series of profiles of the concentration of radioactivity. An elderly woman with diabetes and hypertensive arteriosclerotic heart disease, while recovering from an amputation of the left leg for gangrene, suddenly became severely dyspneic and was found to have profound and persistent hypotension. Massive pulmonary embolism was suspected and a lung scan was obtained. The scan showed marked reduction in blood flow to the right lower lobe and to most of the left lung. The patient succumbed a short time later, and post-mortem examination demonstrated occlusion of the pulmonary arteries corresponding to the sites indicated on the pulmonary scan.

An example of a less acute form of pulmonary embolism has been seen, wherein the plain chest film showed diminished vascular markings at both bases, and the pulmonary arteriogram confirmed partial occlusion of the arteries in these areas. The pulmonary scan confirmed the arteriographic series.

A patient presenting with symptoms suggestive of an episode of pulmonary embolism in the past had a plain chest film that showed diminished vascular markings at the left base, and an arteriogram showed essentially no filling of the left lower lobe. A pulmonary scan was performed and demonstrated a defect in the same area.

In several patients two sites of predilection to embolization have been noted frequently and appear to be almost characteristic of pulmonary embolism. The first site is a partial defect involving the right lower lobe, a lesion often encountered in the experimental series. This is not an unexpected finding, since in most clinical series the right lower lobe is most commonly involved in pulmonary embolism. The second zone frequently observed is a semilunar filling defect (crescent sign) in the periphery of the left midlung field.

In the experimental series it was noted early in the lung scans that removal of the balloon embolus alone did not necessarily cause arterial filling of the involved area in immediate re-scans. In fact, if the embolus had been in place 48 hours or longer, in situ thrombosis frequently occurred distal to the embolus and to a less marked extent proximal to the embolus. However, serial scans showed that with the passage of time subsequent scanning demonstrated slow but progressive return of arterial circulation to the involved part. This has also been observed in man following pulmonary embolism. The pulmonary scan of a 62-year-old woman with thrombophlebitis, chest pain, and fever demonstrated an absence of arterial circulation in the right upper lobe. Gradual improvement in the clinical signs occurred over a period of two months, but there was then a sudden return of symptoms, including hemoptysis. A second scan at that time was performed and showed filling of the previously nonfilled right upper lobe, although reduced filling in the right lower lobe was apparent. A diagnosis of recurrent pulmonary embolism was made and plication of the inferior vena cava was performed. At the time of operation a thrombus was found in the inferior vena cava.

Despite the use of numerous methods directed toward its prevention, pulmonary embolism continues to represent a serious threat to patients following operation. It is also well recognized that pulmonary embolism occurs as a complication of a variety of medical conditions, particularly congestive heart failure. One of the primary problems in the institution of proper therapy in the management of pulmonary embolism is the difficulty encountered in establishing a certain diagnosis. Furthermore, it is seldom possible to make an accurate assessment of the magnitude and localization of embolism. The symptom complex and physical manifestations which occur in pulmonary embolism may closely resemble those of other cardiorespiratory disorders, particularly myocardial infarction. The means available for the diagnosis of pulmonary embolism include the clinical history, physical findings, plain chest film, and the electrocardiogram.

In 1938, Westermark described the radiographic signs of massive pulmonary embolism which may be present in the plain chest film (14). These consist primarily of blanching of the vascular markings in those vessels obstructed by embolism. Torrance has again emphasized these findings in a recent monograph (9). Although this sign and related findings on the plain chest film are helpful, such changes are not absolute and emboli may be missed when complete reliance is placed upon this manifestation alone.

Pulmonary arteriography is the most reliable means of diagnosis of pulmonary embolism. Unfortunately, this procedure has the disadvantage that it is time-consuming and requires experienced personnel. Furthermore, the injection of radiopaque contrast medium into the pulmonary circulation of patients with pulmonary embolism may produce a pronounced hypotension in an already critically ill patient.

Thus, the use of pulmonary arteriography presents serious contraindications and makes desirable the availability of an alternate technic which is both safe and reliable. The feasibility of the use of colloidal materials for the study of liver blood flow was first demonstrated by Dobson and Jones in 1952 (3). They injected particulate material intravenously and measured its disappearance from the blood stream in an effort to measure hepatic flow. In these studies, the particles used were quite small and localized primarily in the liver and spleen, being phagocytized by the reticulo-endothelial cells in these organs. In 1955, Benacerraf and associates (1) described the use of aggregates of human serum proteins labeled with radioactive iodine as an example of particulate matter which might be employed to advantage in the study of phagocytosis. Larger particles of such material can be prepared using carefully controlled conditions. These particles are blocked by the pulmonary arteriolar and capillary beds. Thus, a minute amount of macroaggregated human serum albumin with a low dosage of radioactivity may be injected intravenously with a majority of the particles becoming lodged in the lungs. This allows a scan to be performed which demonstrates the distribution of pulmonary blood flow and clearly delineates areas in which the pulmonary arterial flow is diminished or absent. Quantitative determinations of pulmonary blood flow may be made since the concentration of radioactivity in the lungs in a particular region depends upon the blood supply according to the principle of conservation of material.

Experimental and clinical studies with labeled macroaggregated isotope albumin have been shown to be without significant effect on pulmonary hemodynamics in the amounts employed, and it is without toxicity, radiation hazard, or antigenic effect (5, 10).

Following a number of experimental observations, the technic of pulmonary scanning was introduced for clinical use. More than 100

patients have been studied by this method for a variety of cardiorespiratory disorders. In this communication the use of this technic in the
diagnosis of pulmonary embolism is emphasized, since many patients
with this disorder have an essentially negative chest film. In those
instances in which the plain film indicates a blanching of the vascular
markings, it is difficult to be certain of the site and extent of pulmonary embolism. Lung scanning is of greatest usefulness in establishing the diagnosis of massive pulmonary embolism in a patient with a
clear chest film. In the early studies, pulmonary arteriography was
simultaneously obtained with the scan to prove the correlation. In
every patient the arteriogram confirmed the scan and it is now
believed pulmonary arteriography is not necessary, although it is of
value in distinguishing massive embolism from multiple small emboli.
Pulmonary scanning has proven to be an objective and reliable means
of establishing a firm diagnosis of pulmonary embolism and is especially useful in the selection of patients for direct pulmonary embolectomy employing extracorporeal circulation. In this group of patients it
is particularly important to establish the diagnosis firmly and to thus
exclude other serious causes producing similar clinical manifestations
such as acute myocardial infarction. These studies have also indicated
that patients with pulmonary embolism may show a return of pulmonary arterial flow to areas of the lung previously obstructed by
emboli. This is in agreement with recent experimental studies with
autologous, organized pulmonary emboli (6, 7) and with some recent
respiratory function studies in patients evaluated months following
pulmonary embolism (4). Thus, it now appears clear that if a patient
can withstand the acute insult of pulmonary embolism, there may be
partial lysis or recanalization of the embolus with ultimate return of
pulmonary function toward normal. Pulmonary scanning has also been
useful in determining the magnitude of embolism and in the selection
of the appropriate method of therapy.

References

1. Benacerraf, G., Halpern B. N., Stiffel C., Crushaud S., and Biozzi,
   G. Phagocytose d'une fraction du serum chauffee et iode par le

systeme reticuloendothelial et comportement consecutif de ses cellules a l'egard d'autres colloidas. *Ann. Inst. Pasteur*, 89: 601, 1955.

2. DeBakey, M. K. Critical evaluation of problem of thromboembolism. *Surg. Gynec. & Obst.*, 98: 1, 1954.

3. Dobson, K. L., and Jones, H. B. The behavior of intravenously injected particulate material: Its rate of disappearance from the blood stream as a measure of liver blood flow. *Acta Med. Scand.*, 144, Suppl. 273, 1952.

4. Durner, H., Pernow, B., and Rigner, K. C. The prognosis of pulmonary embolism. *Acta. Med. Scand.*, 168, fasc. 5, 1960.

5. Lio, M. and Wagner, H. N. Studies of the reticuloendothelial system (RES). I. Measurement of phagocytic capacity of the RES in man and dog. *J. Clin. Invest.*, 42: 417,1963.

6. Marshall, R., Sabiston, D. C., Allison, P. R., Bosman, A. R., and Dunnill, M. S. Immediate and late effects of pulmonary embolism by large thrombi in dogs. *Thorax*, 18: 1, 1963.

7. Sabiston, D. C., Marshall, R., Dunnill, M. S., and Allison, P. R. Experimental pulmonary embolism: Description of a method utilization large venous thrombi. *Surgery*, 52: 9, 1962.

8. Taplin, G. V., Dore, K. K., and Johnson, D. F. Clinical studies of reticuloendothelial functions with colloidal suspensions of human albumin I-131. UCLA report (Biology and Medicine), Sept. 1961.

9. Torrance, D. J. *The Chest Film in Massive Pulmonary Embolism.* Springfield, Illinois: Charles C. Thomas Co., 1963.

10. Wagner, H. N., and Sabiston, D. C. Unpublished observations.

11. Wastermark, N. Roentgen diagnosis of long embolism. *Acta. Radiol.*, 19: 357, 1938.

Chapter 29

Diagnosis of Massive Pulmonary Embolism in Man by Radioisotope Scanning: First Report of Use of Urokinase to Treat Pulmonary Embolism[1]

*T*he diagnosis of massive pulmonary embolism is frequently difficult and always uncertain, primarily because the symptoms and
signs may mimic those of some other diseases, such as myocardial
infarction or pneumonia. Ancillary examinations, including X-ray
study of the chest and electrocardiography, are rarely definitive. The
diagnosis can be suspected when sudden dyspnea, pleural pain,
hemoptysis, syncope, or a bloody pleural effusion occurs in patients
who are predisposed to pulmonary embolism—that is, those who are
suffering from congestive heart failure or polycythemia, or who are
bedridden, as during the postoperative or postpartum state.

A high degree of suspicion is no longer adequate. When therapeutic measures were relatively nonspecific, absolute accuracy in diagnosis
was not required. Today, however, the need for improved diagnostic
ability has increased because new means of treating pulmonary thromboembolism are available. These include anticoagulant drugs to prevent further thrombosis, proteolytic agents to dissolve thrombi that
have already formed, and specific surgical therapy, including ligation or
plication of the inferior vena cava, to prevent passage of peripheral
thrombi into the lungs, and pulmonary embolectomy, the removal of
obstructing clots from the pulmonary arteries themselves. The present

---

1. Coauthored by Henry N. Wagner, Jr., M.D., John N. G. McAfee, M.D.,
Donald Tow, M.D. and Howard S. Stern, Ph.D. in 1964.

report describes the development and initial evaluation of a new radioisotope scanning procedure that has been found to be a safe and effective way of diagnosing massive pulmonary embolism in man. In addition to its use in thromboembolic diseases, the method has been employed to obtain information concerning regional pulmonary blood flow in other pulmonary diseases.

In the present series of over 100 patients, autopsy, operation, or selective pulmonary arteriography confirmed the diagnosis of regional pulmonary avascularity in 14 cases in which filling defects were observed in the lung scans. The size of the smallest lesion that could be detected is not known with certainty although it is likely that lesions less than a few centimeters in diameter would be missed with present scanning equipment. Since we have used selective pulmonary arteriography as a means of confirming the diagnosis of pulmonary embolism in the patients who were not studied at autopsy, a reasonable question is what lung scanning offers in the diagnosis on pulmonary embolism that pulmonary arteriography does not. Each technic has its own particular strong points and deficiencies. To be completely satisfactory, pulmonary arteriography must be performed by injection of relatively large volumes of radiopaque material directly into the pulmonary artery. Intravenous injections usually do not give sufficiently good definition of the vasculature. Therefore, cardiac catheterization is required, which is cumbersome at best and may result in the dislodgment of venous thrombi at worst. Furthermore, experience has shown that patients with pulmonary hypertension tolerate injections of X-ray contrast material very poorly. Up until now, lung scanning has not been associated with any known toxicity and does not result in any morbidity. An important advantage is that serial studies can be performed at frequent intervals in the same subject, thereby providing follow-up information at intervals that would not be possible if one had to perform repeated pulmonary arteriography.

Examples of follow-up studies now in progress are evaluation of the natural history of pulmonary embolism, evaluation of the incidence of recurrences of pulmonary embolism after plication or ligation of the vena cava and determination of the efficacy of thrombolytic drugs. The scanning procedure is technically simple, and, at present, we have a scanner available for immediate use as soon as the diagnosis is suspected. In at least 20 patients serious consideration of the diagnosis of massive pulmonary embolism was discarded when lung scans revealed normal pulmonary vasculature. On the other hand, whenever we obtained strong evidence of multiple areas of pulmonary avascularity, selective pulmonary arteriography was performed if the possible necessity of pulmonary embolectomy was considered. Is the scanning procedure sufficiently definitive to permit the diagnosis of massive pulmonary embolism on the basis of the scan alone? The answer to this question is a qualified no, because, as we have previously reported (1), most parenchymal lesions of the lungs result in avascularity of the pulmonary circulation, the blood supply presumably being provided by the bronchial circulation. On the other hand, in a large number of patients, a characteristic pattern has been observed in massive pulmonary embolism. This pattern consists of crescent-shaped defects, particularly at the lateral borders of the lungs.

In the studies in dogs we found that the right lower lobe is by far the most commonly involved lobe when large emboli pass into the lungs. Frequent involvement of the right lower lobe has also been reported in pathological studies in man, and in the present series of patients we have confirmed this finding.

Even in the absence of the characteristic pattern, one should suspect pulmonary embolism if one finds multiple avascular areas on the scan, particularly if no parenchymal lesions are seen on the X-ray film of the chest. This has usually been the case, both in the experimental emboli in dogs and in patients subsequently proved to have massive embolism. Particularly helpful is the finding of a corresponding zone of increased radiolucency, initially reported by Westermark (2) and recently extended by Torrance (3).

On the other hand, if there is a lesion on the film of the chest, from our past experience, regardless of whether the lesion is the result of an infarct, pneumonia, atelectasis, abscess, or tumor, the area will be avascular so far as the pulmonary arterial blood flow is concerned, and an area of decreased radioactivity will be found on the lung scan. In these cases, although of considerable academic interest, the information is of no diagnostic value.

A particular word of caution must be given about lung bullae or cysts. These areas are both avascular and radiolucent on X-ray study of the chest and may therefore mimic the findings in pulmonary embolism. An example of this type of case was previously reported (5).

In summary, radioisotope scanning of the lungs in the first 100 patients and after the intravenous injection of miroaggregated albumin (MAA) labeled I-125 or Cr51 is a safe and effective way of diagnosing massive pulmonary embolism.

In many patients a characteristic pattern of avascularity was observed. This consisted of a decreased pulmonary blood flow to all or part of the right lower and crescent-shaped filling defects on the lateral borders of the lungs.

To date, no hemodynamic, immunologic, or radiation hazard has been observed. The method has been found to be an important adjunct to selective pulmonary arteriography, and has important advantages in being readily available, faster, technically easier, and free of morbidity. Consequently, it was used as a rapid screening procedure and made possible serial studies at frequent intervals in the same patients.

The scanning technic was found to be particularly suitable for the evaluation of the natural history of massive pulmonary embolism, as well as in determination of the effectiveness of surgical procedures, such as vena cava ligation, or of drugs, such as anticoagulants and flbrinolytic agents.

Since this manuscript was submitted for publication, we have continued to use the experimental model in dogs to evaluate the possible effectiveness of urokinase in the treatment of pulmonary thromboembolic disease. The latex balloon containing radiopaque material was left in place for forty-eight hours before we removed it by withdrawing the attached string. Characteristically, this resulted in in situ thrombosis distal to the point of arterial obstruction. The appearance of the scan indicated when the blood supply was normal.

Of 8 dogs that did not receive urokinase, none had restoration of pulmonary blood flow within twenty-four hours. The average time required for spontaneous restoration of flow was more than twenty-two days. Of 12 dogs given 2,000 to 6,000 units of urokinase per kilogram of body weight immediately after removal of the balloon, 7 had complete restoration of blood flow when examined twenty-four hours later.

Autopsy study of these dogs indicated no thrombosis; in contrast, autopsy study of the control dogs revealed the presence of thrombi, fibrosis, and atrophy of the involved arteries. These data in dogs suggest that this dose of urokinase had a significant thrombolytic effect. The scanning technic was of particular value in that it permitted evaluation of the pulmonary circulation without sacrifice of the animals until such time as was indicated by the functional data provided by the scans.

References

1. Wagner, H. N., Jr. et al. Regional pulmonary blood flow in man by radioisotope scanning. *J.A.M.A.*, 187: 601–603, 1964.
2. Westermark, N. On roentgen diagnosis of lung embolism. *Acta radiol.*, 19: 357–372, 1938.
3. Torrance, D. J., Jr. *The Chest Film in Massive Pulmonary Embolism: Foreword by Warde Allan.* Springfield, Illinois: Thomas, 1963. (American Lectures in Roentgen Diagnosis.)

Chapter 30

The Pathophysiology of Pulmonary Embolism: Relationships to Accurate Diagnosis and Choice of Therapy[1]

*P*ulmonary embolism is the most common of the serious disorders affecting the pulmonary circulation. The significance of this condition is further emphasized by recent postmortem studies in which careful examination of the lungs showed evidence of pulmonary embolism in more than half of adult patients who died from all causes. In many patients the diagnosis of fatal pulmonary embolism is often made for the first time at necropsy. The difficulty in establishing a firm diagnosis is explained by the fact that the signs and symptoms of pulmonary embolism often closely resemble those of other serious cardiorespiratory diseases. Increased attention is now being directed toward an accurate diagnosis of pulmonary embolism due, in large part, to the introduction of improved methods for management of this potentially fatal complication. The use of anticoagulants to prevent continued formation of thrombi remains the most frequently employed method of treatment. In those instances in which the degree of arterial occlusion by pulmonary emboli is more serious, surgical interruption of the inferior vena cava is often indicated, while massive pulmonary embolism with severe clinical manifestations is best managed by direct pulmonary embolectomy. While an accurate diagnosis is important in all patients with pulmonary embolism, definite evidence of the presence and magnitude of pulmonary embolism should be mandatory prior to the use of surgical therapy. Interruption of the inferior vena cava may produce specific complications, and the risks in

---

1. Coauthored with Henry N. Wagner, Jr. M.D. in 1965.

the direct removal of pulmonary emboli are clearly recognized. Furthermore, experience has shown that in some patients operated upon with clinical signs and symptoms of pulmonary embolism alone, the diagnosis has been in error. In these instances, the correct diagnosis has usually been some other disease of the heart or lungs and one which may be seriously aggravated by an unnecessary surgical procedure. It is for these reasons that the establishment of a firm diagnosis of both the site and magnitude of the pulmonary embolism is of prime importance.

Physiological consequences of pulmonary embolism. Under normal conditions, the pulmonary circulation receives the total flow of the right ventricle which is approximately equal to systemic cardiac output. One of the primary features of the pulmonary circulation is its low vascular resistance, thereby enabling flow in the pulmonary vascular bed to be increased several fold without significant elevation of pulmonary arterial pressure. Despite much experimental and clinical investigation, opinion remains divided concerning the relative importance of the reflex versus the mechanical effects of pulmonary embolism (33). The occasional finding of a small pulmonary embolus in a patient who dies suddenly raises the possibility that intraluminal occlusion of a relatively small portion of the pulmonary arterial bed can be fatal, presumably by reflex vasoconstriction.

It is well established that pneumonectomy in normal man is usually well tolerated. Studies of tidal volume and oxygen exchange following resection of a lung have shown few changes. Similarly, occlusion of one pulmonary artery in man or the experimental animal by means of an intraluminal balloon is also well tolerated and is accompanied by few cardiodynamic changes. Patients have tolerated this procedure for periods of up to 2 hours (5). In the dog with similar occlusion, pulmonary arterial pressure is increased only 12 to 50 percent, while cardiac output increases as much as threefold (17). Occlusions of this type closely simulate the obstruction produced by the mechanical effects of pulmonary embolism. One must remember, however, that such studies have been conducted in normal subjects. The presence of underlying cardiac or respiratory disease may produce different effects. Sloan and associates (27) studied 18 patients with temporary occlusion of the right or left pulmonary artery by a balloon catheter. Exercise during unilateral occlusion of the pulmonary artery produced a marked rise in pulmonary arterial pressure in those patients with heart disease. Furthermore, an abnormal increase in the arteriovenous oxygen difference was noted and a failure of the cardiac output to increase significantly with exercise. In a recent study, data have been presented which suggest that resection of less than one lung is followed by only slight changes in the pulmonary arterial pressure, whereas removal of greater amounts of pulmonary tissue usually results in an elevation of pulmonary arterial pressure (38).

In experimental studies, embolization of the entire right or left pulmonary artery by large emboli usually produced few serious changes in cardiopulmonary dynamics. Animals survive such procedures without significant difficulty. In recent studies it was shown that large pulmonary emboli in dogs produced no serious effects which could be attributed to reflex action, provided the embolism was confined to one lung. Such procedures did not produce effects on the electrocardiogram, systemic arterial pressure, or central venous pressure (15, 16, 19, 2). In most animals, occlusion of the right or left pulmonary artery was proved by the marked depression of the oxygen consumption in the embolized lung as demonstrated by differential bronchospirometry. Similar findings were noted in another study, with the use of a simplified technique for the production of massive experimental pulmonary embolization, in which regional pulmonary flow was determined by subsequent study by radioactive pulmonary scanning (20).

Clinical and pathological studies also add further support to the importance of mechanical factors in massive pulmonary embolism In a postmortem study of 100 consecutive patients with massive pulmonary embolism at the New York Cornell Medical Center, Gorham (12, 13) found that 85 had occlusion involving one pulmonary artery and, in addition, embolism in the opposite lung. Only 15 patients had emboli restricted solely to one lung, and 12 were more than 54 years of age, a group with an appreciable incidence of underlying cardiac and respiratory disease. In patients with massive pulmonary embolism in whom embolectomy is performed, it is usual to find emboli in more than one pulmonary artery (2, 10). Such evidence supports the concept of the importance of mechanical blockage in the symptom complex in massive pulmonary embolism, reinforcing the data obtained from occlusion of the pulmonary circulation by arterial ligature, intraluminal balloon, pulmonary resection, and experimental emboli.

Despite the foregoing evidence, one cannot ignore the role of reflex factors in the production of the cardiovascular changes associated with pulmonary embolism. Much experimental data suggest that embolization of the lung with small particles (less than 100 microns in diameter) creates reflex effects, producing tachypnea, pulmonary hyptertension, systemic hypotension, and death. However, microembolism of the lung is infrequently encountered clinically, and embolization with larger particles requires considerably more blockage of the pulmonary arterial system to produce serious effects. In a recent study in dogs, Dexter injected graded sizes of polystyrene beads, matched to the size of the lumen of the branches of the pulmonary artery, varying between lobar (4 to 5 mm.) and atrial arteries (0.17 mm.). The number of emboli required to produce pulmonary hypertension corresponded to the number required to obstruct a similar fraction of the vascular bed. Thus it appears that arterial emboli produce pulmonary hypertension by mechanical obstruction and that vasoconstriction results from arteriolar embolism mediated by reflex changes. These studies suggest that the clinical manifestations of pulmonary embolism are usually produced primarily by occlusion of the larger pulmonary arteries.

Pathological consequences of pulmonary embolism. Of equal importance are the pathological changes associated with pulmonary embolism, particularly the fate of the emboli. Allison, Dunnill, and Marshall (1) introduced large radiopaque blood clots into the inferior vena cava or jugular vein of the dog. Motion picture films traced their passage through the heart and into the pulmonary arteries. Repeated studies showed the clots to be absorbed from the pulmonary circulation rapidly. Histologic examination demonstrated that at 4 days a smooth layer of cells covered the clot, and ingrowth of vasa vasorum could be seen arising from the adventitia of the artery. At 21 days the clot had been reduced to a subintimal fibrous plaque, and at 28 days the arterial wall had essentially returned to normal. We repeated these studies, using large thrombi produced in situ in the inferior vena cava of the dog. When these were also injected into the pulmonary arterial circulation, reduced function of the embolized lung occurred but the animals showed a return to normal pulmonary function at approximately 1 month. Similarly, marked regression of the histological changes occurred with these 10-to-14-day old thrombi, as well as with fresh blood clots. More recently, we have employed a technique of pulmonary embolism by using a latex balloon filled with radiopaque medium attached to the end of a long suture (20). Pulmonary thrombosis formed in situ both proximal and distal to the "embolus," and, following removal of the balloon, the distal thrombosis remained. By serial radioisotope scanning, we could measure the time required for restoration of pulmonary arterial blood flow to the involved area of the lung. In a series of control studies, the average time required for restoration of pulmonary arterial blood flow to normal was 23 days (range: 3 to 63 days). Using this experimental model in dogs, we were able to demonstrate that administration of the fibrinolytic enzyme, urokinase, accelerated the return of flow, presumably by lysis of the in situ thrombi. In 7 dogs, the scan had returned to normal within 24 hours, in 3, the blood flow had become normal within a week; in the only other treated dog, flow was not restored. Evidence provided by the scans was supported by pulmonary arteriography and autopsy. Serial scans in patients with pulmonary embolism have also indicated restoration of blood flow after a period of time. The restoration of blood flow was evident.

Clinical manifestations. The clinical manifestations of pulmonary embolism may closely resemble those of a variety of other diseases. While there are characteristic symptoms, such as dyspnea, chest pain, hemoptysis, and hypotension which are often present, these are not sufficiently specific. In 1933, White (37) described a group of consequences of pulmonary embolism which included tachycardia, accentuation of the second pulmonary sound, dilatation of the cervical veins, and an enlarged and pulsating liver, which indicate the presence of right ventricular embarrassment. The chest radiograph may show diminished pulmonary vascular markings, a sign first described in 1938 by Westermark (36) and recently reemphasized in an excellent monograph by Torrance (30). Despite its usefulness, this sign is not sufficiently reliable to allow it to be recognized as a definitive method of diagnosis, particularly if pulmonary embolectomy is being considered.

Electrocardiogram.   The electrocardiogram often shows changes in pulmonary embolism, but it is neither a sensitive nor a specific means of diagnosis. Alterations may include disturbances of rhythm (atrial fibrillation, ectopic beats, heart block), enlargement of the P waves, ST segment depression, T wave inversion (especially in Lead III, VF, and V, V4, and V5. The most common abnormality is ST segment depression which is a result of the accompanying myocardial ischemia. Although frequently confirmatory, it should be emphasized that the electrocardiogram cannot be relied upon for a certain diagnosis of pulmonary embolism.

Serum enzymes.   Changes in serum enzymes may be helpful in the diagnosis of pulmonary embolism. A triad consisting of an elevated serum lactic dehydrogenase (LDH) activity, an increased serum bilirubin concentration, and a normal serum glutamic-oxatacetic transaminase (SGOT) activity has been described (32). The serum LDH is quite frequently elevated and the bilirubin is increased in approximately two thirds of the cases. While this triad of serum enzyme activity is helpful, Sasahara has emphasized that in patients with massive embolism and acute cardiovascular changes the factor of time is often critical and a more rapid means of diagnosis is necessary.

Ventilation-perfusion unbalance.   Pulmonary embolism alters the normal balance between ventilation and perfusion of the lungs. Robin has demonstrated that an increased ventilatory dead space occurs to pulmonary embolization. His method is based upon the premise that occlusion of a major pulmonary arterial branch decreases gaseous exchange in the corresponding segment of the lung, although alveolar ventilation continues. In a ventilated but underperfused segment of lung, the composition of the alveolar air tends to approach that of inspired air and has a low partial pressure of carbon dioxide. During expiration, this air is mixed with that from the normal areas of the lung but reduces the mean alveolar carbon dioxide tension to a degree that can be detected in the expired air. Arterial carbon dioxide tension remains at a nearly normal level because of the presence of normal lung tissue. The difference between the arterial and alveolar carbon dioxide tensions is therefore of aid in the diagnosis of pulmonary embolism.

However, Robin has emphasized that the shunting of ventilation away from underperfused areas has its counterpart in the shunting of blood away from hypoventilated areas and suggests some mechanism of pulmonary autoregulation of the ventilation-perfusion ratio. While this method may be helpful, complete reliance cannot be placed in it.

Radioisotope pulmonary scanning. In a group of recent studies, Wagner and associates have described a method for the diagnosis of pulmonary embolism by radioisotope scanning (34, 35). The method was initially evaluated experimentally in dogs and later in a group of patients with various forms of pulmonary disease, including pulmonary embolism. The principle of the method is measurement of intravenously injected particles labeled with I-131 and Cr51. Particles of human serum albumin, 10 to 100 micra in size, become lodged in the pulmonary capillary bed following intravenous injection. Radioisotope scanning delineates the distribution of pulmonary arterial blood flow to the lungs and reveals areas of decreased perfusion. The technique is of particular value in the patient with massive pulmonary embolism in whom the plain chest film is essentially normal. Areas of reduced pulmonary blood flow have been found in a series of 40 patients. This is particularly significant since, if an infiltrate is seen, experience has indicated that it will be avascular, regardless of its nature. In the majority of patients with massive pulmonary embolus, infiltrates are usually far less than the defect seen on the scan. Serial scanning is also of value in evaluating the return of pulmonary blood flow.

Pulmonary arteriography. Opacification of the pulmonary arteries may be obtained by the injection of a radiopaque medium into an arm vein or by selective arteriography by injection into a catheter placed in the pulmonary artery. The selective injection requires a smaller amount of contrast substance and produces films with greater detail.

The procedure is attended by some risk, particularly in the severely ill patient in whom contrast medium can produce hypotension. Sasahara (21) recently documented the value of pulmonary arteriography in the diagnosis of pulmonary embolism. He emphasized that pulmonary angiography is particularly valuable when the physical findings are scanty and the history obscure.

The importance of objective diagnosis by either pulmonary scanning or pulmonary arteriography is greatest when embolectomy is contemplated. In a number of patients, the clinical diagnosis of pulmonary embolism was incorrect and the patients were subjected to an unnecessary operation. Such patients were made worse, since the majority had some other serious cardiorespiratory disorder. Therefore, the importance of an accurate diagnosis prior to the undertaking of a surgical measure of this magnitude cannot be overemphasized.

Management. The management of patients with pulmonary embolism depends upon the severity of the disease. Therapeutic measures fall into three main groups, (1) anticoagulation to prevent further thrombosis, (2) venous interruption to prevent further emboli from passing into the pulmonary arterial circulation, and (3) direct pulmonary embolectomy.

Anticoagulation. Anticoagulant therapy is of proved value. Treatment should be administered immediately in order to reduce the likelihood of further embolic episodes. Unless there is a specific contraindication to the use of anticoagulants, heparin is usually given initially since it has the advantage of rapidity of action. Heparin can be administered 50 to 100 mg. every 4 hours for the first 48 hours. Concomitantly, Dicumarol, 200 to 300 mg., is given on the first day followed by 50 to 100 mg. daily thereafter. The dose is regulated by the prothrombin activity and should be maintained at 15 to 25 percent of normal. In most instances, coumadin therapy is effective by 48 hours and at that time the heparin may be discontinued. However, continued use of heparin may be preferred rather than the use of coumadin drugs.

Venous ligation. Although pathologists had recognized for many years that sudden death might he due to the presence of pulmonary thrombi, it was thought that these arose in situ in the pulmonary arteries. Virchow first described the true pathogenesis of pulmonary embolism by emphasizing that the thrombi arose primarily in the veins of the pelvis and legs and were transported secondarily to the lungs (14). Since that time, considerable investigation has been directed toward the most common sites of venous thrombosis. Some years ago it was thought that the majority of pulmonary emboli arose in the veins of the leg, primarily in the calf. However, subsequent evidence has shown that the pelvis, inferior vena cava, and right atrium and ventricle may be additional sites.

Venous interruption originally consisted of ligation of the superficial femoral veins, but it soon became apparent that this procedure was largely ineffectual in reducing the incidence of pulmonary embolism. Recently, attention has been directed toward interruption of the inferior vena cava by ligation or by suture plication. While some authors prefer complete occlusion by ligature, others prefer partition or partial obstruction by narrowing the main vena caval channel into several smaller ones (26). Plastic clips have also been introduced which can be placed around the vena cava and partially occlude it by leaving small channels for the returning blood. In general, there appears to be little difference in the two methods and their effect in preventing future episodes of pulmonary embolism. Advocates of plication believe that there are fewer postoperative sequelae, such as edema and chronic phlebitis, with this procedure. Ligature is to be preferred, however, in those patients with multiple emboli who have cor pulmonale or who are thought likely to develop it.

Embolectomy. The direct removal of thrombi from the pulmonary artery was first proposed by Trendelenburg in 1908 (31). His three attempts were unsuccessful but demonstrated that the operation was feasible. Two patients survived the procedure but died later, one of heart failure and the other of hemorrhage. The first successful pulmonary embolectomy was performed by Kirschner in 1924 (15), and Steenburg and associates (29) reported the first successful pulmonary embolectomy in the United States in 1958. In a recent review, 27 successful reports of pulmonary embolectomy by this method have been collected. In the Trendelenburg operation the chest is entered, as an emergency procedure, without extracorporeal circulation, and the pulmonary artery is opened and the pulmonary thrombi are removed. There is little doubt that more patients have died as a result of attempted Trendelenburg operations than have survived them. Clearly, pulmonary embolectomy should be accompanied by the use of extracorporeal circulation whenever possible, and the Trendelenburg procedure can only be justified in extreme emergencies in which it is thought that no time is available for the preparation of cardiopulmonary bypass.

In 1960, Allison (1) reported the treatment of a gravely ill patient with massive pulmonary embolism by open operation with hypothermia. The body temperature was reduced to 290 C and, by means of a trans-sternal approach, the pulmonary artery was opened and a large amount of thrombus removed. This patient was the first to undergo pulmonary embolectomy with protection of vital organs by hypotherm ia. He made an excellent recovery. The ideal method for performance of pulmonary embolectomy is with the use of extracorporeal circulation which supports the circulation and allows pulmonary embolectomy to be done deliberately. In 1961, Sharp was the first to report this operation with the use of cardiopulmonary bypass, and was followed by Cooley and associates who shortly thereafter performed a similar successful pulmonary embolectomy. Since that time more than 30 patients have successfully undergone pulmonary embolectomy with extracorporeal circulation (2, 3, 10, 22, 23). This technique clearly represents the most satisfactory method of management available at this time for those patients who require embolectomy for massive pulmonary embolism.

An alternative technique is thoracotomy with the opening of either the right or left pulmonary artery for extraction of the embolus, the side with greater involvement being chosen. This approach allows continuing cardiorespiratory function during the procedure. Bradley and associates (4) have reported a successful use of this technique.

Pulmonary embolism remains a serious complication which follows a variety of medical and surgical disorders. It is interesting that statistics from the United States and Europe indicate that the incidence of pulmonary embolism has remained essentially unchanged for the past 30 years. Since the signs and symptoms closely resemble those of several other serious cardiorespiratory disorders, accurate diagnosis may be difficult. While the clinical manifestations may be characteristic and may direct initial attention toward the diagnosis of this condition, the findings are usually not sufficiently objective and are frequently unreliable. Neither the plain chest film nor the electrocardiogram are sufficiently specific for reliable diagnosis. An important question is the extent of pulmonary embolism required to produce serious cardiovascular changes, since this aspect of the problem has important connotations in the therapeutic approach. While there were exceptions, there is much evidence that at least half of the pulmonary circulation must be obstructed for the production of cardiovascular collapse. Pulmonary emboli confined to a small portion of the lung have been rarely proved to be responsible for sudden death. The available data suggest that occlusion of the arterial supply of at least half of one lung or more is required for the production of severe signs and symptoms. This fact has been demonstrated in both the experimental animal and in man, In Gorham's series of patients who died with massive pulmonary embolism, 85 percent had occlusion of more than one pulmonary artery. Furthermore, in patients with embolectomy, emboli are usually found in branches of both pulmonary arteries. Pulmonary scanning and arteriography have further established this point. Debate continues concerning the mechanical versus the reflex factors as the underlying basis for the pathophysiological effects which occur in pulmonary embolism. Most evidence favors the mechanical concept as the primary factor in human embolism. While reflex changes may occur, both experimental and clinical findings suggest that mechanical obstruction is of greater importance.

In patients with moderate or severe pulmonary embolism, surgical treatment should he reserved for those with proved emboli in conjunction with anticoagulant therapy. With evidence of more extensive occlusion, inferior vena caval interruption, either by ligation or partition, is often the procedure of choice. In patients with life-threatening massive pulmonary embolism which has been definitely established by arteriography or scanning, thoracetomy with cardiopulmonary bypass for removal of the emboli is usually indicated. When extracorporeal circulation is not available, the Trendelenburg operation may be performed if the clinical manifestations warrant and when it appears that no time is available to permit a better procedure. The opening of one pulmonary artery (the one with the greatest amount of emboli) is an alternative approach which allows entry into one side of the chest with maintenance of respiratory and circulatory function during the procedure. In all operative therapy, emphasis is placed upon the fact that a positive diagnosis should be established prior to the undertaking of a surgical procedure. After the site and magnitude of embolism is determined, the method of therapy can then be chosen on an objective basis.

In summary, pulmonary embolism continues to represent a serious and often fatal complication. Since the clinical signs and symptoms are variable and may closely resemble those of other cardiorespiratory disorders, emphasis is placed upon the importance of establishing an accurate diagnosis. This is of considerable significance in those patients selected for surgical treatment, and the diagnostic method employed should provide evidence not only of the correct diagnosis but also of the site and magnitude of pulmonary embolism. A combined clinical and experimental study has led to the following conclusions: (1) the diagnosis of pulmonary embolism can be quickly and confidently established in patients by pulmonary scanning with the use of radioactive macroaggregated human serum albumin; (2) pulmonary arteriography is necessary in some patients in order to establish an objective diagnosis; (3) serious hemodynamic effects occur after more than half of the pulmonary arterial bed is occluded; (4) pulmonary arterial flow may return to areas of the lung obstructed with arterial emboli with the passage of time; (5) preexisting cardiac or respiratory insufficiency can seriously aggravate the circulatory response to embolism; and (6) the effectiveness of embolectomy in patients with massive, life threatening pulmonary embolism has been demonstrated.

References

1. Allison, P. R., Dunnill, M. S., and Marshall, R. Pulmonary Embolism. *Thorax*, 15: 273, 1960

2. Baker, R. R. Pulmonary Embolism, *Surgery*, 54: 687, 1963.

3. Beall, A. C., Fred, H. L., and Cooley, D. A. *Pulmonary Embolectomy in Current Problems in Surgery*. Chicago: Year Book Medical Publishers, Inc., 1964, pp. 3–47.

4. Bradley, M. N., Bennett, A. L., III, and Lyons C. Successful unilateral pulmonary embolectomy without cardiopulmonary bypass. *New England J. Med.*, 271: 713, 1964.

5. Brofman, B. L., Charms, B. L, Kohn, P. M., Jr., Newman, R., and Rizika, M. Unilateral pulmonary artery occlusion in man. J. *Thoracic Surg.*, 32: 206, 1957.

6. Burnett, W. E., Long, J. H., Norris, C., Rosemond, G. P., and Webster, M. R. The effect of pneumonectomy on pulmonary function. *J. Thoracic Surg.*, 18: 569, 1949.

7. Cooley, D. A., Beall, A. C., Jr., and Alexander, J. K. Acute massive pulmonary embolism. *J.A.M.A.*, 177: 283, 1961.

8. Dale, W. A. Ligation of the inferior vena cava for thromboembolism. *Surgery*, 43: 24, 1958.

9. Dexter, L. Cardiovascular Responses to Experimental Pulmonary Embolism, Symposium on Pulmonary Embolic Disease. To be published.

10. Flemma, R. J., Young, W. G., Jr., Wallace, A., Whalen, R. E., and Freese, J. Feasibility of pulmonary embolectomy. *Circulation*, 30: 234, 1964.

11. Fletcher, A. P., Sherry, S., Alkjaersig, N., Smyrniotis, F. E., and Jick, S. The maintenance of a sustained thrombolytic state in man. II. Clinical observations on patients with myocardial (infarction and other thromboembolic disorders. *J. Clin. Invest.*, 38: 1111, 1959.

12. Gorham, L. W. A study of pulmonary embolism. Part I, *Arch. Int. Med.*, 108: 8, 1961.

13. Gorham, L. W. A Study of Pulmonary Embolism. Part I, *Arch. Int. Med.*, 108: 189, 1961.

14. Hume, M. Pulmonary embolism. *Arch. Surg.*, 87: 709, 1963.

15. Kirschner, M. Ein durch die Tredelenburgsche Operation Geheilter Fall von Embolic der Art Pulmonalis. *Arch. Klin. Chir.*, 133: 312, 1924. (Described in *J. Thoracic Surg.*, 5: 1, 1935.)

16. Marshall, R. Sabiston, D. C., Allison, P. R., Bosman, A. R., and Dunnill, M. S. Immediate and late effects of pulmonary embolism by large thrombi in dogs, *Thorax*, 18: 1, 1963.

17. Marshall, R. J., Wang, Y., Semier, H. J., and Shepherd, J. T. Pulmonary circulation during exercise. *Circulation Res.*, 9: 53, 1961.

18. Robin, E.D., and others. Physiologic approach to diagnosis of acute pulmonary embolism. *New England J. Med.*, 260: 586, 1959.

19. Sabiston, D. C., Marshall, R., Dunnill, M. S., and Allison, P. R. Experimental pulmonary embolism description of a method utilizing large venous thrombi. *Surgery*, 52: 9, 1962.

20. Sabiston, D. C., and Wagner, H. N. The diagnosis of pulmonary embolism by radioisotope scanning. *Ann. Surg.*, 160: 575, 1964.

21. Sasahara, A. A., Stein, M., Simon, M., and Littman, D. Pulmonary angiography in the diagnosis of thromboembolic disease. *New England J. Med.*, 270: 1075, 1964.

22. Sautter, R. D., Lawton, B. R., Magnin, G. E., and Emanuel, D. A. Pulmonary embolectomy: Report of a case with preoperative and postoperative angiograms. *New England J. Med.*, 269: 997, 1963.

23. Sautter, R. D., Lawton, B. R., Magnin, G. E., and Burns, J. L. Pulmonary embolectomy, a simplified technique. *Wisconsin M. J.*, 61: 309, 1962.

24. Sautter, R. D., Fletcher, F. W., Emanuel, D. A., Lawton, B. R., and Olsen, T. G. Complete resolution of massive pulmonary thromboli. *J.A.M.A.*, 189: 948, 1964.

25. Sharp, E. H. Pulmonary embolectomy: Successful removal of a massive pulmonary embolus with the support of cardiopulmonary bypass. A case report. *Ann. Surg.*, 156: 1, 1962.

26. Sheil, A. F. R., and Sabiston, D. C. Experimental venous thrombosis and thrombectomy. *Arch. Surg.*, 87: 408, 1963.

27. Sloan, H., Morris, J. D., Figley, M., and Lee, R. Temporary unilateral occlusion of pulmonary artery in the preoperative evaluation of thoracic patients. *J. Thoracic Surg.*, 30: 591, 1955.

28. Spencer, F. C., Quattlebaum, J. K., Quattlebaum, J. K., Jr., Sharp, E. H., and Jude, J. R. Publication of the inferior vena cava for pulmonary embolism: A report of 20 cases. *Ann. Surg.*, 155: 827, 1962.

29. Steenburg, R. W., Warren, R., Wilson, R. E., and Rudolf, L. E. A new look at pulmonary embolectomy. *Surg., Gynec. & Obst.*, 107: 214, 1958.

30. Torrance, D. J. The Chest Film in Massive Pulmonary Embolism, Springfield, Ill.: Charles C. Thomas, 1963.

31. Trendelenburg, P. Ueber die Operative Behandlung der Embolie der Lungerarteric. *Arch. Klin. Chir.*, 86: 686, 1908.

32. Wacker, W. E. C., and Snodgrass, P. J. Serum LDH Activity in Pulmonary Embolism Diagnosis. *J.A.M.A.*, 174: 2142, 1960.

33. Wagner, H. N., and Jones, R.H. J. Massive pulmonary embolism. *Physiol. Physicians*, 3: 1, 1965.

34. Wagner, H. N., Sabiston, D. C., Ilio, M., McAfee, J. G., Meyer, J. K., and Langan, J. K. Regional pulmonary blood flow in man by radioisotrope scanning, *J.A.M.A.*, 187: 601, 1964.

35. Wagner, H. N., Sabiston, D. C., McAfee, J. G., Tow, D., and Stern, H. S. Diagnosis of massive pulmonary embolism in man by radioisotope scanning. *New England J. Med.*, 271: 377, 1964.

36. Westermark, W. On the Roentgen diagnosis of lung embolism. *Acta Radiol.*, 19: 357, 1938.

37. White, P. D., and Bernner, O. Pathological and Clinical Aspects of the Pulmonary Circulation. *New England J. Med.*, 209: 1261, 1933.

38. Wiederanders, R. E., White, S. M., and Salchek, H. B. The effect of pulmonary resection on pulmonary artery pressures. *Ann. Surg.*, 160: 889, 1964.

Chapter 31 ☞

Radioactive Ventilation Scanning in the Diagnosis of Pulmonary Embolism[1]

P ulmonary perfusion scanning with the use of intravenously injected macroaggregated human serum albumin labeled with I-131 has proved to be a valuable adjunct in the diagnosis of pulmonary embolism (6). With perfusion scanning, the distribution of pulmonary artery blood flow can be determined, and perfusion defects can be localized. Recently a method has been devised by which the distribution of ventilation can be determined in the lungs and ventilation defects localized (4). The purpose of this paper is to describe the technique for evaluating both perfusion and ventilation with the radioisotope scan and to report on the findings in simultaneous ventilation and perfusion scans in dogs with experimental pulmonary embolism.

Adult dogs weighing 40 to 45 pounds were anesthetized with sodium pentobarbital (0.6 mg. per 5 pounds). The inferior vena çava was exposed through a midline incision and the inferior vena cava was isolated from the renal to the iliac veins. All lumbar branches were ligated and divided except one through which a small polyethylene catheter was passed into the inferior vena cava. The vena cava was then occluded with vascular clamps at its bifurcation and also occluded 2 cm. below the renal vessels. After the blood was removed from the isolated segment by aspiration, 1 ml. of concentrated phenol was introduced. The phenol was then aspirated after 1 minute and the occluded segment of vena cava was thoroughly irrigated with several washings of saline solution to remove as much phenol as possible. First the catheter and then the vascular clamps were removed, and the cir-

---

1. Coauthored with Walter G. Wolfe, M.D.

culation was reestablished. The posterior peritoneum and abdomen were then dosed.

Following a period of 10 to 18 days, the original incision was reopened. The details of this technique and of the thrombi obtained have been described previously (5). It was found that the best preparation of a solid thrombus suitable for embolization was present in about 10 days. The inferior vena cava was usually of normal diameter and contained a well-formed thrombus which could be removed intact. These thrombi were measured, weighed, and then placed in a special cannula which was inserted in the vena cava at the origin of the renal veins. A plunger was used to introduce the embolus into the vessel where it passed into the right heart and was injected into the pulmonary arteries.

After injection of the embolus, chest films and pulmonary arteriograms were obtained on each animal. Approximately 4 hours later, a cuffed endotracheal tube was inserted into the trachea and connected to a respirator attached to a micronebulizer. With automatic breathing used and a flow rate of 6 liters per minute, with pressures of 9 to 13 cm of water, a 0.5 per cent dilution of human serum albumin labeled with 1.5 to 2 millicuries of technetium in 4 to 6 cc was then nebulized and inhaled. Exhaled air was trapped in a plastic bag. After completion of the ventilation, the animal's chest was scanned with a scintillation counter. The animal then received an intravenous dose of 100 microcuries of I-131 tagged macroaggregated human serum albumin and the chest was rescanned. The ventilation and perfusion scans were then repeated at intervals until the perfusion scan returned to normal. The animals were then sacrificed and an autopsy performed. The pathologic examination included microscopic studies of lungs and pulmonary arteries.

All animals were studied following the episode of massive pulmonary emboli by pulmonary arteriography, ventilation scans, and perfusion scans. After acute pulmonary embolism, the arteriogram revealed a complete block of the entire left or right main pulmonary artery or of a lower lobe artery. The ventilation scan demonstrated a decreased ventilation in the lung with the pulmonary embolus. Perfusion scan demonstrated absent or decreased perfusion to the involved lung. Repeated ventilation scan 48 hours later demonstrated a return to normal ventilation while the perfusion scan remained essentially unchanged. The perfusion scan gradually returned to normal in approximately 1 month. Autopsy at this time showed the continuing presence of a large amount of embolus within the pulmonary artery.

The use of the ventilation scan with technetium (Tc 99M) (3) used in conjunction with the perfusion scan enables the simultaneous evaluation of ventilation and perfusion. The reason for this is that the photon energy of Tc and I-131 can be easily separated by the ventilation scanner. Also, the use of technetium permits a larger tracer dose and produces superior scans.

These studies indicate that the accurate and objective diagnosis of pulmonary embolism can be made with the arteriogram and perfusion lung scan. The ventilation scan demonstrates that hypoventilation as well as decreased pulmonary artery perfusion accompanies acute pulmonary embolism. The perfusion scan remains abnormal up to a period of I month whereas the ventilation changes are less chronic and return to normal more rapidly. Also, the changes seen in ventilation seem to be in association with the complete occlusion of the pulmonary artery or of a major branch (14). The mechanisms producing acute alteration in ventilation following pulmonary artery occlusion are not fully understood. The ventilation changes demonstrated by the radioactive scan probably are the result of a combination of factors (increase in surface tension, changes in tissue elasticity, and increase in airway resistance). However, it has been demonstrated that occlusion of the pulmonary artery or pneumonectomy does not significantly alter resting ventilation (9, 13).

Several investigators have shown that homolateral bronchial constriction occurs after unilateral pulmonary artery occlusion (2, 9). This can be reversed by the inhalation of 6 per cent carbon dioxide. Humoral agents, such as serotonin, have been implicated as causing bronchospasm following pulmonary embolism (8, 11). Wheezing has been reported in acute pulmonary embolism in patients without antecedent history of bronchospasm (10).

In acute pulmonary embolism, hypoventilation as applied to the side with the embolus may represent a protective effect. With nearly complete occlusion of the pulmonary artery, physiologic dead space is increased and there is less reason to ventilate alveoli that are not being perfused. Therefore, ventilation of the occluded side is directed to the alveoli of the opposite lung. These studies with the ventilation scan demonstrate a significant decrease in ventilation of the embolized side or an increase in ventilation of the lung without an embolus.

Following occlusion of a pulmonary artery, there is a decrease in compliance and ventilation as well as an increase in airway resistance of the ipsilateral lung (7). Embolism of a lung with fine particles leads to reduction of compliance, due to muscular constriction around the alveolar ducts. However, it is uncertain whether occlusion of a main pulmonary artery induces the same kind of reaction. By using the ventilation technique (previously described) with particles the size of 3 to 5 microns, it has been shown with microradiographs that the radioactive material is deposited within the alveoli and, therefore, that decreases in ventilation, as demonstrated by the scan, represent in part a decrease in alveolar ventilation. This is not certain evidence that muscular constriction occurs about the alveolar ducts in occlusion of a main pulmonary artery but it does support this possibility.

The knowledge that decreased pulmonary ventilation, as demonstrated by the scan, reflects a decrease in alveolar ventilation and implicates surfactant and its alteration as one of the reasons for the change demonstrated. It has been demonstrated that with ligation of a pulmonary artery, the surface tension is increased in the involved lung. We have demonstrated that after occlusion of the pulmonary artery with a preparation identical to the one described in this report that surfactant is decreased (16).

It has been postulated that there may be asynchronous ventilation following occlusion of a pulmonary artery and that nonuniform ventilation is more marked with occlusion of a main pulmonary artery than with occlusion of a lobar vessel. This correlates with our findings that alterations of ventilation as demonstrated by the scan appear to be associated with complete occlusion of a pulmonary artery or a major branch.

Finally, the reason for return of ventilation to normal in 48 hours while the perfusion scan is essentially unchanged is not clear. The particle size of I-131 macroaggregates is 10 to 50 microns while erythrocytes are 7 microns in diameter. Therefore, there could be partial perfusion of the distal pulmonary artery with relief of ischemia. Simultaneously carbon dioxide could again accumulate to reverse bronchoconstriction. However, the perfusion scan may remain unchanged due to the failure of macroaggregates to pass the obstruction.

References

1. Burrows, B., Niden, A. H., Mittman, C., Talley, R. G., and Barclary, W .R. Non-uniform pulmonary diffusion as demonstrated by the carbon monoxide technique. Experimental results in man. *J. Clin. Invest.*, 39: 943, 1960.
2. Severinghaus, J. W., Swenson, E. W., Finley, T. N., Lategola, M. T., and William J. Unilateral hypoventilation produced in dogs by occluding one pulmonary artery. *J. Appl. Physiol.*, 16: 53, 1961.
3. Harper, P. V., Lathrop, K. A., Jimenez, F., Fink, R., and Gottschalk, A. Technetium 99m as a scanning agent. *Radiology*, 85: 101, 1965.
4. Pircher, F. J., Temple, J. R, Kirsch, W. J., and Reeves, R. J. Distribution of pulmonary ventilation determined by radioisotope scanning. *Am. J. Roentgenol.*, 94: 807, 1965.
5. Sabiston, D. C., Marshall, R., Dunnill, M., and Allison, P. Experimental pulmonary embolism. Description of method utilizing large venous thrombi. *Surgery*, 52: 914, 1962.
6. Sabiston, D. C., and Wagner, H. N. Diagnosis of pulmonary embolism by radioisotope scanning. *Ann. Surg.*, 160: 575, 1964.
7. Marshall, R., Sabiston, D. C., Allison, P. R., Bosman, A. H., and Dunnill, M. S. Immediate and late effects of pulmonary embolism by large thrombi in dogs. *Thorax*, 18: 1, 1963.
8. Smith, G. and Smith, A. N. Role of serotonin in experimental embolism. *Surg., Gynec. & Obst.*, 101: 691, 1955.
9. Swenson, E. W., Finley, T. N., and Guzman, S. V. Unilateral hypoventilation in man during temporary occlusion of one pulmonary artery. *J. Clin. Invest.*, 40: 828, 1961.

10. Webster, J. R., Saadeh, G. B., Eggum, P. R., and Suker, J. R. Wheezing due to pulmonary embolism. The treatment with heparin. *New England J. Med.*, 274: 931, 1966.

11. Thomas, D. P, Tanabe, G., Khan, M., and Stein, M. Humoral factors mediated by platelets in experimental pulmonary embolism in pulmonary embolic disease. 59–64, edited by Sasahara, A. A., and Stein, M. New York: Grune & Stratton, Inc., pp. 312, 1965.

12. Finley, T. N., Swenson, E. W., Clements, J., Gardner, R. E., Wright, R. and Severinghaus, J. W. Changes in mechanical properties, appearance and surface activity of extracts of the lung following occlusion of its pulmonary artery in the dog. *Physiologist*, 3: 56, 1960.

13. Burnett, W. E., Long, J. H. Norris, C., Rosemond, G. P., and Webster, M. R. The effect of pneumonectomy on pulmonary function. *J. Thoracic Surg.*, 18: 96, 1949.

14. Wolfe, W. G., Pircher, F. J., and Sabiston, D. C. The ventilation scan in the diagnosis of pulmonary embolism. *S. Forum*, 17: 119, 1966.

15. Nadel, J. A., Colebatch, H. J. H. and Olsen, C. R. Location and mechanism of airway constriction after barium sulfate microembolism. *J. Appl. Physiol.*, 19: 387, 1964.

16. Wolfe, W. G., and Sabiston, D. C. The effects of pulmonary embolism on pulmonary surfactant. *Surgery*, 63: 312, 1968.

VII

The Practice of Surgery

I n addition to its strong emphasis on education and patient care, the American College of Surgery is also involved in socioeconomic issues in the broad field of health care.

Chapter 32 ☞

Professional Liability in Surgery: Problems and Solutions

A t the first Convocation of the American College of Surgeons in 1913, President John M.T. Finney said in his Presidential Address:

> The history of surgery in the United States and Canada is opened to a new page. When at some future time the historian comes to write on that page the record of events that have led up to this meeting, he will there record the taking of another step in the progress of medicine in general and of surgery in particular in Canada and the United States. What is consummated here tonight is destined to produce a deep and lasting impression upon medical progress not alone in those countries but indirectly the world over. (1)

In his Presidential Address in 1954, my chief, Alfred Blalock, to whom I owe so much, emphasized the common feature that binds us. He said: "All physicians — whether active practitioners, teachers, investigators or administrators — have a single common objective which unites us all. This is the welfare of the sick" (2).

The American College of Surgeons has traditionally been committed to excellence in patient care and to continuing education. In the opinion of observers worldwide, the quality of the annual Clinical Congress has risen to the rank of first place. The expanding edge of scientific knowledge is revealed in the research papers presented by our bright young surgeons at the sessions of the Forum on Fundamental Surgical Problems. Updates on all important aspects of surgery and the surgical specialties are presented in the various postgraduate courses each year. Topics deserving special emphasis are presented at the general sessions by panels representing different points of view, and the audiovisual presentations illustrate the newer surgical techniques. All

members of the College have an obligation to honor and maintain this
tradition in the future.

In addition to its strong emphasis on education and patient care,
the College has also been interested in a number of socioeconomic
issues in the broad field of health care. At its recent retreat, the Board
of Regents considered seven such topics and prepared position papers
concerning each. In its final conclusion, the report stated: "Of all the
socio-economic issues facing the surgical profession, that of professional liability most urgently calls for resolute action by the College.
The College is unequivocally committed to seeking legislative reform
of the professional liability system on the national and local level in
cooperation with all of its constituencies and all other medical and
non-medical groups striving for a solution for this complex problem."

The Board of Governors has also voted this issue the most important of our current problems, further emphasizing its significance
today. It is this paramount issue that I wish to discuss.

Malpractice in History

To comprehend this complex subject, a knowledge of the history
of professional liability is essential. While the Code of Hammurabi is
generally regarded as the first of the codified principles of law to mention the issue of malpractice, classic Greek culture, as cited by Plato,
held that actions of physicians should be judged only by other physicians. Aristotle emphasized that the only penalty applicable to any real,
or perceived, wrongdoing by a physician was limited solely to injury
of his reputation and to nothing else.

In English law, the first recorded decision concerning civil liability
of a surgeon was an action brought before the King's Bench in 1374
against a surgeon named J. Mort involving the treatment of a patient
who had a wounded hand. In that decision, the defendant was held
not liable because of a legal technicality, but the court ultimately ruled
that if negligence could be proven by such a patient, the law would
provide a remedy. However, of much significance, the court further
held: "If the surgeon does so well as he can and employs all his diligence to the cure, it is not right that he should be held culpable" (3).
It is interesting that even in medieval times attempts were made to

control medical and surgical professional liability by purchasing a renewable "floater" policy by which consultation was mandatory on each high-risk case (4).

In England, plea records were kept and have been maintained to the present. These serve as a body of evidence for subsequent decisions and generally mean that a decision of a higher court has the force of law and is in essence binding on future cases of a similar type. This is the legal doctrine of stare decisis, and to this day one of the most striking features of English Common Law is its adherence to precedent.

In 1423, the Joint College of Physicians and Surgeons of London produced the "Ordinance Against Malpractice" (4). Interestingly enough, it is written in English rather than Latin or French, which were the classic legal languages of the day. This ordinance required a surgeon to report all patients who were desperately ill within three days.

Fortunately for those in the British Isles and Canada far fewer medicolegal suits are filed than in this country. The difference is largely due to the fact that contingent fees are not legal in Britain and that the judges are primarily responsible for court decisions rather than trial by jury. Moreover, the British society is not nearly as litigious as ours. For centuries the British have maintained a strong sense of justice coupled with emphasis on fairness. In the United States the first liability case was filed in 1794, as Cross vs. Guthrey; it also involved a surgical procedure. The husband of a deceased woman sued because of alleged negligence in the performance of a mastectomy (3). The operation was characterized as being conducted "in the most unskillful, ignorant, and cruel manner, contrary to all the well-known rules and principles of practice in such cases, that the patient survived by but three hours, and the defendant had wholly broken and violated his undertaking and promise to the plaintiff to perform said operation skillfully and with safety to his wife." In the end the jury found the physician liable and awarded damages.

An early medicolegal treatise on malpractice was published in 1866 by Dr. John J. Elwell, a professor of criminal law at Western Reserve University. The evidence comprising the elements of medical jurisprudence of that day were carefully reviewed in this monograph. In the preface, Dr. Elwell said: "It is my earnest desire that its mission may be beneficial, by relieving, to some extent, the labors of the attorney, while it sets forth and maintains the rights of the medical and surgical practitioner, not shielding the culpable and guilty, and at the same time bringing the two professions into closer union, producing greater harmony, sympathy and usefulness. It is an extraordinary text even today and is fascinating reading.

In a collective review of the era between 1794 and the Civil War in 1861, historian C. K. Bums could find only 27 malpractice suits that were adjudicated as appeals in the various state supreme courts (6). During the 20-year period from 1935 to 1955, there were only 605 cases, or an average of 30 each year, predominantly in California and New York. After 1955, it became clear that professional liability suits began to rise dramatically and especially during the last decade.

The gathering storm and the impact of these events on the delivery of health care, health-care costs, and health manpower prompted the appointment of the Presidential Commission on Medical Malpractice. This commission carefully reviewed medical liability claims throughout the nation and found that in 1970 there were some 15,000 claims filed. The rapid escalation of this problem is emphasized by the fact that in the 40 years between 1935 and 1975, 80 percent of all medical professional liability suits were filed in the last five years of that period.

The escalation in the total number of professional liability claims beginning about a decade ago has been astonishing. For the years 1975 and 1976, the National Association of Insurance Commissioners identified 14,074 such claims. The next 30-month period included 57,926 claims, or an average of 23,169 per year. In 1983, 77 percent of the carriers surveyed showed 32,324 cases and, if projected, the expected total exceeded 42,000 (7).

Data collected in California show that the impact of verdict awards for the period 1972 to 1983 was remarkable. In 1972, the average award was $200,296. Over the next decade, the total amount of the verdicts rose sharply with the average award to the plaintiff increasing to $649,000 in 1983.

The number of suits in the nation settled in excess of $1 million has shown a striking rise. Data indicate that by 1981 the number of cases settled of this magnitude had risen to more than 50 annually.

Another factor of considerable concern is the inequity in the rates of professional liability policies in relation to geographic location, even within a single state. In New York the rates for general surgeons vary from $21,000 in upstate New York to $47,000 on Long Island, with a differential for neurosurgeons of $44,000 in upstate compared to $98,000 on Long Island. The premiums for other specialties follow a similar pattern with wide variations depending upon the location within the state.

The rapid escalation in the cost of policies was emphasized in 1974 when a single company insured approximately 95 percent of the practicing physicians in the State of Maryland and the premium was raised 46 percent, immediately followed by another 48 percent increase the following year. When the second increase was rejected, the company ceased writing policies in Maryland.

Such problems led to the establishment of physician-owned non-profit companies to provide insurance. The total number of these companies has now risen to 37, serving 39 states throughout the nation. As is true for private insurance companies, the physician-owned companies have been compelled to increase their premiums in order to remain solvent. One state that established a mutual company in 1979 found it necessary to increase the premiums 109 percent in the first five years, with an additional 47 percent increase last year. In another state, the average premium has increased 22 percent each year since inception of the program in 1980.

Despite the staggering increases in premiums, the present system remains totally inadequate for the patient and physician alike. One of the most distressing aspects of current professional liability instance is the small percentage of the insurance premium dollar that is actually awarded to the patient, generally cited as being about 28 cents on the dollar, a very poor commentary on the system.

The total payment of premiums for insurance policies versus the amount paid in claims shifted dramatically in 1978. Prior to 1978, most insurance companies were able to operate without financial losses, but since that time, the situation has changed dramatically. The companies' losses have escalated and while premiums paid increased from $1.2 to $1.57 billion dollars, or 31 percent, between 1977 and 1983, the losses soared to $817 million in 1979 and to nearly $2 billion in 1983. Last year, Best's Insurance Management Report said: "Medical malpractice is reaching the point of no return in terms of producing investment income and the lost revenues that exceed the underwriting costs."

Concomitant with an increase in suits against physicians, the same has occurred to hospitals throughout the nation. Hospitals are now experiencing a rapid increase, and the St. Paul Fire and Marine Insurance Company experience shows a rise in hospital suits of 76 percent between 1979 and 1983.

The present system of infringements upon the medical profession as a direct result of the flagrant abuse of matters dealing with professional liability is emphasized by the understandable reluctance of physicians to accept high-risk cases in which lawsuits are likely. For example, a questionnaire survey done by this College in 1984 showed that more than 40 percent of the members restricted their practice with the intent of avoiding high-risk problems.

Moreover, the American College of Obstetricians and Gynecologists recently testified that 60 percent of the nation's obstetricians have been sued at least once and 20 percent have been sued three times or more. For this reason, 9 percent of its membership has already ceased practicing obstetrics and a significant percentage has been forced to increase fees as much as 30 percent to cover the charges of increased liability insurance. In careful studies, Jury Verdict Research has shown that the most expensive lawsuits settled in favor of the plaintiff are ones that involve birth injuries, with the mean award now at $1.5 million. Moreover, a recent case was settled at $8 million. With this in mind, as well as the uncertainty of the statute of limitations in these cases, more than 25 percent of the physicians in Florida have ceased managing obstetrical patients.

In a recent study, the American College of Obstetricians and Gynecologists surveyed 560 members of its Michigan section. More than half said they either stopped delivering babies as of May 31 or planned to do so because of skyrocketing malpractice costs. The physicians ranked the lack of limit on potential malpractice awards as the top liability-related problem today.

The impact of this problem is further emphasized by recent experiences on the island of Molokai in Hawaii. The physicians ceased practicing obstetrics after learning of a massive increase in their malpractice insurance premiums. Dr. Ralph Hale, chairman of the Department of Obstetrics and Gynecology at the University of Hawaii in Honolulu, says that pregnant women must now travel to Honolulu a week before their scheduled date of delivery and emphasizes that this has caused them and their families considerable psychological and financial disadvantage.

Such problems are paradoxical since the patient with a complex illness who needs the best medical care possible has increasing difficulty in obtaining it. Moreover, the cost of defensive medicine, that is, the ordering of many, often expensive examinations solely for malpractice protection, is variously estimated to cost the nation between a minimum of $15 billion and in a more recent survey up to $40 billion annually.

The recent practice of awarding large sums to those who experience completely unpredictable complications from the standard vaccinations given our children to prevent communicable diseases is another example of poor judicial settlements. This has, quite understandably, resulted in many physicians not wishing to administer these important vaccines. Moreover, of the 13 original pharmaceutical firms producing vaccines in this country, due to the flood of malpractice suits, only two remain in the nation today. This may well constitute a public health hazard in the future for this country as well as for other nations around the world who depend on our vaccines.

At this point it is appropriate to emphasize the necessity for the medical profession to assume a greater positive societal role in the establishment of a fair and realistic solution for compensation of patient injury. It is now reliably estimated that about 5 percent of all hospital admissions have some unexpected adverse event, primarily problems unassociated with professional management. As a matter of fact, only a small number of these cases actually represent malpractice. Moreover, unless malpractice can be clearly established, the settlement should not require a lawsuit or a trial by jury. Therefore, it should be our goal to foster programs to assure that all patients have a form of health insurance to compensate them adequately but in no way to overcompensate for economic losses in such instances.

Lawyers themselves have great concerns about their own malpractice "crisis." The Journal of the American Bar Association recently noted that the legal community is concerned about the 300 percent rate increase that lawyers' liability insurance carriers are passing on to those whom they insure this year. The medical profession should be aware of the fact that less than 10 percent of the legal profession is involved in professional liability litigation, and many are staunch and effective defendants of physicians.

In our efforts to achieve a solution to this vexing problem, many in our profession do not fully comprehend the legal aspects in relation to the law of the land. As a result of the evolution of common law in this country, professional liability law is determined largely by the state legislatures and the courts in the individual states. A significant problem is the fact that there is considerable variation from state to state. Should Congress pass definitive legislation interpreted as being restrictive, it might violate the Constitution on the basis that such legislation may override state law by a federal mandate.

It is for this reason that several members of Congress have introduced bills, each of which sets forth a proposed model statute to be voluntarily adopted by each state legislature in exchange for a grant of federal funds to establish a proper administrative structure for professional liability settlements. Each state would have a limited amount of time, generally three or four years, to establish such a system in order to receive the federal funds.

The positive and highly effective impact of federal incentives passed by Congress to encourage the states to act responsibly and promptly is dramatically shown by the linkage of federally financed highway funds to the states passing appropriate legislation designed to prevent automobile accidents occurring while drivers are under the influence of alcohol. Such legislation from Congress has been successful in making positive and needed changes on important issues, especially when linked to the receipt of federal funds for related projects

considered essential by the respective states. Surely, the professional liability problem is deserving of such attention and of rapid solution.

The prime features of these congressional bills, which are designed
to attack the basic inadequacies in the present professional liability system, include: limitations on contingency fees and other types of attor-
neys' fees, the formation of screening with uniform standards (including the principle of exclusive jurisdiction), the establishment of
standardized risk-management programs, and the setting of specific
time limits on the final decision (that is, six months to a year). Of particular importance is the need for free exchange of information about
all sources of compensation for the plaintiff, with no restrictions, so
that fair judgments can be rendered rather than the huge and frequently unjustifiable settlements often awarded by the courts today. In other
words, collateral sources of funding should be open for both parties to
review. Provisions should be made for dismissal of frivolous claims, and
the plaintiff should be made to pay administrative costs. Finally, periodic payment of claims should be the rule, with payments made over
time rather than in a single large settlement that is often not in the
patient's best interest. While the decisions of the panels can be
appealed, tight restrictions would make it difficult to overturn a panel's
decision.

The United States Congress has recently given recognition to the
groundswell of dissatisfaction and the inequities involved in the current malpractice situation. Bills introduced into both the House of
Representatives and the Senate are designed to stimulate the states to
pass specific and prescribed laws designed to ameliorate the problem.

On July 25, 1985, Congressman W. Henson Moore from
Louisiana rose in the House of Representatives to say: "Our Nation is
faced with a serious crisis. There are few states that are not enduring
some problem with the high cost of medical malpractice insurance
premiums. Fortunately, my State of Louisiana enacted comprehensive
reform about five years ago and consequently we are not faced with
nearly as serious of a crisis as are states like New York, Florida, Massachusetts, and California.

"Nonetheless, this insurance affordability crisis will not go away.
Newspaper headlines, television news reports, and magazine cover sto-

ries continually remind us that the high cost of medical malpractice insurance is forcing some health-care providers out of the practice of medicine. Patients are no longer assured of access to quality health care in the United States."

This bill was introduced in an effort to bring reform to compensation in professional liability cases. Patients are assured compensation for medical bills, loss of wages, cost of rehabilitation, and living expenses. Its potential disadvantage is the fact that it is in a sense a no-fault plan and could therefore become "open-ended," thus requiring excessive funding; it could well become unaffordable.

In the House of Representatives, Congressman Mrazek introduced a bill on June 4, 1985, with the intent "To establish a program in the Department of Justice to fund State medical malpractice programs which comply with Federal standards, and for other purposes." This bill has many features which would quite likely go far in the solution of many aspects of this problem.

In the Senate, Senator Inouye introduced a bill on January 3 designed "To limit the costs resulting from acts of negligence in health care and to improve the level of health care services in the United States, and for other purposes." The American Medical Association has prepared a draft bill on tort reform, and Senator Hatch has introduced this bill in the Senate.

While the effects of all bills designed to achieve tort reform will yield improvement, it should be recognized that patient insurance is also essential for the ultimate solution. This College should support those features in each of the bills that will yield the best long-term solution, and this is apt to require modification and combination of one or more of the current bills now in Congress.

The members of this College are greatly indebted to the Committee on Professional Liability and to its Chairman, Dr. Frank C. Spencer, and to our extraordinary Director, Dr. C. Rollins Hanlon, whose wisdom and leadership remain unequalled. This committee is preparing a position paper that will be of much significance to all Fellows of this College.

In closing these remarks, I wish to call attention to the fact that in 1856, four years before he was elected president, Abraham Lincoln was involved in a malpractice suit (8) and the proceedings were published in the *Daily Pantograph* in Bloomington, Illinois. This suit was the first filed for malpractice in the McLean County circuit court; Dr. Crothers and Dr. Rodgers were the defendants. The plaintiff, Samuel Fleming, had sustained a fractured leg and engaged them to set the bone. The break was a bad one, and the healing process was slow and when completed, as not to be unexpected in an elderly patient, a slight shortening of the limb occurred. The plaintiff felt that the two surgeons had not given the fracture proper attention and sued them for malpractice.

Lincoln defended the two surgeons, both known to be distinguished in their profession, and he actually used a chicken bone to explain the different conditions in bones of young people compared to those of advanced age. He stressed the fact that the bone of a young person has a springy, wiry condition that makes it less apt to break and it has a tendency to knit quickly. In the case of older individuals, however, Lincoln said, the bone is more brittle because lime and other qualities impair the healing process.

In his final statement, Lincoln concluded a brilliant summary by saying: "Mr. Fleming, instead of bringing suit against these surgeons for not giving your bone proper attention, you should go on your knees and thank God, and them, that you have your leg. Most other practitioners with such a break would have insisted upon amputation. In your case, they exercised their skill and ability to preserve it and did so. The slight defect that finally resulted, through nature's method of aiding the work of the surgeons, is nothing compared to the loss of the limb altogether."

It is apparent that this language, ever so concisely structured, and yet with great depth and scope of meaning and conviction, is akin to the style which he was to later use in his Gettysburg Address. It is obvious that Lincoln committed his thoughts and soul to the defense of these surgeons and the jury promptly returned a verdict in favor of the defendants and indeed placed the cost, which reached a large figure, on the plaintiff in this historic case.

Lincoln's great wisdom, analytical thought, accumulation of scientific evidence, and final judicial summation challenge us today to be active participants in the framing of national legislation to be considered, and indeed passed, by the United States Congress as soon as pos-

sible. All of us know that a case such as Lincoln so brilliantly concluded, and indeed won, is not rare but common in these alleged malpractice suits. Such unnecessary suits, which take much of the physician's
time and cause both anguish and pain to patients, family, and physicians alike, should and can be dealt with in a more effective and intelligent way. Through the activities of this College, and most important
through your personal support, these solutions now seem within
reach.

The mounting tide has now swept this issue to the feet of our law-
makers in Washington with the writing of specific bills. Although we
each recognize that the final solution will not be easy and that multiple factors are involved, nevertheless, the tidal wave must be continued
until the appropriate solutions, both for physicians and patients alike,
are found and established. This can be achieved especially through the
thoughtful modification of the far-reaching bills that are currently
being considered in the Congress. Of equal importance will be the
enabling acts, which must be passed by the legislatures of the states.

Every member of the American College of Surgeons can and
should become a part of this vital effort through state legislators and
the congressmen and Senators in Washington. This is a time for
action, not, as some have said, for further study. This College is clearly
on the move and we enlist support from each Fellow, which will be
essential for success.

References

1. Transactions of societies. American College of Surgeons. *Surg. Gynecol. Obstet.*, 18: 124, 1914.
2. Blalock, Alfred. Our obligations and opportunities. *Bull. Amer. Coll. Surg.*, 40: 1, March–April, 1955.
3. Sandor, A. A.: The history of professional liability suits in the United States. *JAMA*, 163: 459, 1957.
4. Cosman, M. P. The medieval medical third party: Compulsory consultation and malpractice insurance. *Ann. of Plas. Surg.*, 8: 152, February, 1982.

5. Elwell, J. J. *A Medico-Legal Treatise on Malpractice and Medical Evidence*. New York: Baker, Voorhis and Company, 1866.

6. Burns, C. R. Malpractice suits in American medicine before the Civil War. *Bulletin of the History of Medicine*, p.42, January-February, 1969.

7. AMA Special Task Force on Professional Liability and Insurance. *Professional Liability in the '80s*. Chicago, Illinois: AMA, 1984.

8. Health, C. Letter to the Editor, "How Abraham Lincoln dealt with a malpractice suit." *N. Engl. J. Med.*, 295: 735, 1976.

Chapter 33

The Antivivisection Movement: A Threat to Medical Research and Future Progress

T he antivivisection movement has again gained momentum and, together with a well-financed network across the nation, it is vigorously supporting enactment of crippling legislation at the national and state levels. Such bills have been introduced and are pending action in the House of Representatives and the U.S. Senate in Washington as well as a number of state legislatures. In an effort to stem the tide, extremely thoughtful editorials in the Washington Post, the Wall Street Journal, and many other national papers and periodicals have presented compelling evidence opposing this effort (1, 2).

The noted Michael B. DeBakey, pioneer surgeon and Chancellor of Baylor College of Medicine, summarized the current drive of the antivivisectionists and the corresponding challenge to the scientific community, stating: "If scientists abandon cat and dog experiments for other models that are not as suitable or as well understood, many potential medical breakthroughs may be severely crippled or halted." He directed his remarks primarily at the Mrazek bill currently before the House of Representatives and the Senate in the nation's capitol. This legislation would ban the use of pound animals for any research supported by the National Institutes of Health, which is the primary source of biomedical research funding throughout the nation. The tragedy of this bill is that not only would it cripple research and retard future progress but these abandoned animals would nevertheless be killed in the pounds. This is an especially grave issue since each animal bred specifically for research costs much more than does a pound animal, a factor which is compounded many times when one considers that the total amount of funding for research has been diminishing in recent years. Were this, or a similar, bill to pass in Congress or in state legislatures, there would clearly be far less research, and a concomitant reduction in new and original contributions to medicine.

Antivivisection has a long background, and from time to time animal rights groups resurface with considerable force and influence, as is currently the situation. Vigorous demonstrations favoring antivivisection have been made at the nation's treasured center of research, the National Institutes of Health in Bethesda, Maryland. Moreover, zealous groups have secretly invaded a number of research laboratories, destroying laboratory equipment and important scientific data.

In its strictest definition, the word vivisection means "cutting or operating on a living animal." However, in the late 1800s, it acquired a broader meaning and was used to refer to animal experimentation in general. Heavily organized movements began in the 1860s and 1870s in the British Isles, and in 1875 the Victoria Street Society was formed by Frances Power Cobbe, a journalist who wrote about feminist, religious, and philanthropic issues.

The Victoria Street Society became the hub of antivivisection activity, and Cobbe succeeded in convincing Lord Shaftsbury, the eminent and powerful reformer of the day, to become the first president of the society. He was obviously chosen for his social prestige as well as his political power. Later that year, the Royal Commission was formed and charged to "establish the extent of experimentation on living animals taking place in Great Britain, the amount of cruelty that might be taking place in connection with the experimentation, and the best means of preventing such cruelty." The Royal Commission recommended a bill that became known as the Cruelty to Animals Act of 1876, which required that any person performing experiments on living vertebrate animals be licensed and that this license be renewed annually The laboratories of these investigators were periodically checked without notice, and each experiment had to be individually approved by the Home Office in London prior to being performed. Moreover, the investigator was required to adhere strictly to the protocol, irrespective of the finding of interesting and unexpected results, which, as all investigators recognize, frequently changes the course of true research.

Lord Lister, the father of antisepsis, wrote to the noted Philadelphia surgeon W.W. Keen: "Our law on antivivisection of 1876 should never have been passed, and ought now to be repealed." Lister underscored the important role animal experimentation played in his own research, which led to major contributions in antisepsis and in making surgery safe for the patient. In writing to the British Medical Journal in 1897, Lister said: "There are people who do not object to eating a mutton chop, people who do not even object to shooting a pheasant with the considerable chance that it may be only wounded and may have to die after lingering in pain, unable to obtain its proper nutriment, and yet who consider it something monstrous to introduce under the skin of a guinea pig a little inoculation of some microbe to ascertain its action. These seem to me to be most inconsistent views."

Physicians, civic leaders, representatives in federal and state government, and the public at large should be familiar with the fact that the vast majority of medical advances of the 20th century have been dependent upon animal research.

The major health problems being faced today are no different and will predictably require the same type of investigation in the experimental animal prior to application in humans. The spectre of poliomyelitis, formerly a dreaded disease, has all but disappeared in the past three decades following the development of the Salk and Sabin vaccines. Both of these vaccines were first administered to monkeys to test their safety as well as efficacy prior to their use in prevention of human poliomyelitis. Moreover, this need for animal use in testing polio vaccine continues today, as is emphasized by Dr. Joseph Bellanti, Director of Georgetown University's Immunology Center: Every new batch of vaccines for polio, and for other childhood diseases, must be tested on animals to make certain that the virus has been adequately inactivated and that it will indeed not transmit active disease to those children who are inoculated. Should the latter occur, it would obviously be a disaster. For every new vaccine produced, live-animal testing provides the answers to a number of vexing problems before the vaccine is used in humans.

Recently, a new genetic-engineered vaccine against hepatitis B has been developed in ovarian cells of the Chinese hamster. This vaccine promises to save the lives of over 2,000,000 humans annually, primarily in third world counties, since the present human-based vaccine is very expensive, whereas the new one will be only a fraction of that cost and can be widely administered in these deprived nations? Is it conceivable that an intelligent, informed, conscientious public could believe it ethical to give a human such vaccines without previous testing in animals to assure safety?

Much publicity has been given the subject of Alzheimer's disease, and currently much research is being directed toward a better understanding of this disorder as well as means of prevention and treatment. Khachaturian, of the National Institute of Aging, says, "Eight years ago we were at ground zero in understanding Alzheimer's disease. There has been incredible progress in research in this area because our investment in basic research concerns brain functions going back to the 1930s. The bulk of that research involved animals and they hold the key to continued progress." Through studies on primates and other animals, investigators have identified the region of the brain, the nucleus basilis of Meynert, which is the site involved in Alzheimer's disease.

Another major affliction and one with a tragic mortality, the acquired immunodeficiency syndrome (AIDS), is increasing in incidence annually. Currently, encouraging studies are being performed in monkeys and chimpanzees, which provide promising signs for an effective vaccine to be developed against this spreading epidemic. Quite clearly, a vaccine is necessary despite the promising pharmacologic agents currently being evaluated in the treatment of this deadly disorder. The first of these drugs, azidothymidine (AZT), has recently been shown to increase the survival of patients with AIDS at the end of the first year of treatment to 50%, as contrasted with randomized control patients receiving placebo who have only a 10% survival rate.

The more than 50 dietary essentials, including vitamins and minerals now recognized as necessary to maintain life, were determined largely by work on experimental animals.

Another major achievement now used throughout the nation lies in the field of dentistry, where fluoridation is a notable example of the application of results of interrelated studies on animals and humans to public improvement. Many research reports have emphasized that fluoridation offers the easiest and most effective method of preventing dental cavities. The adding of fluoride to drinking water is both safe and effective, and strengthens the teeth against the decay-producing effects of acids in the mouth, thus reducing dental cavities. Once again, these studies were first done in experimental animals.

The public is also aware of the many achievements in heart surgery, which have been the direct result of the development of the heart-lung machine. Today, nearly all heart conditions requiring surgery can be successfully treated in often dramatic and near miraculous procedures. It should always be remembered that Dr. John H. Gibbon and his wife, Maly Gibbon, spent 22 years working as a close research team on many hundreds of animals to develop this machine before it was safe for human use. Further, every diabetic should realize that the discovery of insulin in the islet cells of the pancreas is another major medical achievement which had its origin solely in animal experimentation and replacement prior to the use of insulin in humans.

Animals also benefit from animal research. Louis Pasteur developed the vaccine against rabies through experiments on rabbits, and the livestock industry in the United States has benefited greatly from research now used to treat animal infectious diseases. In its editorial, the Wall Street Journal emphasized, "After all, humans are not the only beneficiaries of laboratory research. Today millions of pets can be free of heart disease, leukemia, or kidney failure solely as a result of experiments based on animal research. Some animal-rights activists can't seem to remember that." Indeed the chemotherapeutic agents and antibiotics, key agents in the treatment of a variety of infectious diseases, were first studied in experimental animals prior to their appropriate and safe use in humans.

The effect of the antivivisectionists and their ruthless approaches to investigators and research is best summarized by Dr. Frederick Goodwin of the National Institute of Mental Health, who says: "My people speak more and more of fear, and demoralization concerning their research and the necessity to use animals for meaningful and objective experiments. If you stop funding or drive up costs by layers of regulation, nobody on the outside knows it's happening. Research just quietly dies."

The animal rights groups in this country have become exceedingly strong and are attempting to eliminate all animal experimentation, which would clearly be a disaster for medical science as it exists today. The director of the Kennedy Center for Bioethics states: "We have to look at the consequences of giving animals rights—are you ready to say that we are more obligated not to use those dogs than we are to the thousands of human beings in this country who have heart attacks every year?" The American Heart Association recently issued a special report entitled "Position of the American Heart Association on Research Animal Use." In summary, the report stated: "Millions of Americans today are healthy, and other millions are alive, because of the advances in the prevention and treatment of heart disease." Death rates from the major forms of heart disease have declined steadily since about midcentury and the decline is continuing. Most recently, between 1972 and 1982, the death toll from cardiovascular disease declined 28%.

The decline is largely related to changes in lifestyle and development of methods of treatment, many of which are based upon animal experimentation. To those who are educated and knowledgeable, it is apparent that there are many benefits from appropriate experiments on anesthetized animals since they would otherwise be sacrificed in public pounds. The facts are unmistakable and the reasons self-evident: Such experiments are essential to medical progress. Civilization as we know it today, and indeed survival, may be at stake, given, for example, the necessity to control the AIDS crisis. According to the American Humane Society, 7,000,000 pet animals are abandoned to pounds or shelters each year and of these 5,000,000 are killed there. These animals could be used productively and with professional care in research. The latter is very important and all investigators should be constantly aware of their obligations to conduct experiments with appropriate sensitivity for all animals (4). This issue is an exceedingly crucial one, and there is a compelling need for responsible citizens to join in supporting the principle of animal research in the prevention and treatment of disease for the betterment of all humankind.

References

1. DeBakey, M. E. Medicine needs these animals. *The Washington Post.* Thurs., June 4, 1987, p. A23.
2. Editorial: Science under attack. *The Wall Street Journal.* June 16, 1987
3. McCabe, K. Who will live, who will die? *The Washingtonian.* Aug., 1986. p. 113.
4. Cohen, C. The case for the use of animals in biomedical research. *N. Engl. J. Med.,* 315: 865–870, 1986.

Chapter 34 ⌒

National Health Insurance

T here are many examples of National Health Insurance plans which have been in practice elsewhere for a number of years and allow us the privilege, and indeed the obligation, to determine their outcome. Of great importance is the effect of these plans on quality of medical care, their effect on the public, the changes which have occurred in the medical profession, and their influence upon the national economy. Much is to be learned from these past experiences in other countries and, in point of fact, it would be foolhardy to repeat misadventures which are already a matter of historic record.

In an effort to place in perspective the history of National Health Insurance in the United States, it should he emphasized that as early as 1912 a group of leaders concerned with this problem concluded that, if the middle class and the poor were to have access to good medical care, a health care insurance program should be enacted sponsored by the Federal Government. It is interesting that the AMA supported this view for a number of years. In 1932 a document summarizing this study was published, entitled "Medical Cure for the American People: The Final report of the Committee on the Costs of Medical Care," being supported by eight foundations with a broad membership of both professionals and laymen. The single issue concerned the financing of health care for the nation, but in the end there was much disagreement among the participating groups and little of significance resulted.

The issue of socialized medicine reemerged in 1939 with the introduction of the Wagner-Murray-Dingell Bill, a proposal submitted to the Congress which gained much public attention. However, this campaign failed to attract enough support to secure passage, and ultimately the issue lost momentum. The details of these efforts are carefully chronicled in Hirshfield's *The Lost Reform—The Campaign Health Insurance in the United States from 1932 to 1943,* a valuable treatise concerning the many issues during that decade.

In the late 1940s and early 1950s, President Truman cast his support behind a revised National Health Insurance program. Once again, the opposition, led primarily by the AMA, proved formidable. Unable to enact such legislation, toward the end of his administration President Truman appointed a committee to report on alternative routes that the federal government might follow to improve the nation's health care. The President's Commission on Health Care Needs of the Nation, often called the Magnuson Commission, recommended that, since changing the financial base was not practical, the federal government should increase its flow of resources into the health care system to expand investments in research and facilities. Thus, two major pieces of legislation emerged, the Hill-Burton Act supporting construction of a number of hospitals throughout the country and, secondly, the National Institutes of Health legislation which greatly augmented federal support for biomedical research. In 1960, Congress passed the Kerr-Mills Act, making funds available to the states to enable the delivery of medical care to low-income, aged persons. This ultimately led to the passage during the Johnson administration in 1965 of the Medicare and Medicaid bills, bringing the issue to the present.

If there is a determined effort to prevent past mistakes, it is essential that objective reviews be made of the experiences in other countries of comprehensive National Health Insurance programs. Gunnar Biorck, Professor of Medicine at the Karolinska Institute in Stockholm, is a distinguished international physician and is so recognized everywhere. In a recent publication entitled, "How to be a Clinician in a Socialist Country, he states his views quite concisely by saying that in Sweden "the impact on the freedom of the medical profession on the patient-physician relationship is considerable and destructive to the concepts of a free profession."

One feature which Biorck emphasizes is the fact that administrators have assumed control and that the machinery has thus lost its lubrication. He summarizes by saying, "Looking at another aspect of the socialization of medicine in my country, the introduction of these various regulatory processes has resulted in a cancerous growth in the number of medical administrators at all levels of incompetence."

Professor Biorck then proceeds to describe the steps taken by the government in Sweden to subjugate the profession in this order:

1. Introduce compulsory health insurance and bind physicians to working rules, fee schedules, and paper work.
2. When this is established procedure, bind physicians to a fixed salary for a regulated office week, that is, make them all civil servants.
3. Forbid professional activities outside regulated working hours. (Activities in capacities other than as physicians may be tolerated. No limitations are set on the activities of "quacks." But physicians are forbidden to offer services under this pretense).
4. Increase the output of medical schools to produce an excess of physicians, thus lowering their income level and standard of living.
5. Centralize all postgraduate training and abolish the individual's free choice of future specialty.
6. Abolish the patient's free choice of physician through systems of geographical adherence to certain hospitals and health centers.
7. Introduce political steering of universities and medical schools and of research granting organizations.
8. Abolish grades and marks in graduate and postgraduate studies and de-emphasize professional merits in the selection for future posts.
9. Let appointments to senior posts he made by local political bodies.
10. Socialize and standardize the production and distribution of drugs.
11. Computerize all patient information in one nationwide computer.

Finally, Biorck laments that "the freedom to choose the area of one's work, and the existence of medicine as an art cherished by people who could not help doing what they loved and loving what they did—the socialist strategy in my country, so far, seems to aim at closing this last reserve." He concludes this keynote address with a statement which bears careful attention in the United States: "It is necessary to take such effects into account in the planning for nationalized health services anywhere in the world."

One might ask if Professor Biorck's position is a politically unpopular one in Sweden. The fact is, however, that shortly after presenting this courageous address at the University of Chicago, Professor Biorck was elected a member of the Swedish Parliament, the only physician in that body.

A long-standing friend and honorary member of this Association, Philip Sandblom, formerly Professor of Surgery at the University of Lund, summarized his views concerning Sweden's National Health Insurance Program before the Board of Governors of the American College of Surgeons stating:

"All hospital doctors now become 100 percent salaried employees with regulated working hours. Capacity and ability are not rewarded. The salary is related to the position held, based on a 40-hour week, with extra payment for more hours, but there is no difference with respect to the kind of specialty or the work load. The salary is thus related to the amount of time spent in the hospital, irrespective of the kind of work performed."

"The older generation of surgeons was accustomed to hard work and did not count the hours. The younger generation has begun to realize the futility of high incomes in a situation where three-fourths of it is cut away by extremely high progressive taxation, and so they begin to put a greater value on their free time. This has resulted in a drive for shorter working hours, which is unworthy of the medical profession and contrary to its ancient ethics."

Two years ago at the meeting of the American section of the International Society of Surgery in New Orleans, Professor Charles DuBost of Paris reviewed the status of government medicine in France. He emphasized the many problems which practicing physicians had encountered with the system and repeated over and over the word "mediocrity—mediocrity—mediocrity," indicating that this had become the hallmark of the entire program, and he thought much to the disservice of the French people. Since they have had 30 years experience with socialized medicine, there is much to be learned from the record now available in the British Isles. In 1947 the labor unions, working through the Labor Government of Prime Minister Attlee, and particularly with the Labor leader Aneurin Bevan, enacted the National Health Service Act. The government assumed control of nearly all hospitals and placed most specialists on salaries. Early experience with the program was by and large regarded as favorable, and there is no doubt that a majority of the British medical profession cooperated wherever possible in making the system a success. With the passage of time, however, increasing problems arose, and Sir George Pickering, the noted Regius Professor of Medicine at Oxford, recently lamented in a Nuffield Lecture the decline in learning and in professional etiquette which has occurred. In this address, he emphasized the fact that, with the growth of the trade unions, social change occurred in Britain, since the object of each union was to obtain the greatest slice of the national gross product for its own members without consideration for others. Its weapons were, he said, the strike and the "go-slows," which were bringing management and government to their knees. Sir George feared that all the signs pointed to the fact that medicine seemed apt to contour to this outlook and behavior. He could only hope that the National Health Service might be removed from political influence and that the leaders of the profession might guide it back towards its traditional role of a learned profession and prevent its becoming a technical trade union.

Most are familiar with the section in the *New England Journal of Medicine* entitled, "By the London Post," authored by John Lister, Dean of the British Postgraduate Medical Federation of the University of London. He has long been a very thoughtful spokesman and collects data carefully before drawing conclusions. Originally a supporter of most aspects of the National Health Service, within the past several years he has recognized its ever increasing defects. In a recent letter he stated: "I personally think it is very sad to see an enlightened scheme getting into serious trouble from many points of view. The early years of the N.H.S. were marked by a considerable degree of collaboration between the health department and the medical and nursing profession, both of whom showed good will in running the service. The reorganization of the N.H.S. in 1974 with its increasing numbers of administrators and increasing difficulties in decision making was a serious setback. Furthermore, the abrasive attitude of Mrs. Barbara Castle when she was Secretary of State for Social Services has alienated much of the good will of the medical profession, who now feel that they have a hostile employer.

"The attack on private patients was a major factor in creating this situation. The serious financial state of the country in the last few years has aggravated the situation and led to stringent economy and reallocation of resources with the politicians deciding the priorities for expenditure on health. The rise of professionalism in the allied health services and the misuse of trade union power, particularly in ancillary hospital workers, has led to loss of medical dominance. While many of us realize that complete dominance cannot reasonably continue in the present social environment, there is no doubt that the erosion of medical influence has had a serious effect on the whole service."

John Lister's message is very clear, and it is apparent that each of his points is deserving of thoughtful consideration in formulating future plans in this country. Eoin O'Malley, Professor of Surgery at University College, Dublin, in a recent address in this country entitled "The Doctor's Dilemma," said, "In Ireland, 85–90% of the population is entitled to free hospital service, free being a euphemism to indicate that the service is provided for by taxation." He then reviewed many problems which he had encountered, including the limited number of operations which can now be performed, the long waiting lists which have become commonplace, and the economic necessity for budgetary restrictions to select patients for operation—leading to an admonition to Americans: "The scene is set for the doctor's dilemma of the future. On my side of the Atlantic the curtain has started to rise; I can only hope that on your side the play may never reach the stage."

Another detracting feature of the British National Health Service is the economic burden it places upon the government and the people. In two recent seminars on "The Future of the Private Sector in Medical Care and Education," sponsored by William G. Anlyan[1] at Duke University, this subject among others was reviewed. A number of the participants commented upon the open-endedness of total government health programs, leading to the statement of Mr. J. Enoch Powell in Britain that "in a system of free medicine, the demand for free care is infinite," a concept which is now termed Powell's Law.

Many here will recall that in his Director's memo entitled, "The British National Health Service," written after attending a London seminar on the subject, C. Rollins Hanlon said: "The dangerous

---

1. William G. Anlyan, M.D. is the former Chancellor of Health Affairs at Duke Medical Center.

oppression of a swollen bureaucracy needs no emphasis. The critical challenge to American surgery is how to maintain quality of surgical services without splitting the profession as one sees it so painfully demonstrated in Britain. Accessibility to services may well have been improved, but the casualty of that alteration is quality."

There is also a lesson to be learned from Canada, as recently stated by Philip R. Bromage who recently emigrated to the United States because of the situation of government medicine there. For the previous seven years Dr. Bromage had been Professor and Chairman of the Department of Anesthesiology at McGill University and Chief of Anesthesia at the Royal Victoria Hospital in Montreal. He is now Professor of Anesthesia at Duke and writes: "Socialization of medicine in Canada is based on federal funding and matching provincial funds.

"Each Province, being autonomous in matters of Health and Education, has been free to develop its own pattern of health care delivery.

"The Province of Quebec modeled its scheme on the Castonguay Report of 1968, and its socialization was very thorough. A series of bills were passed in 1970 and 1971 with the following results:

1. A comprehensive health and hospitalization plan, for all citizens.
2. Destruction of the free market in health care delivery, by creating a state (Provincial) monopoly in health insurance. All private health insurance was outlawed, except in minor areas uncovered by the government scheme.
3. Containment of the medical profession in a) social, b) professional, c) fiscal matters, and d) direction of labor.
4. Hospital management was placed in the hands of lay committees, and the medical profession was virtually removed from the process of decision-making.
5. The medical profession was subjected to industrial-type legislation. Negotiations with the government had to be conducted through the Federations of Medical Specialists, and the Federation of Omnipractitioners (i.e., G.P.s). These were union-type organizations set up for the purpose of negotiating terms and conditions of services.
6. A fee-for-service system was negotiated in which every type of medical act was described, priced and coded for computer purposes. The resulting data bank was extremely comprehensive, and it

was used effectively in adjusting scales of remuneration, both in absolute terms, and relatively between the various specialties.

7. Direction of labor. This has been under consideration, but not implemented as yet. Discussions proceed about the advisability of drafting newly qualified M.D.s to under-doctored areas, as partial solution to maldistribution problems.

8. Cost Containment and Reduction of Acute-Care Beds. Hospital global budgets have failed to match rising nonprofessional labor costs in many instances. This has resulted in closure of about 20-21% of acute care beds in many of the major teaching hospitals (the Royal Victoria Hospital, Montreal, had about 200 of its 800 beds closed when I left last year). There is promise of a comparable increase in chronic care beds, but so far this has not been implemented. The phenomenon of reduction of acute care beds appears to be part of a deliberate policy, and is in accord with patterns of socialized medicine elsewhere.

"A policy of regionalization-rationalization has produced some positive results, particularly in the area of obstetrics and neonatal care. Some small units have been closed down, and services have been concentrated in fewer but larger and more effective facilities.

"In summary, a comprehensive health plan has brought many benefits to the public at large in the Province of Quebec. Within this scheme, government policy appears to be emphasizing the importance of public health and chronic care, while de-emphasizing the importance of traditional acute care. At the same time, the medical profession has been removed from the decision-making process of health care management, and the M.D. has been reduced to the status of a skilled artisan (entitled a 'health professional'). At present, he is adequately remunerated, but the quality of the medical environment in which he works appears to be deteriorating."

The most updated figures for the present status of health care insurance in the United States were recently provided by the National Blue Cross-Blue Shield and the American College of Surgeons. The data show that Blue Cross-Blue Shield currently covers 85 million of the present 213 million population in this country. In addition, private insurance companies have in force a total of 86 million health policies, some of which represent partial coverage and in other instances these policies are supplementary to coverage by Blue Cross. HMOs are now responsible for the health needs of 6,330,000 citizens: Medicare covers 25,500,000 and Medicaid provides care for 21,500,000. Thus, the total health care coverage by one form of insurance or another is quite impressive.

Is it not appropriate to ask if the real problem is not Government-sponsored insurance, preferably managed through private sources, for those citizens who have either inadequate or no coverage, and in addition to institute health insurance for those with catastrophic illnesses? Would it not be much preferred to take this approach and attack the part of the system which needs attention rather than revamp the coverage of the great majority of U.S. citizens who already have well-documented adequate health insurance? It would appear logical to direct attention to the indigent, currently estimated to number approximately 20–25 million of the total 218 million population. If to this a comprehensive policy is added to provide federally guaranteed coverage for catastrophic illness to all citizens, the issue will have largely been solved.

Currently the United States devotes approximately 9% of the gross national product to the health care industry, a complex which employs 1 out of 20 of the workers in the nation. The tremendous escalation in cost of medical care offers a further deterrent to a comprehensive national health scheme directed by the federal government. One need only review the experience of the government with Medicare and Medicaid. Since their introduction in 1965, total federal expenditures for health care have increased approximately eight-fold, from approximately $5–$40 billion annually in 1976. It is widely recognized that further increases in the federal health dollar are apt to seriously affect the overall economy and certainly the inflationary spiral. Eli Ginzberg, the noted Columbia economist, has placed the entire political and fiscal situation in sharp profile in a recently published monograph entitled, "Limits of Health Reform." He emphasizes that the American people have taken extreme positions only when the system comes under great challenge and cites, for example, that when Congress was thoroughly annoyed with the arrogance of the monopolies in 1890 it passed the Sherman Antitrust Act. Similarly, the banking difficulties in

1907 led to the Aldridge Commission and the passage of the Federal
Reserve Act in 1913. Moreover, it required the Great Depression of
the 1930s to make possible the unprecedented government acts which
characterized the New Deal. However, at present Ginzberg feels that it
is out of the question to plan a federal bureaucracy of the size, scope,
and expense of a National Health System.

To add further to this problem, in a recent report to the House
Ways and Means Committee, the Comptroller General of the United
States evaluated performance of the Social Security Administration
compared with that of private fiscal intermediaries in dealing with
institutional providers of Medicare services. The data which were
obtained are of much interest and show how much more it appears to
cost the Federal Government for identical services. The cost of processing a bill by the Division of Direct Reimbursement of the Social
Security Administration is $9.23 per bill, while the total cost for this
processing per bill for the Maryland Blue Cross is $4.94, and the
Chicago Blue Cross is $5.18 for the same service.

In a recent editorial concerning the debate over whether or not
the VA Hospital system should be absorbed into the private sector,
Arnold Relman, editor of the *New England Journal of Medicine*, posed a
very direct question both to the Federal Government and to the
American people when he asked, "The political realities may very well
ordain otherwise, but wouldn't it be a triumph for common sense if
our government were to approach the regulation and reform of its
own Veterans Administration hospital system with the same zeal that
characterizes its present plan for the private sector?"

In summary, before embarking upon a federally sponsored program of National Health Insurance, Relman's question and many others like it require adequate and convincing answers. At this point, it
seems likely that the nation will do well to interfere minimally with
the approximately 80% of Americans whose health care costs are
already largely covered by private insurance and simultaneously to
devise a plan to fully insure by federal support both the indigent and
the total population for catastrophic illness. Such an approach appears
likely to provide a very acceptable solution.

Epilogue ⤿

It is now over forty years after David C. Sabiston, Jr. became Chair of Surgery at Duke University School of Medicine and eleven years after he retired. While scholars will probe Sabiston's contributions to American medicine for years to come, now is an appropriate time for a first look back at Sabiston's legacy to Duke and to the profession of medicine in general. While David Sabiston achieved in many areas as outlined in the Introduction at the beginning of the book, I think over time, his lasting legacies will be his dedication to teaching and modeling of professionalism, his belief in the surgeon as scholar, his accomplishments in cardio-pulmonary research, and his early recognition of and response to the HIV-1 epidemic. While his dedication to teaching and professionalism, his belief in the surgeon as a scholar, and his research accomplishments are well documented throughout "The Heart of Medicine", Sabiston never wrote of his contribution to AIDS-related research. I had the good fortune to interview David Sabiston over the course of several months in 2001-2003 on this and related topics, and from these discussions and my own experience, I will tell the story of Sabiston's leadership in early AIDS research at Duke.

Duke Surgery residents are superb scientists, and many of them trained in the early 1980s with an outstanding researcher in Surgery, Dani Bolognesi. Bolognesi trained with Joseph Beard, another pioneer at Duke in surgical research in the 1950s and 60s who developed the equine infectious anemia virus vaccine. Bolognesi was one of a number of outstanding M.D. and Ph.D. investigators that Sabiston hired to work in surgery in order for there to be a rich diversity of laboratories in which his residents could train and develop. In the early 1980s, it was very unusual for a Department of Surgery to be so committed to basic research in residency training, and to have an outstanding cohort of scientists on the faculty.

In 1982 Bolognesi was working on cancer vaccines and I was working on a new human retrovirus that caused leukemia, the Human T Cell Leukemia/Lymphoma Virus, Type I (HTLV-1). As the AIDS epidemic unfolded, Bolognesi and I became members of the original NIH National Cancer Institute Gay-Related Immunodeficiency Disease (GRID) Task Force led by Robert Gallo, and our work on this problem exponentially increased over the next four years. As we learned about the new AIDS virus, we realized we needed new biocontainment facilities and additional laboratory space. Bolognesi went to a number of Duke administrators to request space and resources for the work, and Sabiston, who immediately recognized the enormity of the problem, quickly responded "What do you need me to do?" Bolognesi asked Sabiston to raise the money to pay for a new biosafety level 3 research laboratory where safe research on the new retroviruses that caused AIDS and cancer could be conducted. Sabiston went to meet with one of his friends, the president of Dupont, and together they worked out an agreement whereby Duke would receive $2,000,000 towards a building for cancer and other viruses, $3,000,000 for collaborative research in the building, and David Sabiston committed $5,000,000 of Surgery reserves to the project. Thus, the Surgical Oncology Research Facility (SORF) was built on the Duke campus. Out of that facility came the early leadership of the US HIV vaccine development effort (Bolognesi, Kent Weinhold, Thomas Matthews and Haynes), the drug Azidothymidine (AZT) (Weinhold and Bolognesi) and the HIV fusion inhibitor, T-20 or Fuzeon (Thomas Matthews and Bolognesi). Bolognesi founded and organized the Duke AIDS Center out of the SORF, and out of the immune reconstitution work in the AIDS Center came the development of thymus transplantation for a congenital immunodeficiency disease, DiGeorge Syndrome (Louise Markert and Haynes).

It is also important to understand the environment in which Sabiston made his enormous commitment to AIDS research in 1985. At this time, only a handful of investigators and clinicians were interested in working on AIDS. That Sabiston made the commitment that he did so early on in the epidemic is all the more extraordinary.

Finally, the Duke Human Vaccine Institute was organized at SORF in 1990 by Bolognesi and myself, and now has 10 investigators, a staff of 55, and an annual research budget of over $16,000,000. Therefore, two major centers and an institute, two AIDS drugs, AIDS vaccine candidates, a curative treatment for DiGeorge Syndrome, a generation of mentored faculty both in and outside Sabiston's department, and saved lives of AIDS and DiGeorge Syndrome patients are the direct products of David Sabiston's vision, wisdom and generosity. David Sabiston's legacy will live on in the lives of his patients, surgical trainees and faculty, and as well will live on in the lives of patients that have benefited from Department of Surgery research.

Barton F. Haynes, M.D.
June 2005

Sources of Chapters

Chapters 1 and 2: Taped Interview, AOA Honor Medical Society Leaders in American Medicine, November 30, 1994 by Paul A. Ebert, M.D.; Sabiston, D. C., Jr. A conversation with the editor. *Amer. J. Cardiology,* 82: 358–372, 1998.

Chapter 3: Wilkins, R. H., Sabiston, D. C., Jr. The Duke University Medical Center. *J. Neurosurg.,* 78:301–304, 1993.

Chapter 4: Sabiston, D. C., Jr., Hart, D. Leader in the development of the Duke University Medical Center. *North Carolina Med. J.,* 44: 441–442, 1983.

Chapter 5: Sabiston, D. C., Jr. The Department of Surgery at the Duke Medical Center. *The American Surgeon,* pp. 2–8, Jan. 1970.

Chapter 6: Sabiston, D. C., Jr. Major contributions to surgery from the South. *Ann. Surgery,* 181: 487–507, 1975.

Chapter 7: Sabiston, D. C., Jr. The first hundred years: Annals of surgery and a century of progress. *Ann. Surgery,* 201: 1–3, 1985.

Chapter 8: Sabiston, D. C., Jr. Surgeons and the Nobel Prize, *Ann. Surgery,* 2:10–13, April 1991.

Chapter 9: Sabiston, D. C., Jr. Trendelenburg's classic work on the operative treatment of pulmonary embolism. *Ann. Thoracic Surg.* 35: 570–574, 1983.

Chapter 10: Sabiston, D. C., Jr., A. O. Whipple Surgical Society. *Surgery,* 74: 471–473, 1973.

Chapter 11: Sabiston, D. C., Jr. Presidential Address: Alfred Blalock. *Ann. Surgery*, 188: 255–270, 1978.

Chapter 12: Sabiston, D. C., Jr., Bahnson, H.T. *Clin. Cardiol.*, 17: 49–50, 1994.

Chapter 13: Sabiston, D. C., Jr. Medicine as a career. *Caduceus*, 1: 2–6, 1966.

Chapter 14: Sabiston, D. C., Jr. A consortium in surgical education. *Surgery*, 66: 1–14, 1969.

Chapter 15: Sabiston, D. C., Jr. The training of academic surgeons for the future: The challenge and the dilemma, in *Academic Medicine, Present and Future*. Eds. John Z. Bowers, M.D. and Edith E. King, *Proceedings of the Rockefeller Archive Center Conference*, Pocantico Hills, North Tarrytown, N.Y., May 25–27, 1982.

Chapter 16: Sabiston, D. C., Jr. The Effect of the Three-year Medical School Curriculum on Undergraduate Surgical Education: A Professor's Point-of-View. *Bullentin of the American College of Surgeons*, Chicago, IL., p. 58:18–29, Sept., 1973.

Chapter 17: Sabiston, D. C., Jr.: In Gifford, J.F., Jr. (Ed.). *Undergraduate Medical Education and the Elective System: Experience with the Duke Curriculum, 1966–1975, William G. Anlyan, M.D., Ewald W. Busse, M.D., Thomas D. Kinney, M.D.* Durham, NC: *Duke University Press*, pp. 109–118, 1978.

Chapter 18: Sabiston, D. C., Jr. Specialization in surgery, *Johns Hopkins Medical Journal*, 133: 224–225, 1973.

Chapter 19: Sabiston, D. C., Jr. The university teaching hospital. In Longue, J.T. (Ed.) *Selected papers on American Medical Education for Foreign Scholars, 1957–1968*. Washington: Association of American Medical Colleges, 1969.

Chapter 20: Sabiston, D. C., Jr. The coronary circulation. *The Johns Hopkins Medical Journal*, 134: 314–329, 1994.

Chapter 21: Sabiston, D. C., Jr. Coronary endarterectomy. *The American Surgeon*, 26: 217–226, 1960.

Chapter 22: Sabiston, D. C., Jr. Observations on the coronary circulation, with tribute to my teachers, *J. Thorac. Cardiovasc. Surg.*, 90: 321–340, 1985.

Chapter 23: Sabiston, D. C., Jr., Gregg, D. C. Effect of cardiac contraction on coronary blood flow. *Circulation,* 15: 14–20, 1957.

Chapter 24: Sabiston, D. C., Jr. , Neill, C. A., Taussig, H. B. The direction of blood flow in anomalous left coronary artery arising from the pulmonary artery. *Circulation,* 23: 591–597, 1960.

Chapter 25: Lang, E. K., Sabiston, D. C., Jr. Coronary arteriography in the selection of patients for surgery. *Radiology,* 76: 32–38, 1961.

Chapter 26: Jones, R. N., Curtis, S. E., Wechsler, A. S., Young, W. G. Jr., Oldham, H. N., Wolfe, W. G., Whalen, R., Morris, J. J., Floyd, W. L., Sabiston, D. C., Jr. The diminishing mortality of coronary artery bypass grafting for myocardial ischemia. *North Carolina Med. J.,* 42: 637–641, 1981.

Chapter 27: Jones, R. N., Austin, E. H., Peter, C. A., and Sabiston, D. C., Jr. Radionucleotide angiocardiology in the diagnosis of congenital heart disorders. *Ann. Surgery,* 193: 710–718, 1981.

Chapter 28: Sabiston, D. C., Jr., Wagner, H. N. The diagnosis of pulmonary embolism by radioisotope scanning. *Ann. Surgery,* 160: 575–588, 1964.

Chapter 29: Wagner, H. N., Sabiston, D. C., Jr., McAfee, J. G., Tow, D., Stern, H. S. Diagnosis of Massive Pulmonary Embolism in Man By Radioisotope Scanning. *New Eng. J. Med.,* 271: 377–384, 1964.

Chapter 30: Sabiston, D.C., Jr. and Wagner, H.N. The pathophysiology of pulmonary embolism: Relationship to accurate diagnosis and choice of therapy. *J. Thoracic and Cardiovas. Surg.,* 50: 339–356, 1965.

Chapter 31: Wolfe, W. G., Sabiston, D. C., Jr., Radioactive ventilation scanning in the diagnosis of pulmonary embolism. *J. of Thoracic and Cardiovas. Surgery,* 55: 149–159, 1968.

Chapter 32: Sabiston, D. C., Jr. Professional liability in the 1980s: Problems and solutions. Presidential Address, The American College of Surgeons. *Bulletin Am. Coll. Surgery,* 70: 6–11, 1985.

Chapter 33: Sabiston, D. C., Jr. The antivivisection movement: A threat to medical research and future progress. *North Carolina Med. J.,* 48: 653–655, 1987.

Chapter 34: Sabiston, D. C., Jr. Panel of National Health Insurance. *Ann. Surgery.,* 188: 571–586, 1978.

Index